Perinatal Programming

Andreas Plagemann (Ed.)

Perinatal Programming

The State of the Art

Edited by Andreas Plagemann

DE GRUYTER

Editor
Prof. Dr. med. Andreas Plagemann
Charité
Universitätsmedizin Berlin
Klinik für Geburtsmedizin
AG "Experimentelle Geburtsmedizin"
Augustenburger Platz 1
13353 Berlin

Gemeinschaft zur Förderung von
vorgeburtlicher und frühkindlicher Vorsorge
und Prävention e.V. (GFVP)
Krantorweg 63
13503 Berlin

ISBN 978-3-11-024944-6
e-ISBN 978-3-11-024945-3

Library of Congress Cataloging-in-Publication Data

Perinatal programming : the state of the art / edited by Andreas Plagemann.
    p. ; cm.
Includes bibliographical references.
ISBN 978-3-11-024944-6 (alk. paper)
1. Perinatology. I. Plagemann, Andreas.
[DNLM: 1. Prenatal Exposure Delayed Effects. 2. Perinatology—trends. WQ 210]

RG600.P47 2011
618.3'2—dc23   2011022261

Bibliographic information published by the Deutsche Nationalbibliothek
The Deutsche Nationalbibliothek lists this publication in the Deutsche Nationalbibliografie;
detailed bibliographic data are available in the Internet at http://dnb.d-nb.de.

© 2012 Walter de Gruyter GmbH & Co. KG, Berlin/Boston

Printing and Binding: Hubert & Co. GmbH & Co. KG, Göttingen
Cover image: Photodisc/Marili Forastieri/Thinkstock
♾ Printed on acid-free paper
Printed in Germany
www.degruyter.com

Contents

Foreword

Perinatal Programming – The State of the Art

The traditional view on the origins of health and diseases is changing rapidly. More and more it becomes clear that there is no static interaction between genes and the environment during the life span but that plastic conditioning of the biological 'hardware' occurs, especially during critical periods of life in the womb and neonatal period, co-determining the long-term fate of an organism. This 'setting' of fundamental life functions and dispositions for diseases has been introduced as *perinatal programming* and might be the most important mechanism in the developmental origins of health and disease, beyond classical teratogenesis and aging. Because it opens fundamentally new perspectives of preventing diseases before they start to develop genuine prophylaxis seems to become possible, and this should be of enormous benefit for the individual as well as for societies in the future.

Overall, five major topics have evolved in the current biomedical discussion on this issue, namely the 'left hand side' and the 'right hand side' of the 'U-shaped curve' on long-term risk in relation to decreased or increased birth weight and its determinants, general environmental exposures, hormonal and nutritional influences on programming, the role of epigenetics, and general mechanistic concepts and perspectives in the field. These overall aspects consequently framed the program of a scientific symposium, which was organized and hosted by the 'Experimental Obstetrics' research group of the Charité, Berlin, on the occasion of the 300th anniversary of the Charité, University Medicine Berlin, and the 200th anniversary of the Humboldt University of Berlin, Germany, in 2010. Plenary lectures from worldwide recognized speakers, most of them providing pioneer work for decades, highly valuable 'hot-topic' presentations, the attendance of plenum participants from some 30 countries and five continents, and respective 'pro-and-con' discussions in the plenum on each of the major topics made this congress a 'landmark-meeting'.

To present this critical come-together in the developmental origins approach to a broader scientific community and readership, review chapters on selected congress contributions compose this volume on *Perinatal Programming – The State of the Art*. Epidemiological, clinical, experimental, and conceptual work is summarized, linking periconceptional, fetal, and neonatal exposures, such as, mal- and overnutrition, stress, infection, xenobiotica, glucocorticoid medication, and so forth, to increased long-term risk of developing metabolic, cardiovascular, allergic, mental, reproductive, malign, and, in general, disorders and diseases associated with modern lifestyle, even independently from classical genetic dispositions. Consequently, all of this may open important new chances and challenges of perinatal medicine for a primary prevention of long-term health risks globally and, moreover, sharpens our view on fundamental mechanisms of developmental processes and ontogenesis, in general.

I am very grateful to many people for enabling this volume. First, I would like to thank the authors for their engaged cooperation, providing pioneer work up to very timely issues, which make this book a 'State-of-the-Art' summary. Especially, I would like to thank my long-term scientific co-worker Thomas Harder, MD, MScE, for many hours of highly reliable editorial work on the book manuscript. Many thanks must go to Elke Rodekamp, MD, for valuable assistance in organizing the respective meeting. Last but not least, I would like to express my personal gratitude to Günter Dörner, MD, for many years of creative collaboration and discussions on the overall topic, and Joachim W. Dudenhausen, MD, FRCOG, and Cornelius Frömmel, MD, for enabling the continuation of our research work at the Charité, Berlin, during recent years.

Aiming to promote the idea and field of epigenetic, environmentally determined early development, ontogenesis, and, consequently, prevention, I would like to express my sincere hope that this book will find a wide circulation and reflection.

Andreas Plagemann
Berlin, August 2011

Abbreviations

5-CSRTT	5-choice serial reaction time test
ADHD	attention deficit hyperactivity disorder
AGA	appropriate for gestational age
AgRP	agouti-related peptide
alpha-MSH	alpha-melanocyte-stimulating hormone
AMPH	amphetamine
APRs	adaptive, predictive responses
ARC	arcuate hypothalamic nucleus
ARH	arcuate nucleus of the hypothalamus
BMI	body mass index
C	controls
CART	cocaine and amphetamine-regulated transcript peptide
CIS	carcinoma in situ
CNS	central nervous system
COMT	catechol-O-methyltransferase
CPT	Continuous Performance Task
CRH	corticotropin-releasing hormone
CR	conditioned response
CS	conditioned stimulus
CVD	cardiovascular disease
DCs	dendritic cells
DIO	diet-induced obesity
DISC-1	disrupted in schizophrenia-1
DMH	dorsomedial hypothalamic nucleus
DNMTS/P	delayed nonmatch to sample/position
DOHaD	developmental origins of health and disease
E	embryonic
EC	embryonal carcinoma
ECG	electrocardiogram
EFSA	European Food Safety Authority
ERPs	event-related potentials
FIPS	Fetal programming – IUGR – Placental markers – Study
fMRI	functional magnetic resonance imaging
FSH	follicle-stimulating hormone
GCK	glucokinase gene
GD	gestational day
GD	gestational diabetes
GDM	gestational diabetes mellitus
GFAP	glial fibrillary acidic protein
GK	Goto-Kakizaki

GR   glucocorticoid receptors
GW   gestational week
GWAS   genome wide association studies
HCG   human chorionic gonadotropin
HFD   high-fat diet
HPA   hypothalamus-pituitary-adrenal axis
HPRT   hypoxanthine guanine phosphoribosyl transferase
HRV   heart rate variability
IGT   impaired glucose tolerance
IL   interleukin
IR   insulin resistance
iRNA   noncoding RNAs
ITGCN   intratubular germ cell neoplasia unclassified
IUGR   intrauterine growth restriction
KB   Kamin blocking
LBW   low birth weight
LH   luteinizing hormone
LHA   lateral hypothalamic area
LI   latent inhibition
LIG   ligated dams
LL   large litters
LMIC   low and middle income countries
LOI   Lee obesity index
LP   low protein
LPN   low protein nutrition
LPS   lipopolysaccharide
MCH   melanin-concentrating hormone
MFI   mean food intake
MMA   methyl malonic acid
MR   mineralocorticoid receptors
MRDM   malnutrition-related diabetes mellitus
MRI   magnetic resonance imaging
NCDs   noncommunicable diseases
NEIS   neuro-endocrine-immune system
NHPs   nonhuman primates
NPY   neuropeptide Y
NRG-1   neuregulin-1
ODM   offspring of diabetic mothers
OGTT   oral glucose tolerance test
OR   odds ratio
PBMC   peripheral blood mononuclear cells
PCP   phencyclidine
PCS   Pune Children's Study
PGC   primordial germ cell
PMAS   prenatal maternal anxiety and stress
PMNS   Pune Maternal Nutrition Study
PolyI:C   polyriboinosinic-polyribocytidilic acid

POMC	proopiomelanocortin
PPAR-α	peroxisome proliferator activator alpha
PPI	prepulse inhibition
PVH	paraventricular hypothalamic nucleus
RU	relative units
SGA	small for gestational age
SL	small litters
SNS	sympathetic nervous system
sOB-R	soluble leptin receptor
SOP	sham-operated dams
ssRNA	single-stranded RNA
STAI	State Trait Anxiety Inventory
STZ	streptozotocin
T2D	type 2 diabetes
TCR	T-cell receptors
TGF	transforming growth factor
tHcy	total homocysteine
TIN	testicular intraepithelial neoplasia
TLR	toll-like receptors
TLR3	toll-like receptor 3
TNF	tumor necrosis factor
TRH	thyreotropin-releasing hormone
UAL	uterine artery ligation
US	unconditioned stimulus
USPEE	US-pre-exposure effect
VMH	ventromedial hypothalamic nucleus
WHO	World Health Organization

1 The past and future of perinatal medicine

Joachim W. Dudenhausen

Although perinatal medicine is as old as humanity, this designation was not used until the second half of the 20th century. However, during thousands of years, healers, shamans, doctors, priests, physicians, and midwives strove to help the women that were in the childbirth process. Up to the 19th century, some reliable sources were known about affections of women, for example, from Soranus of Ephesus and Galen. The 19th century was marked by progress of surgery, the increased use of anesthesia, and the fight against puerperal fever. Scientists such as Adolphe Pinard, who invented the instrument that carries his name; Christian Doppler, who established the physical effect known after his name; and Etienne Tarnier, who invented the traction forceps in obstetrics, are representatives of these decades.

Since 1950, an increase of basic and clinical investigation on normal and risk pregnancy has occurred in the developed world. New knowledge about physiology and pathophysiology of the pregnant woman, fetus, and newborn and the development of new techniques and methods led to the birth of a new interdisciplinary subspecialty: perinatal medicine.

In the scientific era of medical knowledge, perinatal medicine can be said to have five highlight moments: (1) the auscultation of the fetal heart beats by Le Jumeau de Kergaradec in 1821; (2) the entering of the amniotic cavity by Bevis in 1952; (3) the introduction of labor monitoring and fetal heart rate monitoring by Roberto Caldeyro-Barcia in 1956 and Konrad Hammacher in 1962; (4) the study of fetal acid-base balance and chemical monitoring of the fetus during labor by Erich Saling in 1962 in Berlin; and (5) the use of ultrasonography in obstetrics by Ian Donald in 1965. The international cooperation in perinatal medicine of these days in the middle of the 20th century was demonstrated at the symposium 'Effects of Labor on the Fetus and the Newborn' held October 1–3, 1964, in Montevideo/Uruguay (▶Fig. 1.1).

Besides Montevideo, New York, and other cities of the world, the focus on child health in obstetrics was developed in Berlin. We credit Erich Saling with the focus on the child and the collaboration with pediatricians, which thereby created perinatal medicine (Saling, 1966, 1968).

In the second half of the last century perinatal scientists like Günter Dörner in Berlin have found that intercellular messengers such as neurotransmitters, hormones, and cytokines are capable of programming central nervous controllers during perinatal brain organization (Dörner et al., 1986).

In the meantime, perinatal medicine is becoming one of the biggest interdisciplinary new fields of human medicine. Not only are obstetricians and neonatologists exploring the up-to-now unknown intrauterine space intensively, but also other disciplines of medicine are joining them and discovering the intrauterine compartment from their point of view in order to find out which features are of particular importance for the later stages of human health.

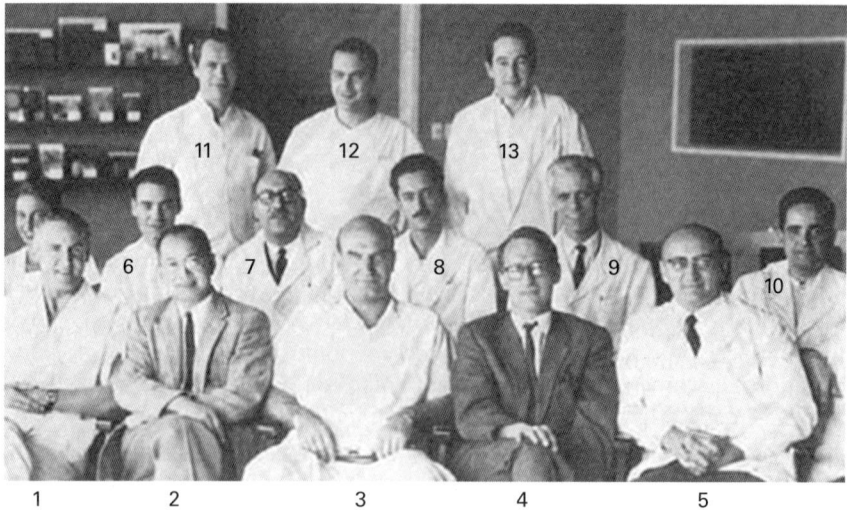

Fig. 1.1: Participants of the symposium 'Effects of Labor on the Fetus and the Newborn', October 1–3, 1964, in Montevideo/Uruguay. First row from left to right: (1) L. Stanley James; (2) E.H. Hon (USA); (3) R. Caldeyro-Barcia (Uruguay); (4) F. Kubli; (5) E.Z. Saling (Germany); Second row: (6) J. Esteban-Altirriba (Spain); (7) D. Fonseca; (8) L. Escarcena; (9) S.V. Pose; (10) C. Mendez-Bauer (Uruguay); Third row: (11) L.O. Alvarez; (12) O. Althabe; (13) R. Schwarcz (Argentina).

Each year, 600,000 women around the world die during pregnancy, in childbed, or as a result of unsafe abortion. Of these deaths, 99% occur in developing countries. Over the past 15 years, this figure has remained the same – this is an outrage that nobody can accept, and the tragedy of it is that the majority of these deaths could have been and could be avoided.

Poverty is one of the most serious causes of illness, and illness is one of the most serious causes of poverty. An absolute necessity for interrupting this cycle is better education. Therefore, information campaigns and prevention are cornerstones of our work in perinatal medicine. We must work toward strategies and their deployment all over the world to provide mothers and children with access to better education and, thereby, to improve their health status (Dudenhausen, 2009).

Looking around our world, we are all aware that the problems and challenges we face in perinatal medicine differ from one region to the next. At the same time, there are other tasks that we must address on a global level. The various regions of the world, with their different health care systems and different demands for health care, are looking for different solutions from us in perinatal medicine. Looking at the basic sciences, the insights we gain today may serve the global solutions of tomorrow. That is why we should meet and discuss ideas to get inspiration so that we get to a point where high-tech medicine influences basic care levels and where clinicians and scientists learn from each other.

From another perspective, perinatal medicine is confronted with changes in human reproductive behavior. The changes in established social structures and the accessibility of medical contraception have contributed to these changes. What is the status of reproduction today? In the past two centuries, the world population has seen a huge increase. On the other hand, in certain regions of the world, families are started at an increasingly later age, and fewer children are born. In 1970, the average age of a woman in Europe giving birth to her first child was 24 years; in 2002, it was 29 years.

While families are started later, they are completed earlier: in the 1960s, during the time of the so-called baby boom in Germany, an average family had three to four children. In 2005 the fertility rate was 1.3 children. Whether we regret or welcome this decline in the birth rate, the fact is that its consequences will affect perinatal medicine in the future. The application of reproductive medicine, the numbers of multiple pregnancies, intrauterine programming, and primary prevention in obstetrics are all aspects that will be the main focus in the future.

References

Dörner G, McCann SM, Martini L, editors. Systemic hormones, neurotransmitters and brain development (Monogr: Neural Sci. Vol. 12). Basel: Karger; 1986.

Dudenhausen JW. Opening remarks by the congress president, "Take responsibility for the future". 9th World Congress of Perinatal Medicine. Berlin, October 21–November 4, 2009.

Saling E. *Das Kind im Bereich der Geburtshilfe.* Stuttgart: Thieme; 1966.

Saling E. *Foetal and Neonatal Hypoxia.* London: Arnold; 1968.

2 Perinatal brain programming and functional teratology

Günter Dörner

Three hundred years ago the Charité was founded, 200 years ago the Humboldt University was founded, and about 100 years ago Selmar Aschheim (▶Fig. 2.1A, left) began here in our laboratories to investigate problems of reproductive and sexual endocrinology. These studies, carried out in collaboration with Bernhard Zondek (▶Fig. 2.1A, right), led to the detection of large amounts of estrogens in the urine of pregnant women and, hence, to the isolation and elucidation of the chemical structure and synthesis of estrogens by Butenandt and Doisy, who received the Nobel Prize. Moreover, the discovery of gonadotrophins (human chorionic gonadotropin [HCG], follicle-stimulating hormone [FSH], and luteinizing hormone [LH]) and the development of the first bioassay for detection of early pregnancy were achieved (Aschheim-Zondek-Test).

In 1945 Walter Hohlweg came from Steinach in Vienna and the Schering AG Berlin as successor of Aschheim to the Charité, and in 1951 he founded the Institute of Experimental Endocrinology (▶Fig. 2.1B). During that time, my teacher Hohlweg (▶Fig. 2.1C, left) made a number of outstanding discoveries in sexual endocrinology, for example, (a) the discovery of a gonadotrophin regulating sex center in the brain, (b) the first development of orally active estrogens and progestagens in collaboration with H. Inhoffen, and (c) the detection of the ovulation-inducing positive estrogen feedback effect for LH (Hohlweg-Effect)

After erection of the Berlin wall in 1961, Hohlweg returned to his home country, Austria, and I was appointed Professor and Director of the Institute of Experimental Endocrinology. During decades of research, we could demonstrate by extensive experimental, clinical, and epidemiological investigations that hormones, neurotransmitters, and cytokines are not only regulators of fundamental processes of life; in critical, mostly pre- and early postnatal developmental periods, they are organizers and programmers of their own life-long controllers within the neuro-endocrine-immune system (NEIS). By neurotransmitters and neurohormones, the brain – as central nervous controller of the NEIS – acts on the endocrine and immune system. The endocrine system interacts via hormones with the nervous and immune system, while the immune system, by cytokines and antibodies, acts on the nervous and endocrine system (▶Fig. 2.2).

Life is based on ontogenetic interactions between genes and the environment. In higher organisms these interactions are controlled by the NEIS. Here, neurotransmitters, hormones, and cytokines are mediators between the environment and the genes and can decisively affect gene expression. Most of all, during critical pre- and early postnatal organization periods, neurotransmitters, hormones, and cytokines codetermine, by means of their environment-dependent quantities, the life-long qualities of their own controllers. Thus, a pre- and early postnatal programming and self-organization of the brain and NEIS does occur, that is, an environment-dependent predetermination of their functional and tolerance ranges for the total life (ontogenetic basic rule). Accordingly, we could demonstrate that unphysiological concentrations of neurotransmitters, hormones,

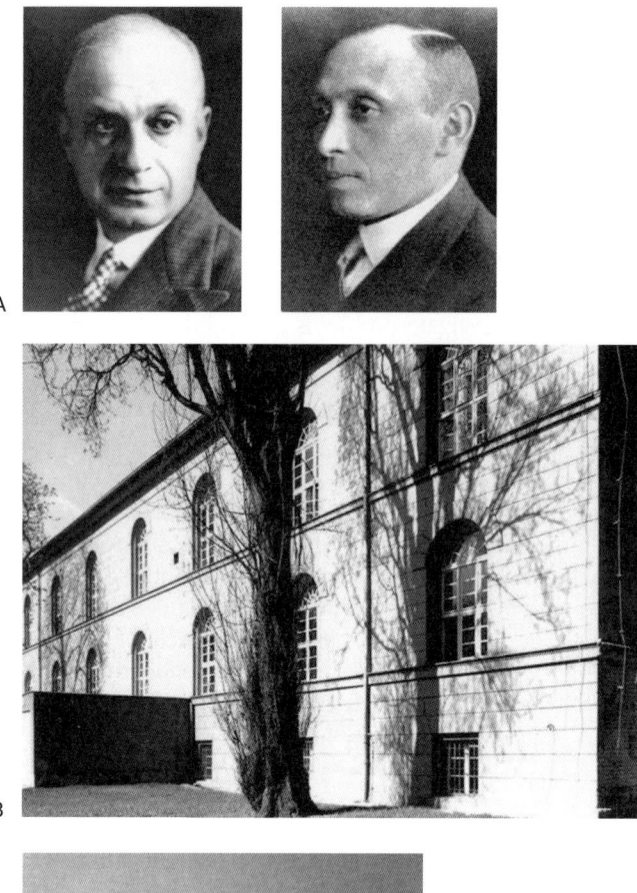

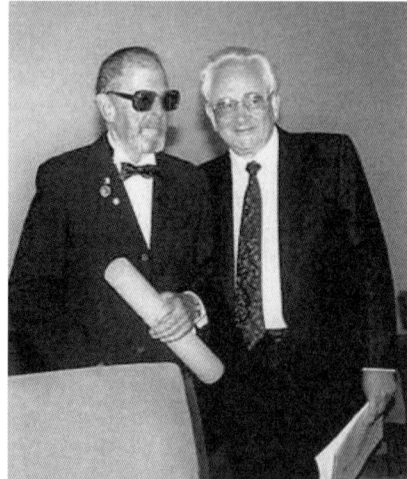

Fig. 2.1: (A) Selmar Aschheim (left) and Bernhard Zondek (right). (B) The building of the Institute of Experimental Endocrinology of the Charité (1951–2008). (C) Walter Hohlweg (left) and Günter Dörner (right) on the occasion of the award of the 'doctor honoris causa' to Hohlweg at Humboldt University Berlin in 1990.

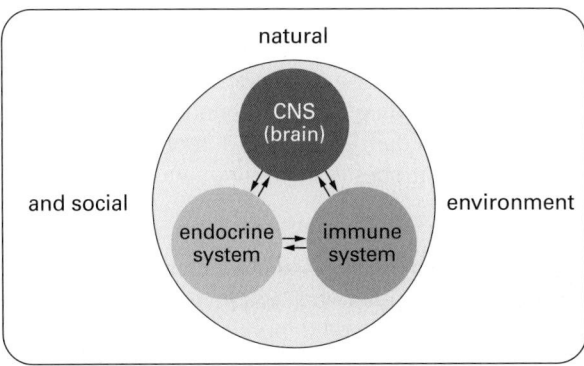

Fig. 2.2: The Neuro-endocrine-immune system (NEIS).

and cytokines during brain organization give rise to dysfunctions and important diseases in later life, which means they can act as endogenous functional teratogens. Consequently, developmental neuro-endocrine-immunology and functional teratology were introduced (Dörner 1975, 1976).

In addition to the ontogenetic basic rule mentioned before, in the last 3 decades I have published 10 ontogenetic theses and recommendations for a neuro-endocrine-immune prophylaxis. They propagate most of all a pre- and early postnatal optimization of the natural and psychosocial environment. Consequently, unphysiological concentrations of neurotransmitters, hormones, and cytokines can be prevented as endogenous functional teratogens of the NEIS. Such prevention is also possible by timely correction of genetically conditioned unphysiological concentrations of these chemical messengers (Dörner 1975, 1976; Dörner et al., 2001).

As early as 1974, I reported about our epigenetic findings at an International Conference on 'Neurobiology of CNS-Hormone Interactions' in Chapel Hill, North Carolina, USA, and in 1976 in Halle, Germany, as member of the German Academy Leopoldina. In the USA, our scientific results were remarkably acknowledged and were used as a basis to promote the foundation of epigenetic centers and of a task force for improved cooperation between geneticists and environmental physicians.

In East-Germany, we could achieve the following results:

1. Introduction of a 'baby-year'. That means, since 1976 mothers could take a 1-year long maternity leave with continuation of the full salary after the birth of a second or following child, since 1986 already after the birth of the first child, and after the birth of the third child even for 1½ years. Due to these measures, mental and psychosocial capacities of children could be significantly increased. In animal experiments, we could demonstrate that early postnatal maternal psychosocial deprivation is followed by a decrease of the neurotransmitter acetylcholine during brain organization and life-long diminished mental capacity (Dörner et al., 2008).
2. By means of improved diagnosis and therapy of gestational diabetes we could prevent fetal hyperinsulinism and reduce the prevalence of childhood-onset diabetes to less than one-third. In animal experiments, we had shown that perinatal hyperinsulinism can result in diabetes mellitus, and this effect appeared to be even

heritable through the maternal line (Dörner and Plagemann, 1994). Most recently, diabetes mellitus was recognized by the World Health Organization (WHO) as the first and only noncommunicable disease to be considered as threat to mankind.

3. By means of increased breast-feeding rates in connection with the 'baby-year' and prevention of overnutrition during the first 3 months of postnatal life we could reduce the development of obesity in children and juveniles by more than one-third (Dörner et al., 2008).

Recently, the president of the general health insurance company in Germany (AOK) reported that the successive diseases of childhood- and juvenile-onset obesity may cost about 70 billions Euros annually for the Federal Republic of Germany.

On the other hand, we could not prevent the application of the insecticide DDT, which resulted in a clear reduction of birth rates in East-Germany, caused by significantly increased disturbances of spermiogenesis as well as increased rates of polycystic ovaries.

Furthermore, I suggested four decades ago that we should recognize hetero-, bi-, and homosexuality as natural variations of sexual orientation because they are based on various sex-hormone and neurotransmitter concentrations during sexual brain organization. Hence, homosexuality could and should no longer be prosecuted and considered as a disease.

Thus, I achieved the total cancellation of prosecution of homosexuality in East-Germany and, by counselling the parliament, also in New Zealand during the 1980s. This was followed by a worldwide liberalization of the legislation for homosexuality during the following decades. In 1989, at the World Conference for Perinatal Psychology and Medicine in Jerusalem, I also proposed the cancellation of homosexuality from the register of diseases of the WHO, and this was realized soon afterwards. Magnus Hirschfeld introduced his unfulfilled guiding principle 'per scientia ad iustitiam', which I would like to extend to 'per scientia ad veritatem, sanitatem, et iustitiam' (per science to truth, health, and justice).

As early as in 1985, we organized in East-Berlin an International Symposium titled 'Systemic Hormones, Neurotransmitters and Brain Development'. The proceedings of this conference already contain some of the most important findings on 'Developmental Neuro-Endocrine-Immunology' to understand the importance of environment-dependent developmental processes for human epigenesis and global health (Dörner et al., 1986).

Already in this context, I have published the following 10 ontogenetic theses and recommendations for promotion of health and prevention or correction of unphysiological concentrations of systemic hormones and/or neurotransmitters during brain organization, that is, by prevention or correction of the following unfavorable conditions during pre- and/or early postnatal life: (1) iodine deficiency; (2) hyperinsulinism, mostly induced by gestational diabetes; (3) hypoxia; (4) stress; (5) placental insufficiency and other gestational disorders; (6) quantitative and/or qualitative malnutrition; (7) radiation and pollution by environmental chemicals; (8) abuse of drugs, hormones, alcohol, and nicotine; (9) psychosocial deprivation; and (10) abnormal levels of systemic hormones and/or neurotransmitters, induced by genetic defects (e.g., congenital hypothyroidism, congenital adrenal hyperplasia, phenylketonuria, and other inborn errors of metabolism) (Dörner, 2000).

In June 2000, Bill Clinton, Craig Venter, and Francis Collins declared the rough chemical elucidation of the human gene code as a great turning point in the history of mankind. Shortly before, in January of the same year, I had emphasized at a Parliamentary Evening in Berlin the importance of the pre- and early postnatal natural and psychosocial environments, which, during the critical organization period of the NEIS, codetermine the life-long capacities of body and mind, especially by perinatal programming of the brain as controller of the NEIS.

Meanwhile, the great importance of the epigenetic code for ontogenesis, which I have postulated since the 1970s as the beginning of the transition from structural to functional genomics, becomes also generally acknowledged by the geneticists. It is finally based on methylation of DNA, histone modifications, and RNA-interference by micro-RNA.

In 2001 – some years after the publication of our 10 theses for perinatal promotion of health and prevention of important diseases – the International Society for Developmental Origins of Health and Disease was founded.

In November 2009, the sixth World Congress of this Society was organized, titled 'From Developmental Biology to Global Health', similar to what we had postulated since the 1970s.

In 2003, the European Society for Primal Health Care was founded, which has supported our recommendations for a pre- and early postnatal neuro-endocrine-immune prophylaxis in all European countries.

Today, I can ascertain that due to primary neuro-endocrine-immune prophylaxis the ontogenesis of millions of human beings could meanwhile be improved. Furthermore, by improving ontogenesis, socio- and phylogenesis are also improved and *vice versa* (▶Fig. 2.3). Consequently, primary neuro-endocrine-immune prophylaxis is not only a possibility for prevention of medical maldevelopments, but also of sociocultural and even economic maldevelopments.

Recently, on the occasion of my 80th birthday, I received a letter from the President of the Leopoldina Prof. Volker ter Meulen, in which the hope was expressed that our ontogenetic theses, which represent the basic rules for protection and optimal development of progressing life, may also be taken into account for future legislation.

I would like to mention, that our successful research work was only possible with excellent co-workers, for example, Andreas Plagemann, Fritz Stahl, Franziska Götz, Wolfgang Rohde, Rolf Lindner, and Renate Tönjes; special technical assistants and

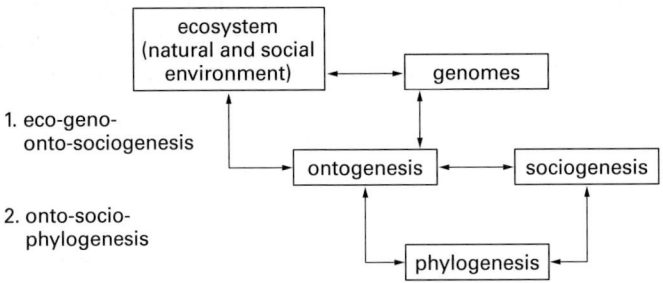

Fig. 2.3: Environment- and gene-dependent human ontogenesis, sociogenesis, and phylogenesis.

secretaries; and my dear wife. In addition, the Society for Human Ontogenetics was founded in cooperation with Karl-Friedrich Wessel and Günter Tembrock.

Finally, I have to emphasize that the worldwide acknowledgement of the importance of perinatal brain programming, functional teratology, and primary neuro-endocrine-immune prophylaxis and their beneficial clinical utilizations was only possible by the excellent research work of outstanding experts in many countries. I am very pleased that many of them gave lectures at this International meeting on 'Perinatal Programming – The State of the Art' and celebrate with us the bi- and tricentenary of Humboldt-University and Charité.

References

Dörner G. Perinatal hormone levels and brain organization. In: Stumpf WE, Grant LD, eds. *Anatomical Neuroendocrinology*. Basel: Karger; 1975: 245–52.

Dörner G. *Hormones and Brain Differentiation*. Amsterdam, Oxford, New York: Elsevier; 1976.

Dörner G. Ten ontogenetic theses for promotion of health and primary prevention of important diseases by a prenatal and early postnatal neuro-endocrine-immune prophylaxis. *Neuroendocrinol Lett* 2000;21: 265–7.

Dörner G, Götz F, Rohde W, Plagemann A, Lindner R, Peters H, Ghanaati Z. Genetic and epigenetic effects on sexual brain organization mediated by sex hormones. *Neuroendocrinol Lett* 2001;22: 403–9.

Dörner G, McCann SM, Martini L, eds. Systemic hormones, neurotransmitters and brain development (Monogr: Neural Sci. Vol. 12). Basel: Karger; 1986.

Dörner G, Plagemann A. Perinatal hyperinsulinism as possible predisposing factor for diabetes mellitus, obesity, and enhanced cardiovascular risk in later life. *Horm Metab Res* 1994;26: 213–21.

Dörner G, Rodekamp E, Plagemann A. Maternal deprivation and overnutrition in early postnatal life and their primary prevention: Historical reminiscence of an "ecologic experiment" in Germany. *Hum Ontogenet* 2008;2: 51–9.

3 Experimental models of low birth weight – insight into the developmental programming of metabolic health, aging and immune function

Chantal A. A. Heppolette, Donald Palmer, and Susan E. Ozanne

The thrifty phenotype hypothesis states that nutrition in utero can program irreversible metabolic changes in the fetus and subsequently influence the risk of developing metabolic syndrome and associated diseases in adulthood. These include cardiovascular disease, type 2 diabetes and hypertension. Animal studies using nutritional, surgical and pharmacological manipulations, have shown that a suboptimal fetal environment can result in fetal growth retardation, subsequent low birth weight and alterations in body composition and metabolism. These predispose offspring to a poor metabolic profile in later life, especially when they experience rapid early postnatal growth and an obesogenic environment. Recent evidence suggests a wider range of conditions resulting from such developmental programming. These include mental health, osteoporosis, immune function and even the aging process. It is also now apparent that a wider range of exposures during gestation in addition to nutrition, can influence long term health and not necessarily through changes in fetal growth. This paper reviews the current evidence for the role of developmental programming in metabolic diseases, aging and immune function.

3.1 Developmental programming and the metabolic syndrome in humans

The global pandemic of metabolic diseases such as type 2 diabetes (T2D), obesity and cardiovascular disease (CVD) have devastating consequences on human morbidity, mortality and quality of life, in addition to the economic strain on healthcare systems. The population shift towards a demographic of a higher obesogenic phenotype in the relatively short time span of two generations, suggests that it is driven by environmental factors rather than genetic contributions. Whilst current environment for the individual is accepted as having a crucial impact on their health, accumulating evidence suggests that early environmental factors such as nutritional and environmental imbalances *in utero* and in early postnatal life play a vital role in determining the long-term health of an individual.

3.2 The thrifty phenotype hypothesis

Epidemiological studies by Anders Forsdahl in Norway were the first to suggest a causative link between early life environmental factors and disease in later life (Forsdahl,

1977). Here a positive correlation was found between mortality from atherosclerotic heart disease in individuals aged between 40 and 69, and infant mortality (used as an index of quality of life) in the same county (Forsdahl, 1977). Later studies by Barker outlined the detrimental effect of poverty, poor nutrition and maternal health on infant mortality and risk for cardiovascular disease (CVD) (Barker and Osmond, 1986). Through studies of UK cohorts Barker and colleagues demonstrated a link between low birth weight and subsequent CVD, indicative of an important role played by the fetal environment (Barker, 1995).

The thrifty phenotype hypothesis (or Barker hypothesis to which it is often referred) was proposed in 1992 by Hales and Barker to provide a mechanistic framework by which the early environment, and in particular early nutrition affects long-term health. It is outlined in ▶Fig. 3.1.

It suggests that a growing fetus when subjected to limited nutrition undergoes an adaptive response, whereby the growth of crucial organs such as the brain is maintained at the expense of the viscera such as the endocrine pancreas. In addition metabolism is programmed to promote nutrient storage to maximise its chance of survival. Consequentially the structure and function of the body is altered (Hales and Barker, 1992). However these adaptations can become detrimental if the postnatal environment differs to that experienced *in utero*. This is especially evident when malnutrition *in utero* is followed by adequate or over-nutrition postnatally. The reduced endocrine pancreatic mass and altered muscle and fat metabolism are unable to deal appropriately with relative over-nourishment and conditions including the metabolic syndrome, type 2 diabetes (T2D), cardiovascular disease (CVD) and hypertension can ensue (Hales and Barker, 1992). The metabolic syndrome involves the onset of visceral obesity, hypertriglyceridemia, low HDL-cholesterol, hypertension, fasting hyperglycemia and insulin resistance.

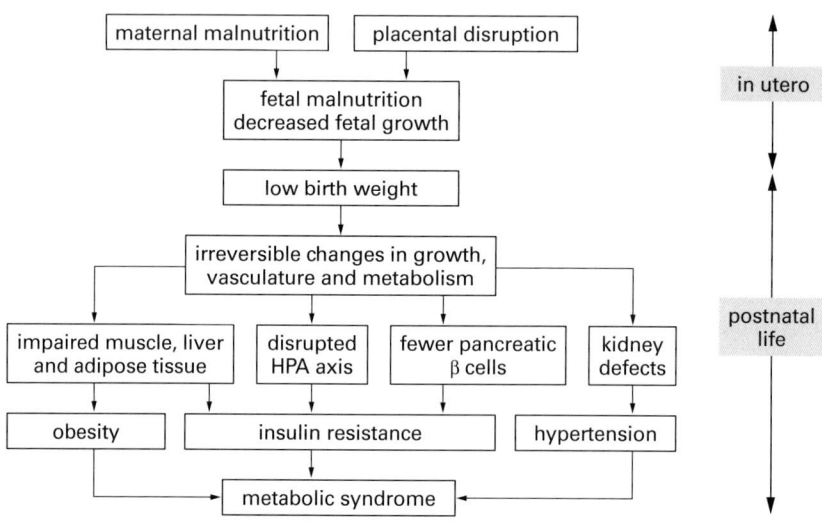

Fig. 3.1: The thrifty phenotype hypothesis.

3.2.1 Significance of low birth weight

Birth weight is a key indicator of growth *in utero*. In normal pregnancy birth weight is highly variable and influenced more heavily by the intra-uterine environment than the genome (Carr-Hill et al., 1987). This is demonstrated by studies showing that the birth weights of half siblings have a correlation coefficient of 0.1 when sharing the same father and 0.58 when sharing the same mother (Carr-Hill et al., 1987). The growth rate of a fetus is limited by its supply of nutrition and oxygen, so maternal malnutrition and placental disruption can therefore result in low birth weight. Additional markers of malnutrition include disproportionate head circumference, body length and weight.

Low birth weight is considered a significant risk factor for T2D, CVD and the metabolic syndrome (Hales and Barker, 2001; Lindsay and Bennett, 2001). The Hertfordshire study of 64 year old males, was the first to demonstrate that low birth weight increases the susceptibility towards T2D and metabolic syndrome, where no threshold level of birth weight was evident (Hales et al., 1991). Such findings have been repeated in numerous countries worldwide. The Dutch famine, which occurred from November 1944 to May 1945, provided direct evidence that maternal nutrition can influence fetal growth and long term health. This demonstrated that individuals *in utero* at this time had lower birth weights and increased plasma glucose concentration and increased fasting pro-insulin concentration, amounting to increased insulin resistance by age 50 (Ravelli et al., 1998). Their growth had accelerated after the famine when their nutritional environment was restored. This is indicative of catch-up growth which predisposes individuals towards metabolic syndrome (Ravelli et al., 1998). It has since been demonstrated that famine during early gestation alters fetal lipid metabolism whereas when this insult occurs during mid to late gestation, glucose/insulin metabolism is affected (Ravelli et al., 1998). The Leningrad famine occurred between 1941 and 1944 so the period of malnutrition was prolonged and accelerated catch-up growth did not occur (Stanner and Yudkin, 2001). Consequentially the association between famine exposure and altered glucose/insulin metabolism was not statistically significant, although this study was also weak in statistical power (Stanner and Yudkin, 2001). An association between catch-up growth and increased mortality from CVD has also been demonstrated (Eriksson et al., 1999). Further studies from UK cohorts showed similar associations between low birth weight and adult central adiposity using DEXA scanning (Kensara et al., 2005).

Twin studies provide a key insight into the significance of *in utero* environmental influences on birth weight on developmental programming as they negate confounding genetic and maternal factors. Even though on average twins are born of a lower weight compared to singleton counterparts, they do not have a higher incidence of cardiovascular-related mortality (Christensen et al., 2001; de Geus et al., 2001). However a recent study of monozygotic and dizygotic twins born between 1926 and 1958 revealed a negative correlation between birth weight and blood pressure independent of genetic factors (Bergvall et al., 2007). In a retrospective study in Denmark involving monozygotic and dizygotic twins discordant for T2D and impaired glucose tolerance, birth weights were lower in those individuals who suffered from T2D and impaired glucose tolerance (Poulsen et al., 1997). Twin studies have also demonstrated a negative relationship between birth weight and unhealthy body composition characteristics such as waist-to-hip ratio, skin-fold thickness and reduced muscle mass (Loos et al., 2001).

3.2.2 High birth weight and maternal obesity in humans

Elevated birth weight can be equally detrimental to the health of the child in later life as low birth weight (Catalano et al., 2003). There is growing interest in maternal hypernutrition given the rise in birth weights and incidence of "large for gestational age" (LGA) babies in developed countries (Surkan et al., 2004). Studies in more contemporary populations have shown that a U- or J-shaped association can exist between birth weight and obesity and T2D in later life. This especially occurs in cultures where T2D is prevalent in the population, for example in the Pima Arizonian Indians (McCance et al., 1994).

Various factors are considered influential in overweight births including maternal obesity, maternal hypernutrition, maternal hyperglycaemia and pre-pregnancy maternal body composition (Sacks et al., 2006). Children born of mothers who were obese prior to pregnancy have a tendency towards being overweight in childhood, and this is a key predictor of obesity in adulthood (Field et al., 2005). Although this could be explained by genetic inheritance, a further study reported that moderate weight gain between successive pregnancies resulted in more complications such as LGA births (Villamor and Cnattingius, 2006). Offspring of obese women and those with gestational diabetes, are themselves more likely to have greater neonatal fat, develop insulin resistance, become obese in later life and have an increased risk of metabolic syndrome (Catalano et al., 2003). Sibling pair studies in the Pima Arizonian Indian population, where siblings were discordant for maternal diabetes, show a strong offspring diabetic and obesogenic trait acquired in pregnancy (Dabelea and Pettitt, 2001).

3.2.3 Effects of early postnatal nutrition

In addition to the environment *in utero*, nutrition and subsequent growth during the early postnatal period can also have significant effects on long-term health. McCance was the first to observe an effect of early infant malnutrition on susceptibility to infection in rats (McCance, 1962). Since then there have been numerous animal studies demonstrating that early nutrition can permanently influence blood lipids levels, insulin levels, blood pressure, body fat proportion, atherosclerosis, behaviour, learning and longevity (Hahn, 1984; Lewis et al., 1986; McCance, 1962; Ozanne and Hales, 2004). Human studies have been implemented in order to investigate the nutritional programming effects of breast milk and formula milk on long term health (Lucas, 2005). Preterm infants fed human breast milk have reduced incidence of necrotizing enterocolitis in comparison to those fed formula milk (Lucas and Cole, 1990). This effect was most dramatic in infants born after 30 weeks of gestation when other risk factors were diminished (Lucas and Cole, 1990).

Cardiovascular disease is affected by both the type and composition of milk during lactation, which in turn influences postnatal growth (Lucas, 2005). Retrospective studies have shown that breast-fed infants have reduced risk of CVD, hypercholesterolemia, obesity, T2D and hypertension compared to formula fed infants (Lucas, 2005). Such effects could be due to socio-biological confounding factors so intervention trials have been implemented in order to overcome these. Here pre-term infants whose mothers chose not to breast feed, were randomly assigned to either human milk from donor mothers or formula milk (Singhal et al., 2004). Those infants fed human milk for at least one month had reduced blood pressure, LDL cholesterol, leptin resistance and insulin resistance in comparison to those fed formula milk (Singhal et al., 2004). These effects were still observed 13–16 years post intervention and the greater the consumption of breast milk during the neonatal period, the lower the risk factor status in later life (Singhal et al., 2004). In summary these observational studies and intervention trials provide compelling evidence suggesting that the intake of breast milk in infancy reduces the risk of metabolic syndrome in later life.

These trials also compared the effects of enriched and standard formula on preterm infants and found that infants fed the growth-promoting enriched formula showed increased cardiovascular risk factors in later childhood (Singhal et al., 2004). However preterm infants fed enriched formula had better neurocognitive functioning and reduced risk of degenerative bone disease in later life compared to those fed standard formula (Lucas, 2005). In a separate study full term infants who were small for gestational age were given growth-promoting formula and had elevated diastolic blood pressure 6–8 years following the study, compared to those fed standard formula (Singhal and Lucas, 2004). More recently a clinical trial was performed where full term infants whose mothers chose to formula feed, were randomized to receive formula milk with either high or low protein content. Those fed the high protein milk had greater weight gain, which suggests that low protein feeding in infancy may protect against later obesity (Koletzko et al., 2009).

3.3 Evidence for developmental programming of the metabolic syndrome from animal models

Animal models can further our understanding of developmental programming and have provided direct evidence for the effect of the early environment on long term health. Such models include maternal calorie restriction, low protein, hypernutrition and obesity, vitamin restriction, hyperglycemia, hypoxia, iron restriction, psychological stress, intrauterine artery ligation and dexamethasone treatment amongst others. Despite the multitudinal possible insults to the fetus, the phenotypic outcomes are fairly similar, suggesting common mechanisms underlying these changes.

3.3.1 Calorie restriction and malnutrition

Maternal malnutrition during critical periods of development *in utero* has various effects on offspring, including predisposing towards the development of the metabolic syndrome. The concept of implementing maternal malnutrition to programme adult disease began with Winick and Noble who observed that malnutrition during fetal development resulted in reduced pancreatic cell number (Winick and Noble, 1966). The timing of the insult is crucial, as revealed by animal models where malnutrition during early gestation results in small well proportioned babies, but neonates with malnutrition during late gestation have normal weight with altered proportions (Widdowson and McCance, 1975).

Maternal calorie restriction (CR) can alter the programming of adipocyte metabolism and body composition which later predisposes towards obesity (Bispham et al., 2005). For example sheep of low birth weight have a higher neonatal fat proportion, compared to sheep of higher birth weight (Greenwood et al., 1998). This is especially evident when the insult of nutrient restriction is administered during the period of optimal placental growth, again implying a sensitive time window for exposure (Budge et al., 2005). 30% reduction in food intake during gestation in rodents severely impairs fetal growth and predisposes towards adulthood hypertension, elevated fasting plasma insulin concentration, glucose intolerance and heightened food intake in later life (Vickers et al., 2000). Wistar rats fed a 50% calorie restricted diet from day 15 of pregnancy gradually lost glucose tolerance, and insulinopenia and loss of β-cell mass was evident with age (Garofano et al., 1999). Severe (70%) maternal CR in Wistar rats led to altered plasma insulin at birth and hypertension in adulthood (Woodall et al., 1996).

Effects are exacerbated when an intra-uterine calorie restricted diet is followed by postnatal hypernutrition (Budge et al., 2005). For example rodents subjected to moderate (50%) and severe (70%) prenatal caloric restriction, have high fat deposition when given a hypercaloric or high fat diet postnatally (Vickers et al., 2000).

3.3.2 The maternal low protein (MLP) diet

The availability of protein is a key determinant of fetal growth. Amino acids determine pancreatic β cell differentiation, replication and insulin secretion and as insulin acts as a crucial growth factor in the fetus, protein indirectly influences the rate of fetal growth (Hales and Barker, 1992). The earliest investigation into the Maternal Low Protein (MLP) diet was led by Weinkove who demonstrated that perinatal and postnatal low protein diets produced permanently impaired insulin secretion (Weinkove et al., 1974). Since then MLP diets have been used to explore the links between fetal malnutrition and impaired growth and subsequent CVD, T2D and associated pathologies. For example, a low protein diet during gestation results in a programmed increase in postnatal production of enzymes for glucose synthesis even when the postnatal diet is normal (Desai et al., 1995). Rats fed a MLP diet during gestation have low birth weight, evidence of growth restriction *in utero*. If followed by the same diet during lactation permanent growth-restriction results and this is maintained into adulthood (Desai et al., 1996).

An MLP diet restricts fetal growth and has a permanent effect on offspring health (Langley and Jackson, 1994). As in human studies, MLP insults have sensitive time windows. Maternal protein restriction during pregnancy and lactation results in hypertension and an age-dependent loss of glucose tolerance which is especially evident in male offspring (Petry et al., 2001). This is associated with β-cell dysfunction and insulin resistance. More recently Kwong *et al* showed that rat dams fed a low protein diet of 9% from conception through to implantation followed by standard chow resulted in offspring developing elevated glucose levels by day 4 and hypertension in adulthood (Kwong et al., 2000).

The MLP rat model has been modified giving recuperated (Recup) and postnatal low protein (PLP) diets which enable us to identify critical time windows of nutritional programming (Ozanne, 2001). In this model recuperated rats are fed a low protein diet of 8% during pregnancy which results in low birth weight, then cross-fostered during lactation to a mother fed a control diet containing 20% protein (Desai et al., 1996). By weaning at 21 days these Recup animals have similar body weights to controls as they have undergone catch-up growth (Jennings et al., 1999). This increases stress in the individual and its long-term effects include elevated fasting glucose concentration, β-cell dysfunction and increased susceptibility to T2D and vascular dysfunction (Tarry-Adkins et al., 2008). Postnatal low protein (PLP) rats are fed a normal protein diet (20%) during pregnancy then cross-fostered during lactation to a mother fed a low protein diet (8%) until weaning where their diet is restored to normal levels (Ozanne and Hales, 2004). These offspring undergo slow early growth during the suckling period and long-term effects include enhanced insulin sensitivity, reduced insulin and glucose concentration, dampened albuminuria and reduced susceptibility to CVD (Tarry-Adkins et al., 2008).

3.3.3 Maternal iron deficiency

Iron deficiency anemia occurs when iron absorption is insufficient, usually due to depleted dietary levels, resulting in reduced formation of hemoglobin. Maternal hemoglobin levels are associated with offspring birth weight and preterm birth in a U-shaped relationship (Rasmussen, 2001). A similar relationship is likely to occur between haemoglobin levels and perinatal mortality although this is not yet fully established. Iron deficiency anemia results in defective placental vascularisation and dysregulation of maternal and fetal hormones such as IGF-1 and cortico-releasing hormone, which when elevated, can induce preterm labor and pre-eclampsia, and inhibition of IGF-1 production, resulting in defective fetal development (Rasmussen, 2001). This was shown in a rodent model of maternal iron restriction, where offspring also had elevated blood pressure by 40 days of age, in addition to having low birth weights (Lewis et al., 2002). Further maternal iron restriction studies have shown increased glucose tolerance and fasting serum triglyceride in 3 month old rats subjected to maternal iron restriction although these effects were not maintained through to late adulthood (Lewis et al., 2001).

3.3.4 Intrauterine artery ligation

The fetal environment in humans is severely impaired by placental disruption caused by maternal smoking, pre-eclampsia and abnormal placenta development (Baschat and Hecher, 2004). Uteroplacental insufficiency is occurring more commonly in western society and results in disrupted fetal growth and subsequently low birth weight (Baschat and Hecher, 2004). Thus animal models have been engineered to study such effects on offspring. For example fetuses from maternal bilateral uterine artery ligations were hypoxic, hypoglycemic, with dampened insulin and IGF-1 levels (Ogata et al., 1986). Uteroplacental insufficiency also leads to poor development of the pancreas, liver and kidney, and can result in T2D and gender-specific development of hypertension in adult life (De Prins and Van Assche, 1982; Merlet-Benichou et al., 1994; Moritz et al., 2009; Vuguin et al., 2004).

3.3.5 Maternal glucocorticoid exposure

Fetal development is free from glucocorticoid exposure until the late trimester, where upon glucocorticoids stimulate the maturation of tissues and organs (Fowden and Forhead, 2004). Early or overexposure to glucocorticoids results in growth retardation and subsequently low birth weight in offspring (Reynolds et al., 2001). This environment is mimicked in animal studies by the administration of dexamethasone, a potent synthetic glucocorticoid. Resultantly elevated levels of glucocorticoids especially during the final trimester of gestation, predispose offspring towards insulin resistance, glucose intolerance and hypertension (Benediktsson et al., 1993; Lindsay et al., 1996; Nyirenda et al., 1998). Glucocorticoids may also provide a link between maternal calorie restriction, maternal protein restriction and fetal growth retardation. In these models, glucocorticoid levels are elevated (Langley-Evans et al., 1996). However it is important to consider that maternal exposure to dexamethasone can dampen maternal food intake (Woods and Weeks, 2005).

3.3.6 Models of maternal hypernutrition and maternal obesity

Several studies have demonstrated the significance of hypernutrition during gestation and lactation on the subsequent development of obesity in offspring. An early study in baboons showed that overfeeding during the pre-weaning stage resulted in an irreversible increase in adiposity in female offspring via adipocyte hypertrophy (Lewis et al., 1986). A further study observed an increase in fat pad weight by weaning age in the offspring of rats fed a 40% fat diet during pregnancy and lactation (Guo and Jen, 1995). Such changes persist into adulthood demonstrated by the increase in body weight and visceral fat depot at 6 months in offspring of rat dams fed a 24% fat diet (Khan et al., 2004).

Maternal obesity has also been linked to the programming of other metabolic diseases. Offspring exposed to maternal obesity/hypernutrition *in utero* and during lactation develop hypertension, increased adiposity, insulin resistance and glucose intolerance (Samuelsson et al., 2008). A recent study in sheep showed that maternal obesity before and during gestation led to impaired glucose and insulin regulation, in addition to changes in adiposity in offspring in later life (Long et al., 2010). The effects of maternal obesity on the cardiovascular system of offspring have also been observed, with the occurrence of hypertension, vascular dysfunction, hypercholesterolemia and hyperlipidemia (Drake and Reynolds, 2010; Samuelsson et al., 2008).

3.4 Developmental programming of aging

Characteristics of the metabolic syndrome are age-associated and there is now evidence for the existence of developmental programming of aging. The maternal low protein model in rodents has shown reduced longevity, accelerated aging, and accelerated pancreatic islet and kidney telomere shortening in animals that undergo fetal growth restriction and accelerated postnatal catch-up growth as a result of maternal protein restriction (Jennings et al., 1999; Ozanne and Hales, 2004; Tarry-Adkins et al., 2008). In contrast slow growth during lactation in rodents results in extended longevity, increased antioxidant enzymes, suppressed renal telomere shortening, and fewer aortic DNA single strand breaks (Chen et al., 2009a; Ozanne and Hales, 2004; Tarry-Adkins et al., 2008). Such findings suggest that pathways of cellular senescence and aging are responsive to environmental cues early in life and that the rate of aging is irreversibly established at such early time points.

3.5 Developmental programming and immunity

Although initial focus of developmental programming was on nutrition and its effects on metabolic disease, this has since been expanded to include a range of early exposure types and numerous health outcomes. One such area of growing interest is the effects of the early environment on the immune system. An efficient and functional immune system is considered vital for the protection against infection, autoimmune diseases and tumor growth. These conditions however are more prevalent in the elderly due to age-dependent immune deterioration, termed immunosenescence (Aw et al., 2008).

3.5.1 Developmental programming of adaptive immunity in humans

Epidemiological data from human studies have shown that in rural Gambia the birth season can predict infection-related adult mortality (Collinson et al., 2003). Those born during the hungry season where food supplies are limited are more prone to infection and have a smaller thymic volume in comparison to those born in the harvest season (Collinson et al., 2003). This is also evident in Guinea-Bissau where a reduction in thymic weight is associated with increased infection-related mortality (Aaby et al., 2002). Reports from the Philippines and Pakistan showed a positive correlation between birth weight and subsequent antibody response to a polysaccharide antigen (McDade et al., 2001). A longer period of breast-feeding was also shown to increase thymic volume in infants, which is indicative of increased immune capacity (Moore et al., 2009).

3.5.2 Developmental programming of adaptive immunity in animal models

Various animal studies have shown that maternal malnutrition during gestation can have detrimental effects on thymus development in the offspring. For example sheep offspring whose mothers were malnourished during gestation, have reduced thymic mass (Osgerby et al., 2002). Thymic mass and architecture was defective in rat offspring given half the feed *in utero* with consequential dampened cellular and humoral immune responses at 4 months of age (Schuler et al., 2008). Prenatal malnutrition can also reduce the secretion of the thymic active hormones such as thymopoietin in rat and human offspring (McDade et al., 2001; Schuler et al., 2008).

More recently Odaka and colleagues showed that a maternal high fat diet in mice can cause immune dysfunction in the offspring (Odaka et al., 2010). A significant reduction in thymic cortical thickness and splenocyte count was observed in animals born from mothers that were given a high fat diet during gestation. In addition it was observed that these animals had an increased level of TNFα production together with an alteration of specific antibody responses (Odaka et al., 2010). The maternal low protein model has also demonstrated immune effects in offspring. Thymi from mice exposed to maternal protein restriction during lactation (PLP) were approximately 50% heavier at 3m than at 21d, whereas control animals demonstrated no difference in thymic weight during this period (Chen et al., 2009b). PLP thymi also had increased expression of SIRT1, an important factor in mediating the positive effects of CR on lifespan, and a reduction in p16, a robust biomarker of cellular ageing (Chen et al., 2009b). This implies a reduction in thymic aging in animals that undergo slow early postnatal growth. Prenatal stress is another method of insult with immune programming implications. Shown in rodent and pig studies, thymus size, morphology and function is altered by maternal psychological stress (Hashimoto et al., 2001; Tuchscherer et al., 2002). Prenatal stress can also lead to defective T lymphocyte cell counts and specific antigen responses (Gotz et al., 2007; Sobrian et al., 1997).

3.5.3 Developmental programming of innate immunity

Atopic diseases are considered to have a high genetic component but growing evidence suggests a role for the prenatal environment in influencing the development of conditions such as eczema, hayfever and asthma (Los et al., 2001). Recent studies in Danish and Swedish twins suggest low birth weight to be a significant risk factor for the development of childhood asthma (Kindlund et al., 2010). Conversely studies on Swedish twins discordant for childhood atopic eczema revealed a positive association between birth weight and disease incidence (Lundholm et al., 2010). Maternal intake of foods high in *n*-3 polyunsaturated fatty acids like fish protects against the development of such atopic diseases which are positively associated with the maternal intake of foods high in *n*-6 polyunsaturated fatty acids, such as vegetable and sunflower oils (Calder et al., 2010). These studies indicate that the human innate immune system is susceptible to programming, particularly when associated with allergic reactions, although low and high fetal growth can have opposing outcomes on different allergies.

In rodents maternal food restriction during gestation and lactation results in elevated basal inflammation but reduced cytokine responses in offspring (Desai et al., 2009). Maternal obesity increases macrophage accumulation, inflammatory cytokines and factors of the inflammatory signaling pathway in placenta of sheep offspring during mid-gestation (Zhu et al., 2010). Maternal psychological stress also inhibits the innate immune system of offspring, with effects including impaired functioning of macrophages, natural killer cells and neutrophils (Bellinger et al., 2008).

3.6 Conclusions

Observations from both human and animal studies have revealed a variety of maternal insults capable of programming a wide range of health outcomes in later life which are outlined in ▶Fig. 3.2.

Suboptimal fetal nutrition alters fetal growth resulting in metabolic and structural changes in tissues at birth. These are further exacerbated by early postnatal hypernutrition. Changes in the epigenotype have been suggested to play a role in mediating long term effects of developmental programming. In addition to the already substantial evidence supporting the role of developmental programming in the metabolic syndrome and associated pathologies, there is now growing support for the effect of early life environment on developing other conditions. Most diseases affected by developmental programming are age-related. Consistent with this observation, growing evidence suggests an effect of prenatal and early postnatal exposures on the structure and function of the immune system, which have already been reported to become impaired with age

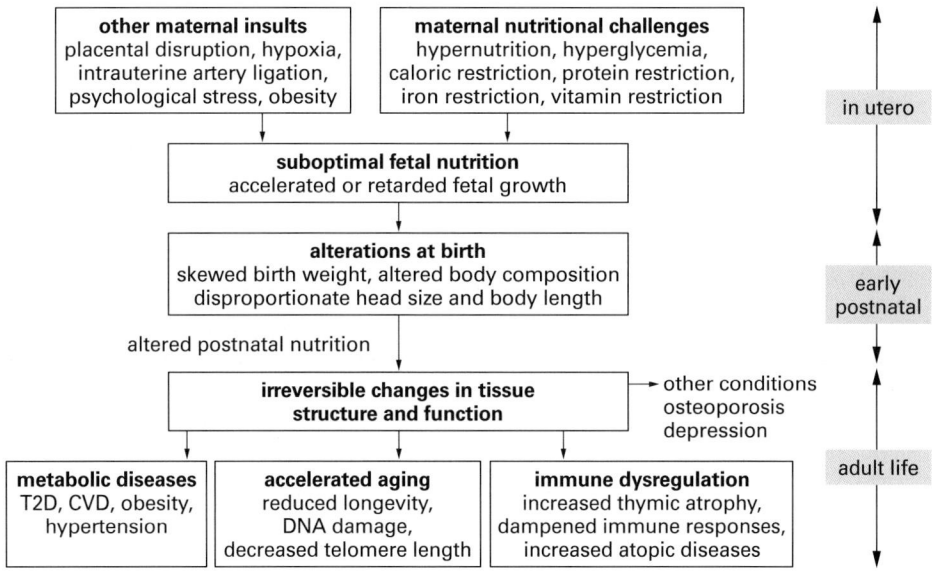

Fig. 3.2: Overview of the origins and impacts of developmental programming.

under normal conditions. Therefore targeting early life as a critical period for optimization of nutrition and environment exposures has the potential to maximize the chances of the population to age healthily.

References

Aaby P, Marx C, Trautner S, Rudaa D, Hasselbalch H, Jensen H, Lisse I. Thymus size at birth is associated with infant mortality: a community study from Guinea-Bissau. *Acta Paediatr* 2002;91: 698–703.

Aw D, Silva AB, Maddick M, von Zglinicki T, Palmer DB. Architectural changes in the thymus of aging mice. *Aging Cell* 2008;7: 158–67.

Barker DJ. Fetal origins of coronary heart disease. *BMJ* 1995;311: 171–4.

Barker DJ, Osmond C. Infant mortality, childhood nutrition, and ischaemic heart disease in England and Wales. *Lancet* 1986;1: 1077–81.

Baschat AA, Hecher K. Fetal growth restriction due to placental disease. *Sem Perinatol* 2004;28: 67–80.

Bellinger DL, Lubahn C, Lorton D. Maternal and early life stress effects on immune function: relevance to immunotoxicology. *J Immunotoxicol* 2008;5: 419–44.

Benediktsson R, Lindsay RS, Noble J, Seckl JR, Edwards CR. Glucocorticoid exposure in utero: new model for adult hypertension. *Lancet* 1993;341: 339–41.

Bergvall N, Iliadou A, Johansson S, de Faire U, Kramer MS, Pawitan Y, Pedersen NL, Lichtenstein P, Cnattingius S. Genetic and shared environmental factors do not confound the association between birth weight and hypertension: a study among Swedish twins. *Circulation* 2007;115: 2931–8.

Bispham J, Gardner DS, Gnanalingham MG, Stephenson T, Symonds ME, Budge H. Maternal nutritional programming of fetal adipose tissue development: differential effects on messenger ribonucleic acid abundance for uncoupling proteins and peroxisome proliferator-activated and prolactin receptors. *Endocrinology* 2005;146: 3943–9.

Budge H, Gnanalingham MG, Gardner DS, Mostyn A, Stephenson T, Symonds ME. Maternal nutritional programming of fetal adipose tissue development: long-term consequences for later obesity. *Birth Defects Res C Embryo Today* 2005;75: 193–9.

Calder PC, Kremmyda LS, Vlachava M, Noakes PS, Miles EA. Is there a role for fatty acids in early life programming of the immune system? *Proc Nutr Soc* 2010;69: 373–80.

Carr-Hill R, Campbell DM, Hall MH, Meredith A. Is birth weight determined genetically? *BMJ* 1987;295: 687–9.

Catalano PM, Thomas A, Huston-Presley L, Amini SB. Increased fetal adiposity: a very sensitive marker of abnormal in utero development. *Am J Obstet Gynecol* 2003;189: 1698–1704.

Chen JH, Martin-Gronert MS, Tarry-Adkins J, Ozanne SE. Maternal protein restriction affects postnatal growth and the expression of key proteins involved in lifespan regulation in mice. *PLoS One* 2009a;4: e4950.

Chen JH, Tarry-Adkins JL, Heppolette CA, Palmer DB, Ozanne SE. Early-life nutrition influences thymic growth in male mice that may be related to the regulation of longevity. *Clin Sci* (Lond) 2009b;118: 429–38.

Christensen K, Wienke A, Skytthe A, Holm NV, Vaupel JW, Yashin AI. Cardiovascular mortality in twins and the fetal origins hypothesis. *Twin Res* 2001;4: 344–349.

Collinson AC, Moore SE, Cole TJ, Prentice AM. Birth season and environmental influences on patterns of thymic growth in rural Gambian infants. *Acta Paediatr* 2003;92: 1014–20.

Dabelea D, Pettitt DJ. Intrauterine diabetic environment confers risks for type 2 diabetes mellitus and obesity in the offspring, in addition to genetic susceptibility. *J Pediatr Endocrinol Metab* 2001;14: 1085–91.

de Geus EJ, Posthuma D, Ijzerman RG, Boomsma DI. Comparing blood pressure of twins and their singleton siblings: being a twin does not affect adult blood pressure. *Twin Res* 2001;4: 385–91.

De Prins FA, Van Assche FA. Intrauterine growth retardation and development of endocrine pancreas in the experimental rat. *Biol Neonat* 1982;41: 16–21.

Desai M, Crowther NJ, Lucas A, Hales CN. Organ-selective growth in the offspring of protein-restricted mothers. *Br J Nutr* 1996;76: 591–603.

Desai M, Crowther NJ, Ozanne SE, Lucas A, Hales CN. Adult glucose and lipid metabolism may be programmed during fetal life. *Biochem Soc Trans* 1995;23: 331–5.

Desai M, Gayle DA, Casillas E, Boles J, Ross MG. Early undernutrition attenuates the inflammatory response in adult rat offspring. *J Matern Fetal Neonatal Med* 2009;22: 571–5.

Drake AJ, Reynolds RM. Impact of maternal obesity on offspring obesity and cardiometabolic disease risk. *Reproduction* 2010;140: 387–98.

Eriksson JG, Forsen T, Tuomilehto J, Winter PD, Osmond C, Barker DJ. Catch-up growth in childhood and death from coronary heart disease: longitudinal study. *BMJ* 1999;318: 427–31.

Field AE, Cook NR, Gillman MW. Weight status in childhood as a predictor of becoming overweight or hypertensive in early adulthood. *Obes Res* 2005;13: 163–9.

Forsdahl A. Are poor living conditions in childhood and adolescence an important risk factor for arteriosclerotic heart disease? *Br J Prev Soc Med* 1977;31: 91–5.

Fowden AL, Forhead AJ. Endocrine mechanisms of intrauterine programming. *Reproduction* 2004;127: 515–26.

Garofano A, Czernichow P, Breant B. Effect of ageing on beta-cell mass and function in rats malnourished during the perinatal period. *Diabetologia* 1999;42: 711–8.

Gotz AA, Wittlinger S, Stefanski V. Maternal social stress during pregnancy alters immune function and immune cell numbers in adult male Long-Evans rat offspring during stressful life-events. *J Neuroimmunol* 2007;185: 95–102.

Greenwood PL, Hunt AS, Hermanson JW, Bell AW. Effects of birth weight and postnatal nutrition on neonatal sheep: I. Body growth and composition, and some aspects of energetic efficiency. *J Anim Sci* 1998;76: 2354–67.

Guo F, Jen KL. High-fat feeding during pregnancy and lactation affects offspring metabolism in rats. *Physiol Behav* 1995;57: 681–6.

Hahn P. Effect of litter size on plasma cholesterol and insulin and some liver and adipose tissue enzymes in adult rodents. *J Nutr* 1984;114: 1231–4.

Hales CN, Barker DJ. Type 2 (non-insulin-dependent) diabetes mellitus: the thrifty phenotype hypothesis. *Diabetologia* 1992;35: 595–601.

Hales CN, Barker DJ. The thrifty phenotype hypothesis. *Br Med Bull* 2001;60: 5–20.

Hales CN, Barker DJ, Clark PM, Cox LJ, Fall C, Osmond C, Winter PD. Fetal and infant growth and impaired glucose tolerance at age 64. *BMJ* 1991;303: 1019–22.

Hashimoto M, Watanabe T, Fujioka T, Tan N, Yamashita H, Nakamura S. Modulating effects of prenatal stress on hyperthermia induced in adult rat offspring by restraint or LPS-induced stress. *Physiol Behav* 2001;73: 125–32.

Jennings BJ, Ozanne SE, Dorling MW, Hales CN. Early growth determines longevity in male rats and may be related to telomere shortening in the kidney. *FEBS Lett* 1999;448: 4–8.

Kensara OA, Wootton SA, Phillips DI, Patel M, Jackson AA, Elia M. Fetal programming of body composition: relation between birth weight and body composition measured with dual-energy X-ray absorptiometry and anthropometric methods in older Englishmen. *Am J Clin Nutr* 2005;82: 980–7.

Khan I, Dekou V, Hanson M, Poston L, Taylor P. Predictive adaptive responses to maternal high-fat diet prevent endothelial dysfunction but not hypertension in adult rat offspring. *Circulation* 2004;110: 1097–1102.

Kindlund K, Thomsen SF, Stensballe LG, Skytthe A, Kyvik KO, Backer V, Bisgaard H. Birth weight and risk of asthma in 3–9-year-old twins: exploring the fetal origins hypothesis. *Thorax* 2010;65: 146–9.

Koletzko B, von Kries R, Closa R, Escribano J, Scaglioni S, Giovannini M, Beyer J, Demmelmair H, Gruszfeld D, Dobrzanska A, Sengier A, Langhendries JP, Rolland Cachera MF, Grote V, European Childhood Obesity Trial Study Group. Lower protein in infant formula is associated with lower weight up to age 2 y: a randomized clinical trial. *Am J Clin Nutr* 2009;89: 1836–1845.

Kwong WY, Wild AE, Roberts P, Willis AC, Fleming TP. Maternal undernutrition during the pre-implantation period of rat development causes blastocyst abnormalities and programming of postnatal hypertension. *Development* 2000;127: 4195–4202.

Langley-Evans SC, Phillips GJ, Benediktsson R, Gardner DS, Edwards CR, Jackson AA, Seckl JR. Protein intake in pregnancy, placental glucocorticoid metabolism and the programming of hypertension in the rat. *Placenta* 1996;17: 169–72.

Langley SC, Jackson AA. Increased systolic blood pressure in adult rats induced by fetal exposure to maternal low protein diets. *Clin Sci* (Lond) 1994; 86: 217–22; discussion 121.

Lewis DS, Bertrand HA, McMahan CA, McGill HC, Carey KD, Masoro EJ. Preweaning food intake influences the adiposity of young adult baboons. *J Clin Invest* 1986;78: 899–905.

Lewis RM, Forhead AJ, Petry CJ, Ozanne SE, Hales CN. Long-term programming of blood pressure by maternal dietary iron restriction in the rat. *Br J Nutr* 2002;88: 283–90.

Lewis RM, Petry CJ, Ozanne SE, Hales CN. Effects of maternal iron restriction in the rat on blood pressure, glucose tolerance, and serum lipids in the 3-month-old offspring. *Metabolism* 2001;50: 562–7.

Lindsay RS, Bennett PH. Type 2 diabetes, the thrifty phenotype – an overview. *Br Med Bull* 2001;60: 21–32.

Lindsay RS, Lindsay RM, Waddell BJ, Seckl JR. Prenatal glucocorticoid exposure leads to offspring hyperglycaemia in the rat: studies with the 11 beta-hydroxysteroid dehydrogenase inhibitor carbenoxolone. *Diabetologia* 1996;39: 1299–1305.

Long NM, George LA, Uthlaut AB, Smith DT, Nijland MJ, Nathanielsz PW, Ford SP. Maternal obesity and high nutrient intake before and during gestation in the ewe results in altered growth, adiposity, and glucose tolerance in adult offspring. *J Anim Sci* 2010;88: 3546–53.

Loos RJ, Beunen G, Fagard R, Derom C, Vlietinck R. Birth weight and body composition in young adult men – a prospective twin study. *Int J Obes Relat Metab Disord* 2001;25: 1537–1545.

Los H, Postmus PE, Boomsma DI. Asthma genetics and intermediate phenotypes: a review from twin studies. *Twin Res* 2001;4: 81–93.

Lucas A. Long-term programming effects of early nutrition – implications for the preterm infant. *J Perinatol* 2005;25 Suppl 2: S2–6.

Lucas A, Cole TJ. Breast milk and neonatal necrotising enterocolitis. *Lancet* 1990;336: 1519–23.

Lundholm C, Ortqvist AK, Lichtenstein P, Cnattingius S, Almqvist C. Impaired fetal growth decreases the risk of childhood atopic eczema: a Swedish twin study. *Clin Exp Allergy* 2010;40: 1044–53.

McCance DR, Pettitt DJ, Hanson RL, Jacobsson LT, Knowler WC, Bennett PH. Birth weight and non-insulin dependent diabetes: thrifty genotype, thrifty phenotype, or surviving small baby genotype? *BMJ* 1994;308: 942–5.

McCance RA. Food, growth, and time. *Lancet* 1962;280: 671–6.

McDade TW, Beck MA, Kuzawa CW, Adair LS. Prenatal undernutrition and postnatal growth are associated with adolescent thymic function. *J Nutr* 2001;131: 1225–31.

Merlet-Benichou C, Gilbert T, Muffat-Joly M, Lelievre-Pegorier M, Leroy B. Intrauterine growth retardation leads to a permanent nephron deficit in the rat. *Pediatr Nephrol* 1994;8: 175–80.

Moore S, Prentice A, Wagatsuma Y, Fulford A, Collinson A, Raqib R, Vahter M, Persson L, Arifeen S. Early-life nutritional and environmental determinants of thymic size in infants born in rural Bangladesh. *Acta Paediatr* 2009;98 1168–75.

Moritz KM, Mazzuca MQ, Siebel AL, Mibus A, Arena D, Tare M, Owens JA, Wlodek ME. Utero-placental insufficiency causes a nephron deficit, modest renal insufficiency but no hypertension with ageing in female rats. *J Physiol* 2009;587: 2635–46.

Nyirenda MJ, Lindsay RS, Kenyon CJ, Burchell A, Seckl JR. Glucocorticoid exposure in late gestation permanently programs rat hepatic phosphoenolpyruvate carboxykinase and glucocorticoid receptor expression and causes glucose intolerance in adult offspring. *J Clin Invest* 1998;101: 2174–81.

Odaka Y, Nakano M, Tanaka T, Kaburagi T, Yoshino H, Sato-Mito N, Sato K. The influence of a high-fat dietary environment in the fetal period on postnatal metabolic and immune function. *Obesity* 2010;18: 1688–94.

Ogata ES, Bussey ME, Finley S. Altered gas exchange, limited glucose and branched chain amino acids, and hypoinsulinism retard fetal growth in the rat. *Metabolism* 1986;35: 970–7.

Osgerby JC, Wathes DC, Howard D, Gadd TS. The effect of maternal undernutrition on ovine fetal growth. *J Endocrinol* 2002;173: 131–41.

Ozanne SE. Metabolic programming in animals. *Br Med Bull* 2001;60: 143–52.

Ozanne SE, Hales CN. Lifespan: catch-up growth and obesity in male mice. *Nature* 2004;427: 411–2.

Petry CJ, Dorling MW, Pawlak DB, Ozanne SE, Hales CN. Diabetes in old male offspring of rat dams fed a reduced protein diet. *Int J Exp Diab Res* 2001;2: 139–43.

Poulsen P, Vaag AA, Kyvik KO, Moller Jensen D, Beck-Nielsen H. Low birth weight is associated with NIDDM in discordant monozygotic and dizygotic twin pairs. *Diabetologia* 1997;40: 439–46.

Rasmussen K. Is there a causal relationship between iron deficiency or iron-deficiency anemia and weight at birth, length of gestation and perinatal mortality? *J Nutr* 2001;131: 590S–601S; discussion 601S–603S.

Ravelli AC, van der Meulen JH, Michels RP, Osmond C, Barker DJ, Hales CN, Bleker OP. Glucose tolerance in adults after prenatal exposure to famine. *Lancet* 1998;351: 173–7.

Reynolds RM, Walker BR, Syddall HE, Andrew R, Wood PJ, Whorwood CB, Phillips DI. Altered control of cortisol secretion in adult men with low birth weight and cardiovascular risk factors. *J Clin Endocrinol Metab* 2001;86: 245–50.

Sacks DA, Liu AI, Wolde-Tsadik G, Amini SB, Huston-Presley L, Catalano PM. What proportion of birth weight is attributable to maternal glucose among infants of diabetic women? *Am J Obstet Gynecol* 2006;194: 501–7.

Samuelsson AM, Matthews PA, Argenton M, Christie MR, McConnell JM, Jansen EH, Piersma AH, Ozanne SE, Twinn DF, Remacle C, Rowlerson A, Poston L, Taylor PD. Diet-induced obesity in female mice leads to offspring hyperphagia, adiposity, hypertension, and insulin resistance: a novel murine model of developmental programming. *Hypertension* 2008;51: 383–92.

Schuler SL, Gurmini J, Cecilio WA, Viola de Azevedo ML, Olandoski M, de Noronha L. Hepatic and thymic alterations in newborn offspring of malnourished rat dams. *J Parenter Enteral Nutr* 2008;32: 184–9.

Singhal A, Cole TJ, Fewtrell M, Deanfield J, Lucas A. Is slower early growth beneficial for long-term cardiovascular health? *Circulation* 2004;109: 1108–13.

Singhal A, Lucas A. Early origins of cardiovascular disease: is there a unifying hypothesis? *Lancet* 2004;363: 1642–5.

Sobrian SK, Vaughn VT, Ashe WK, Markovic B, Djuric V, Jankovic BD. Gestational exposure to loud noise alters the development and postnatal responsiveness of humoral and cellular components of the immune system in offspring. *Environ Res* 1997;73: 227–41.

Stanner SA, Yudkin JS. Fetal programming and the Leningrad Siege study. *Twin Res* 2001;4: 287–92.

Surkan PJ, Stephansson O, Dickman PW, Cnattingius S. Previous preterm and small-for-gestational-age births and the subsequent risk of stillbirth. *N Engl J Med* 2004;350: 777–85.

Tarry-Adkins JL, Martin-Gronert MS, Chen JH, Cripps RL, Ozanne SE. Maternal diet influences DNA damage, aortic telomere length, oxidative stress, and antioxidant defense capacity in rats. *Faseb J* 2008;22: 2037–44.

Tuchscherer M, Kanitz E, Otten W, Tuchscherer A. Effects of prenatal stress on cellular and humoral immune responses in neonatal pigs. *Vet Immunol Immunopathol* 2002;86: 195–203.

Vickers, MH, Breier BH, Cutfield WS, Hofman PL, Gluckman PD. Fetal origins of hyperphagia, obesity, and hypertension and postnatal amplification by hypercaloric nutrition. *Am J Physiol Endocrinol Metab* 2000;279: E83–7.

Villamor E, Cnattingius S. Interpregnancy weight change and risk of adverse pregnancy outcomes: a population-based study. *Lancet* 2006;368: 1164–70.

Vuguin P, Raab E, Liu B, Barzilai N, Simmons R. Hepatic insulin resistance precedes the development of diabetes in a model of intrauterine growth retardation. *Diabetes* 2004;53: 2617–22.

Weinkove C, Weinkove EA, Pimstone BL. Micro assays for glucose and insulin. *S Afr Med J* 1974;48: 365–8.

Widdowson EM, McCance RA. A review: new thoughts on growth. *Pediatr Res* 1975;9: 154–6.

Winick M, Noble, A. Cellular response in rats during malnutrition at various ages. *J Nutr* 1966;89: 300–6.

Woodall SM, Johnston BM, Breier BH, Gluckman PD. Chronic maternal undernutrition in the rat leads to delayed postnatal growth and elevated blood pressure of offspring. *Pediatr Res* 1996;40: 438–443.

Woods LL, Weeks DA. Prenatal programming of adult blood pressure: role of maternal corticosteroids. *Am J Physiol* 2005;289: R955–62.

Zhu MJ, Du M, Nathanielsz PW, Ford SP. Maternal obesity up-regulates inflammatory signaling pathways and enhances cytokine expression in the mid-gestation sheep placenta. *Placenta* 2010;31: 387–91.

4 Cardiovascular consequences of IUGR: Experimental aspects

Simon C. Langley-Evans

Intrauterine growth retardation (IUGR) resulting in low weight at birth (LBW) has long been a focus of interest in the context of early life programming of disease. The etiology of IUGR in humans is complex, but LBW has widely been interpreted as a marker of maternal under-nutrition. Varied approaches adopted to limit fetal nutrition in animals have been shown to have consistent cardiovascular outcomes across small and large animal species. Offspring of animals subject to any form of nutrient restriction during pregnancy manifest raised blood pressure in later life and this may be associated with impaired endothelium-dependent and independent vasodilation, atherosclerosis and greater susceptibility to ischemia-reperfusion injury. From a mechanistic perspective it seems likely that a sub-optimal environment during organogenesis and tissue maturation results in remodelling of structures involved in cardiovascular functions and regulation of those functions. Unfortunately there is remarkably little data that considers the perhaps transient changes to expression of genes, proteins and pathways in embryonic and fetal life that may establish permanent changes in tissue structure and function. It is clear, however, that maternal undernutrition establishes strong cellular memories of the initial insults, which continue to exert their influence across multiple generations and in cell culture. Nutritional effects upon epigenetic markers across the genome are suspected to play a key role in establishing such a memory, but to date, few candidate genes with a clear cardiovascular function have been shown to be targets for such effects.

4.1 Intrauterine growth retardation and maternal undernutrition.

Data obtained from historical cohorts of men and women from developed and developing countries, is suggestive of associations between early life factors and risk of cardiovascular disease. In the late 1980's Barker and colleagues reported that among men and women born in Hertfordshire (UK) during the period 1911–1932, coronary heart disease mortality (Barker et al., 1989), blood pressure (Barker et al., 1990), occurrence of the metabolic syndrome and type 2 diabetes (Hales et al., 1991) were all more prevalent in individuals who were of lower weight at birth. This was a fascinating observation and like other similar findings from other cohorts, suggested that factors which influence growth *in utero* may also irreversibly influence organ development and physiological function. A key aspect of these observations was that programming of function occurred within the normal range of birthweights and was not dependent upon occurrence of preterm birth or what would be regarded as clinically relevant intrauterine growth retardation (IUGR), resulting in low birthweight (LBW, weight less than 2.5 kg at birth).

Whilst fetal growth and eventual weight at birth are heavily determined by genetics, and by a wide variety of maternal environmental and lifestyle factors (▶Fig. 4.1), most attention for researchers interested in the early life origins of disease was focused upon undernutrition as a possible driver of early life programming. This was an interesting choice as the relationship between maternal nutritional status and fetal growth appears to be weak in humans (Harding, 2004). Even in populations subjected to severe famine situations, average birth weights vary by no more than 20–25%, and when considering variation in birth weight across the normal range, the influence of maternal nutrition is greatly outweighed by factors such as social class, maternal size and maternal physical activity. There are few robust studies where estimated intakes of energy or nutrients can be related to birth weight or proportions (e.g. length, head circumference, ponderal index) in humans (Doyle et al., 1992; Langley-Evans & Langley-Evans, 2003; Mathews et al., 1999).

Attempts to demonstrate relationships between maternal nutrient intake in pregnancy and long-term cardiovascular function in the resulting offspring are few and far between in the literature (Campbell et al., 1996; Gillman et al., 2004; Godfrey et al., 1994) and this is only to be expected given the nature of the problem and the time-span required for a properly conducted evaluation. Where such data does exist it can be difficult to interpret. For example Campbell et al. (1996) reported that blood pressures of middle aged men were related to their mother's protein intake, but with the association going in opposite directions dependent upon carbohydrate consumption. As stated above, there is little in the literature to demonstrate firm associations between maternal nutrient intakes and birth weight within the normal range. The lack of clear information relating limited nutrient intake to long-term consequences should not be surprising given the near impossibility of the task of accurately estimating even macronutrient intakes, let alone micronutrient intakes, in population studies. Although attractive, searching for evidence that maternal intake of protein, or iron or zinc in relation to programming of

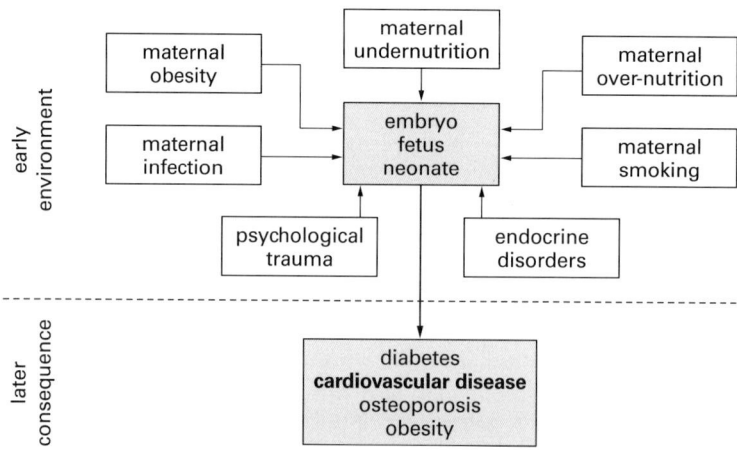

Fig. 4.1: Influences upon early development which are associated with disease in later life. Maternal nutritional status is one of a number of different influences upon fetal development which may adversely impact upon later physiological function and risk of disease in adulthood.

disease in humans is perhaps misguided and in this context we could learn a lot from the errors made in cancer epidemiology over the last 30 years. A focus on trying to break diet-cancer relationships down into simple effects of single nutrients failed to take into account the ways in which nutrients interact with each other, with the genes carried by individuals and with other risk factors in the environment (Gerber, 2001). It is overly simplistic to assume that intakes of a single nutrient are representative of the whole range of dietary and environmental exposures experienced by individuals. In the cancer field this ultimately led to misguided trials of interventions using antioxidant nutrients with disastrous effects upon some participants (Bjelakovic and Gluud, 2007) and it is now recognized that whole dietary patterns give a better representation of associated risk. The human diet comprises varied mixtures of foods, each providing different combinations of nutrients, prepared in a variety of different ways. This means that within each food and within each meal, there is considerable scope for interactions between nutrients, and between nutrients and the non-nutrient components of food-stuffs (Gerber, 2001). As such it will be the combinations of factors in the habitual diet of any pregnant woman that determine the responses of her developing child, rather than intakes of specific nutrients or foods.

Despite these problems with epidemiological approaches to investigation of early life programming of cardiovascular functions, a wide diversity of experimental models have been developed to demonstrate the biological plausibility of programming by maternal undernutrition. Such models have enabled the downstream consequences of specific manipulations of either maternal nutritional status or fetal growth to be characterized and provide useful vehicles for studies which aim to identify the mechanistic basis of early life programming.

4.2 Long-term cardiovascular consequences of undernutrition: Animal models of programming

Although animal models may over-simplify the relationship between maternal nutritional status and long-term programming, they carry the major advantages of control over confounding factors and the ability to sample invasively and across the whole lifespan. Models of programming have been reported using a wide range of species including small animals (rats, mice and guinea pigs), large animals (sheep and pigs) and non-human primates. Diverse nutritional manipulations have been applied during pregnancy, pregnancy and lactation and for specific periods within pregnancy. Some strategies have been designed specifically to elicit IUGR, including ligation of the uterine artery (Persson & Jansson, 1992) or placental reduction (Owens et al., 2007), whilst others have been used to model a variety of forms of undernutrition, including global food restriction (Kind et al. 2002; Vickers et al., 2003; Woodall et al., 1996), micronutrient deficiency (Gambling et al., 2005) and macronutrient restriction (Langley & Jackson, 1994; ▶Fig. 4.2). Despite the diversity of approach, the common phenotypic endpoint which has been reported in all cases, is raised blood pressure. Vickers and colleagues (2003), for example, reported that offspring of rat dams fed just 30% of *ad libitum* food intake were born extremely growth retarded and by 100 days of age were hypertensive. The programming effect of maternal undernutrition on blood pressure was exacerbated by postweaning feeding of the offspring with a hypercaloric diet. Gambling et al., (2005)

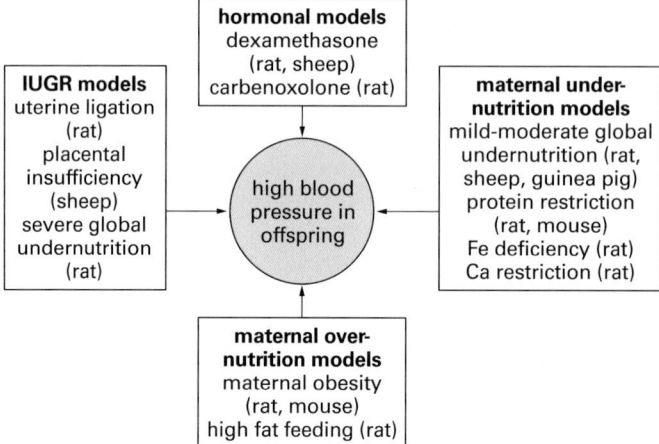

Fig. 4.2: Animal models of cardiovascular programming. A variety of approaches have been taken to model the developmental origins of disease. Programming of blood pressure is the primary marker of early life influences upon the cardiovasculature, and this can be demonstrated by manipulation of fetal growth or fetal hormone exposure to generate IUGR. In contrast to these extreme approaches, the imposition of both under- and over-nutrition during pregnancy will program hypertension in the resulting offspring.

modelled maternal iron deficiency anemia by feeding rats a low iron diet prior to and during pregnancy. Offspring from these pregnancies exhibited higher blood pressure in early adulthood.

The most extensively characterized of all animal models of programming by undernutrition involves the feeding of a low protein diet during pregnancy (Langley and Jackson, 1994). Offspring of dams subjected to this relatively mild insult are of normal birthweight but exhibit higher blood pressure than controls from the age of weaning onwards (Langley-Evans et al., 1996a; 1996b; 1996c). The causes of this hypertension appear to be multifactorial and may be partly driven by a deficit of nephrons in the kidney (Langley-Evans et al., 1999), by increased peripheral vascular resistance and defects of the renin-angiotensin system (McMullen et al., 2004). It is clear that vascular function is abnormal as isolated vessels exhibit blunted vasorelaxation in response to acetylcholine and other evidence of endothelial cell dysfunction (Torrens et al., 2006). When the hearts from low protein exposed animals are mounted on Langendorff perfusion apparatus and function is monitored ex vivo, they exhibit differences in responses to β-agonists and have an impaired recovery following ischemia-reperfusion events (Elmes et al., 2007;2008). Many of these effects show sex differences, but the overall phenotype that is programmed by maternal protein restriction is consistent with abnormal cardiovascular physiology.

High blood pressure and endothelial cell dysfunction are merely risk factors for cardiovascular disease and are not in themselves disease states. As most of the animal models that have been used to assess early life programming of the cardiovascular system are based upon rodents, there is very little evidence that maternal undernutrition

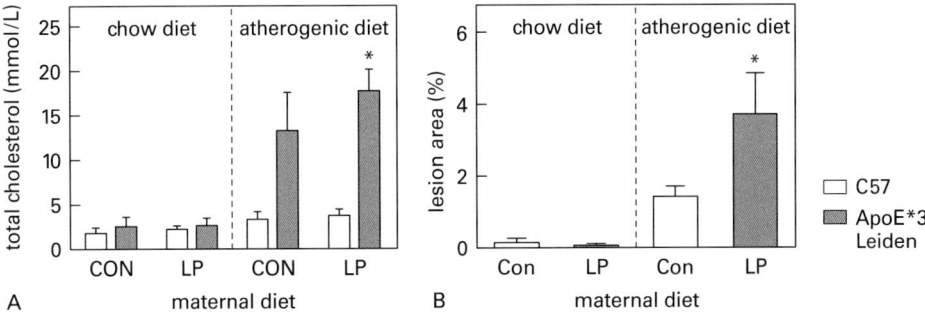

Fig. 4.3: Programming of atherosclerosis by maternal protein restriction. Female C57 or Apo E*3 Leiden offspring (n = 5–7 per group) of C57 mice fed control (CON) or low protein (LP) diets throughout pregnancy were fed either a standard chow or a high-fat, high cholesterol atherogenic diet from weaning for three months. Apo E*3 Leiden mice fed atherogenic diet had an exaggerated increase in total plasma cholesterol and developed larger atherosclerotic lesions at the aortic root if exposed to protein restriction in utero. Data are shown as mean ± SEM, *indicates P < 0.05 compared to control group. Data redrawn from Yates et al. (2008).

results in endpoints that are representative of the observed associations between early life factors and coronary heart disease and coronary mortality in humans. The transgenic apo E*3 Leiden mouse carries a mutated version of the human apo E3 gene and develops atherosclerosis if fed a cholesterol containing atherogenic diet. This is a useful model to consider influences upon the development of atherosclerotic disease (Yates et al., 2008). When male apo E*3 Leiden mice were mated with wild type females and the pregnancies were maintained on a low protein diet, the resulting apo E*3 Leiden offspring had an exaggerated increase in total plasma cholesterol and developed larger atherosclerotic lesions than mice exposed to the control diet *in utero* (▶Fig. 4.3). This provided the first direct evidence that coronary heart disease can be programmed by protein restriction in fetal life.

Not all, if any, of these experimental studies in animals can be truly said to be representative of nutritional problems that are seen in humans. Whilst iron deficiency anemia is endemic among pregnant women in some parts of the world, it would be rare to see it in isolation, as poor iron status is inevitably associated with "fellow travellers", such as vitamin A, zinc and folate deficiencies. Similarly it can be argued that protein restriction of the magnitude used in rodent studies does not really reflect the range of protein intakes across the social classes in women in developed or even developing countries (▶Fig. 4.4). These concerns are largely unimportant as the animal models serve a far more important function in that they demonstrate the biological plausibility of the developmental programming hypothesis. The observation that an iron deficient diet appears to programme a similar phenotype to a low protein diet or a maternal diet that is high in fat or providing only 70% of *ad libitum* calories, and across different species, is of huge significance. The existence of common responses to diverse insults suggests that only a limited range of mechanisms are likely to underpin the programming of physiological function.

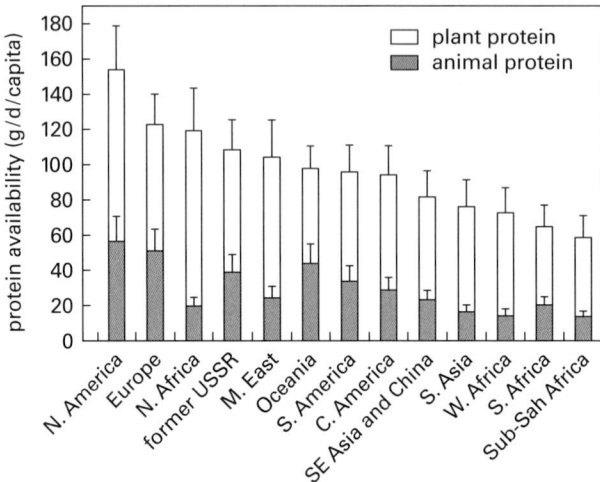

Fig. 4.4: Availability of animal and plant protein by world region. Per capita availability of protein from plant and animal sources calculated from the 2004 Food and Agriculture Organisation, global food balance sheets. Availability data represent an over-estimation of actual population intakes, which will vary considerably within each region. It is clear that significant numbers of adults will be at risk of marginal protein intake in developing countries by virtue of low availability of protein rich foods and a heavy reliance on lower quality plant sources. This can be regarded as justification for the use of a low protein diet model of nutritional programming, but it is important to note that similar populations will simultaneously be blighted by deficiencies of vitamin A, iron, zinc and iodine. Taken from Langley-Evans (2009).

4.3 The mechanistic basis of cardiovascular programming

In considering the mechanisms which link fetal experience to risk of disease in adult life there are two key questions that need to be addressed. Firstly, what are the direct responses to maternal insult which initiate the progression to compromised physiological and metabolic function? Secondly, what are the processes which subsequently take the individual to a disease state?

4.3.1 Primary responses

A simplistic view of the association between maternal undernutrition and later disease might feature the statement that a simple lack of nutrients impacts upon the growth of organs during rapid phases of cell proliferation and development. Observations from a number of animal experiments demonstrate that this is not the case. In sheep and in rats, restriction of maternal nutrition during the pre-implantation phase can result in long-term cardiovascular consequences (Kwong et al., 2000; Sinclair et al., 2007; Watkins et al., 2008). Manipulation of nutritional status at this stage precedes the period when a fetal nutrient supply is established by a considerable period of time. This implies that some other signal must be passed between mother and fetus, perhaps conveying some endocrine or metabolic indicator of sub-optimal nutritional status.

It is clear that whatever the nature of this signal, it is capable of leaving a long-term memory of the nutritional insult within the embryonic/fetal cells. Feeding ewes a diet that was deficient in methyl donors during the periconceptual period resulted in male offspring that were heavier and fatter, elicited altered immune responses to antigenic challenge, were insulin-resistant, and had elevated blood pressure (Sinclair et al., 2007). In rats, there is clear evidence that hypertension and renal insufficiency programmed by a maternal low protein diet can be transmitted to subsequent generations via either the maternal or paternal line (Harrison et al. 2008). Primary cell cultures derived from neo-natal cardiomyocytes also exhibit altered glucose uptake if derived from rats exposed to a low protein diet in utero (Austin and Langley-Evans, 2011).

The existence of the cellular memory of early life events that is implied by the above observations is often attributed to programmed changes in DNA methylation and his-tone acetylation (Lillycrop et al., 2007, Burdge et al., 2009). DNA methylation is a potent suppressor of gene expression, either through blocking access of transcriptional machinery to the chromatin structure surrounding specific gene promoters, or through interference with the binding of transcription factors to DNA, whilst acetylation of histones promotes gene expression. Epigenetic marks are believed to be stably inher-ited and this may therefore allow phenotypic traits, acquired as a result of nutritional programming, to be passed on to subsequent offspring, or to cells which are divid-ing in culture. Changes in such marks in response to periods of undernutrition may provide important mechanisms through which expression of genes and proteins are perturbed by nutritional signals, beyond the period when the signal is withdrawn. For example, we have recently shown that maternal protein restriction in the rat results in hypomethylation of the adrenal AT1b receptor, with an associated increase in gene expression (Bogdarina et al., 2010; ▶Fig. 4.5). This is a similar finding to that of Lillycrop et al. (2005) who reported differential methylation of the glucocorticoid receptor and peroxisome proliferator activated receptor α following protein restriction.

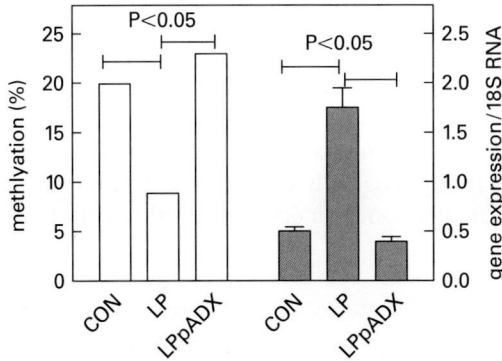

Fig. 4.5: DNA methylation and gene expression of the rat adrenal AT1b receptor. Pregnant rats were fed control (CON) or low protein (LP) diets until delivery. Half of the LP group were subjected to pharmacological adrenalectomy using metyrapone up until d14 gestation (LPpADX). Methylation of the AT1b promoter was determined by bisulphite treatment and gene expression by quantitative RT-PCR in adrenal glands from offspring aged 7 days. Data are shown as mean ± SEM for n = 5 observations. Data redrawn from Bogdarina et al. (2010).

In terms of endocrine imbalance during pregnancy, most attention has focused upon a possible contribution of glucocorticoids to nutritional programming (Seckl, 2004). During normal rat pregnancy the expression of the enzyme 11ß-hydroxysteroid dehydrogenase (11ßHSD2) in placenta plays a critical role in maintaining a gradient of active glucocorticoids, with maternal corticosterone concentrations being up to 1000-fold higher than fetal. This is an essential function that allows the fetal hypothalamic-pituitary-adrenal axis to develop independently of maternal influences. Experiments in which synthetic glucocorticoids, which are poor substrates for 11ßHSD2, are administered to pregnant rodents, result in offspring which develop hypertension (Benediktsson et al., 1993) and similar effects are produced when 11ßHSD2 activity is inhibited in pregnancy (Langley-Evans, 1997; Lindsay et al., 1996). Studies of human and animal pregnancies have shown that low birthweight is associated with reduced activity of 11ßHSD2 in placenta (Benediktsson et al., 1993, Shams et al. 1998). Our own work, supported by independent laboratories has shown that both enzyme activity and 11ßHSD2 mRNA expression are down-regulated (Bertram et al., 2001; Langley-Evans et al., 1996d) in pregnancies associated with undernutrition (both global undernutrition and protein restriction). This has led to the suggestion that nutritional programming may be partly mediated by an associated disruption of the maternal-fetal glucocorticoid gradient. This may in itself disturb the normal developmental pattern of gene expression, since glucocorticoids are important regulators of gene expression which promote growth retardation and early tissue maturation. It is important to appreciate that a glucocorticoid-driven theory of nutritional programming would not be exclusive of a role for nutritional modulation of epigenetic regulation. When rats fed a low protein diet were treated with metyrapone to inhibit maternal synthesis of endogenous glucocorticoids, methylation and expression of the AT1b receptor were normalized along with offspring blood pressure (Bogdarina et al., 2010) (▶Fig. 4.5).

The above processes, or other signals that maternal nutritional status is less than optimal, will inevitably alter the expression of a wide range of genes. To date, there has been little research aimed at identifying which genes and processes are most affected during key phases of growth and maturation. It is a major challenge to identify these primary targets for programming stimuli as, firstly, there has not been an effective characterization of exactly when programming is initiated, and secondly because the period during which expression is altered need only be transient. For example a relatively short period in which genes which favour cell proliferation are suppressed would result in an organ that is morphologically compromised. Similarly a brief activation of genes could promote greater commitment of progenitor cells to a particular lineage.

4.3.2 Secondary processes

Two decades ago Alan Lucas (1991) attributed programming to a change in the number or type of cells that are present within an organ. An organ that matures with altered morphology as a result of a programming insult might be expected to have a reduced capacity to perform physiological function. Although today this concept is often ignored, with epigenetic processes being favoured as drivers of programming, the idea that tissue remodelling takes place remains attractive and is supported by a number of experimental observations.

Many organs in humans have completed their development by the time of birth and in rodents, although the developmental window extends a short way into postnatal life, much of tissue growth and maturation is complete by the time of birth. If insults impact upon cell proliferation or differentiation during periods of rapid growth, then it would be expected that organs will mature at a lower size and with a reduced functional capacity. There are numerous examples of this available from experimental models that are associated with programming of high blood pressure. In the pancreas of rats exposed to low protein diets *in utero* there are fewer islets, smaller islets and reduced vascularisation of the islets that are present (Snoeck et al., 1990). The same maternal insult is also associated with altered size and neuronal densities in hypothalamic centres that regulate food intake (Plagemann et al., 2000), with reduced vascularisation of the brain cortex (Bennis-Taleb et al., 1999), alterations to the bone growth plate (Mehta et al., 2002) and differences in muscle fibre types (Mallinson et al., 2007).

Tissue remodelling is perhaps best demonstrated by consideration of the numbers of nephrons present in the kidney. Nephron number appears to be highly sensitive to variation in the quality and quantity of nutrients in the maternal diet (Langley-Evans et al., 1999; Vehaskari et al., 2001). Rat offspring from dams fed either low protein diets or subjected to iron deficiency exhibit reductions in nephron number that are of the order of 20–30% (▶Fig. 4.6). Similar observations have been made in sheep that experienced maternal food restriction in early fetal life (Gopalakrishnan et al., 2004). Lower nephron number appears to be a consequence of disruption of tissue differentiation, since organ size is generally reported to be normal despite the significant nephron deficit. Interestingly there are studies of humans which indicate that LBW is associated with lower nephron number, and that the presence of a reduced nephron complement is associated with hypertension (Hughson et al., 2006). Remodelling of the kidney can

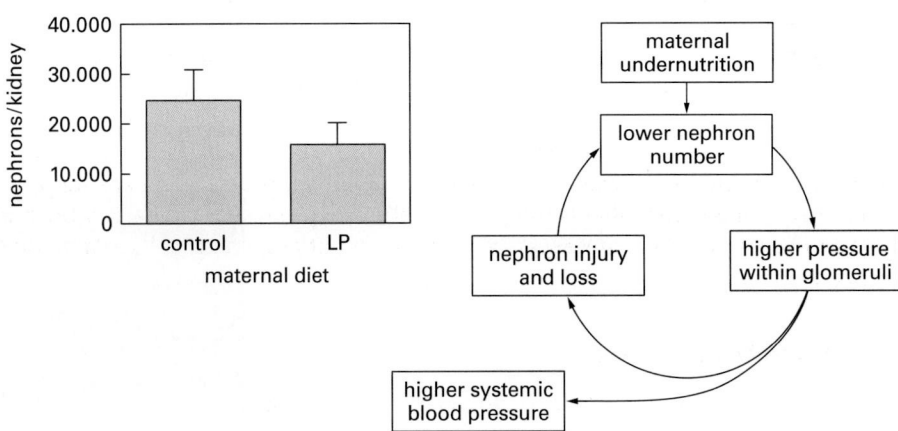

Fig. 4.6: Maternal protein restriction results in low nephron number in the rat. Nephron number in rats exposed to control or low protein (LP) diets in utero. Data are shown as mean ± SEM for 10 observations per group. Lower nephron number at birth, as a result of maternal undernutrition, results in higher systemic blood pressure as a consequence of a vicious cycle of rising intra-renal pressures to maintain renal function and progressive nephron loss.

therefore be regarded as a consequence of exposures that drive IUGR and as a driver of the cardiovascular disease that is observed subsequent to IUGR.

Subsequent to the irreversible modification of organ structure through tissue remodelling, it is relatively simple to determine how physiological processes become disturbed. For example, changes to renal morphology, with a reduction in the number of functional nephrons would produce local increases in blood pressure to maintain renal function (▶Fig. 4.6). This would eventually result in greater systemic pressure (Brenner and Chertow, 1993). Renal injury is also an endpoint of this process and the offspring of rats fed a low protein diet in pregnancy exhibit an earlier onset of impaired renal function, associated with morphological evidence of tissue damage (Joles et al., 2010; ▶Fig. 4.7). Similarly remodelling of centres in the hypothalamus such that sympathetic outflow is altered could also impact upon homeostatic control over blood pressure. Changing the profile of cell types within a tissue may result in altered patterns of hormone receptor expression and responsiveness. These in turn may establish altered expression of genes, proteins and pathways which will therefore appear to have been programmed by early life experience. The existence of disease or disordered physiological processes may exacerbate such changes.

Targets such as these have often been the subject of mechanistic investigations, and the identification of specific genes, proteins and pathways that appear programmed by early undernutrition is certainly a cause for some excitement. For example, we, and others, have reported that fetal exposure to protein restriction results in the early up-regulation of peroxisome proliferator activated receptor α, the expression of which is suppressed with ageing (Erhuma et al., 2007; Lillycrop et al., 2005). Although this appears to provide an explanation of the programming of metabolic disturbance, it has not

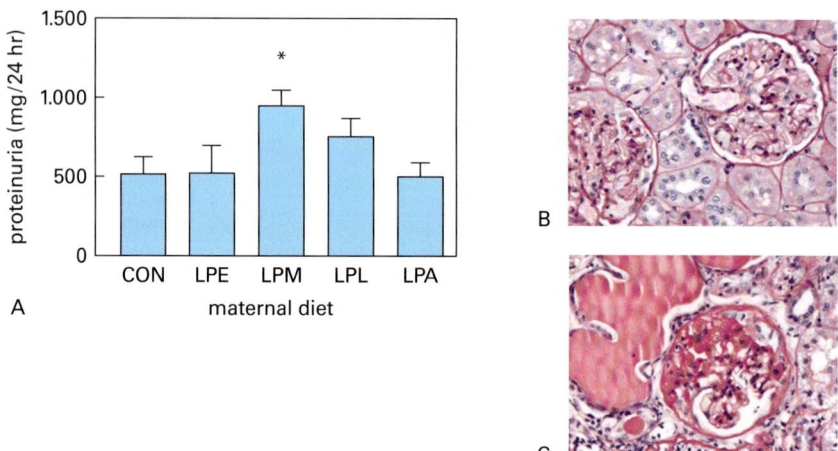

Fig. 4.7: Renal injury following prenatal protein restriction. 18 month old male offspring of rats fed a low protein diet from d0–7 (LPE), d8–14 (LPM), d15–22 (LPL) or throughout pregnancy (LPA) exhibit greater protein excretion than control animals (A). Data (mean ± SEM for n = 6–8 observations) redrawn from Joles et al. (2010). *P < 0.05 vs control. Histological examination reveals significant injury to glomeruli and tubules of 18 month old rats exposed to low protein diet in utero (C) compared to age-matched controls (B).

been possible to establish whether the changes in gene and protein expression directly cause, or are a consequence of the metabolic phenotype. It is important to remember, that these processes are almost certainly not the primary drivers of programming. The events and processes that initially drive tissue remodelling are the true mechanisms through which the maternal diet programs disease. Those processes may be difficult to identify as they may only operate in short, discrete periods of embryonic and fetal life and those windows of opportunity have yet to be isolated.

4.4 Research priorities

It is perhaps surprising that more than twenty years after the initial epidemiological findings of Barker and colleagues from the Hertfordshire cohort were published, and fifteen years after the publication of the first robust animal model of cardiovascular programming (Langley and Jackson, 1994), that we have not identified the primary processes that link exposure to maternal undernutrition, to disease in later life. The main laboratories in the developmental origins of adult disease field have spent much of that time collecting evidence of phenotype in multiple experimental models, and characterising the nature of the responses to early life undernutrition. The study of the pathways that lead to disease, consequent to early life programming events is clearly of interest and may potentially be exploited from a therapeutic perspective, but I would contend this is not the most important issue. It is clear from studies of animals that even short periods of exposure to a nutritional insult can have effects upon the embryo or fetus that will persist for the rest of the lifespan and may even be passed on to subsequent generations. It is of primary importance to identify what the processes are that are responsible for this. What, for example, causes quite profound tissue remodelling following a relatively mild shift in maternal nutritional status? It is critical to know if the effects observed in animals also hold true for humans and to know whether the processes that may act upon the embryo also hold true for a late gestation fetus or a neonate. Whilst in the past our fascination lay in the fact that early insults could exert permanent effects upon whole body physiology, our attention needs to shift back towards what is happening at the time of the insult. If we can acquire knowledge of why epigenetic markers are so responsive to the prevailing environment *in utero* then we can begin to address questions about whether programming effects can be reversed or somehow manipulated to produce positive health outcomes in later life.

References

Austin RM, Langley-Evans SC. Cultured neonatal rat cardiomyocytes display differences in glucose uptake and sensitivity to dexamethasone related to meternal diet. *J DOHAD* 2011;2: 50–4.

Barker DJ, Winter PD, Osmond C, Margetts B, Simmonds SJ. 1989. Weight in infancy and death from ischaemic heart disease. *Lancet* 1989;2: 577–80.

Barker DJ, Bull AR, Osmond C, Simmonds SJ. Fetal and placental size and risk of hypertension in adult life. *BMJ* 1990;301: 259–62.

Benediktsson R, Lindsay RS, Noble J, Seckl JR, Edwards CRW. Glucocorticoid exposure in utero – new model for adult hypertension. *Lancet* 1993;341: 339–41.

Bennis-Taleb N, Remacle C, Hoet JJ, Reusens B. A low-protein isocaloric diet during gestation affects brain development and alters permanently cerebral cortex blood vessels in rat offspring. *J Nutr* 1999;129: 1613–9.

Bertram C, Trowern AR, Copin N, Jackson AA, Whorwood CB. The maternal diet during pregnancy programs altered expression of the glucocorticoid receptor and type 2 11 beta-hydroxysteroid dehydrogenase: Potential molecular mechanisms underlying the programming of hypertension in utero. *Endocrinology* 2001;142: 2841–53.

Bjelakovic G, Gluud C. Surviving antioxidant supplements. *J Natl Cancer Inst* 2007;99: 742–3.

Bogdarina I, Haase A, Langley-Evans S, Clark AJ. Glucocorticoid effects on the programming of AT1b angiotensin receptor gene methylation and expression in the rat. *PLoS One* 2010;5: e9237.

Brenner BM, Chertow GM. Congenital oligonephropathy and the etiology of adult hypertension and progressive renal injury: Symposium in Honor of Neal S Bricker: The Pathophysiology of Chronic Renal Disease. Denver, Co, 1993, 171–5.

Burdge GC, Lillycrop KA, Jackson AA. Nutrition in early life, and risk of cancer and metabolic disease: alternative endings in an epigenetic tale? *Br J Nutr* 2009;101: 619–30.

Campbell DM, Hall MH, Barker DJ, Cross J, Shiell AW, Godfrey KM. Diet in pregnancy and the offspring's blood pressure 40 years later. *Br J Obstet Gynaecol* 1996;103: 273–80.

Doyle W, Wynn AHA, Crawford MA, Wynn SW. Nutritional counselling and supplementation in the second and third trimester of pregnancy: a study in a London population. *J Nutr Med* 1992;3: 249–56.

Elmes MJ, Gardner DS, Langley-Evans SC. Fetal exposure to a maternal low protein diet is associated with altered left ventricular pressure response to ischaemia reperfusion injury. *Br J Nutr* 2007;98: 93–100.

Elmes MJ, Haase A, Gardner DS, Langley-Evans SC. Gender differences in sensitivity to β-adrenergic agonist in the isolated adult rat heart following prenatal protein restriction. *Br J Nutr* 2008;101: 725–34.

Erhuma A, Salter AM, Sculley DV, Langley-Evans SC, Bennett AJ. Prenatal exposure to a low-protein diet programs disordered regulation of lipid metabolism in the aging rat. *Am J Physiol Endocrinol Metab* 2007;292: E1702–14.

Gambling L, Maloney CA, Andersen HS, McArdle HJ. Maternal iron deficiency during pregnancy in the rat induces high blood pressure, obesity and dyslipidaemia in her offspring. *Pediatr Res* 2005;58: 1024.

Gerber M. The comprehensive approach to diet: a critical review. *J Nutr* 2001;131: 3051S-5S.

Gillman MW, Rifas-Shiman SL, Kleinman KP, Rich-Edwards JW, Lipshultz SE. Maternal calcium intake and offspring blood pressure. *Circulation* 2004;110: 1990–5.

Godfrey KM, Forrester T, Barker DJ, Jackson AA, Landman JP, Hall JS, Cox V, Osmond C. Maternal nutritional status in pregnancy and blood pressure in childhood. *Br J Obstet Gynaecol* 1994;101: 398–403.

Gopalakrishnan GS, Gardner DS, Rhind SM, Rae MT, Kyle CE, Brooks AN, Walker RM, Ramsay MM, Keisler DH, Stephenson T, Symonds ME. Programming of adult cardiovascular function after early maternal undernutrition in sheep. *Am J Physiol* 2004;287: R12–20.

Hales CN, Barker DJ, Clark PM, Cox LJ, Fall C, Osmond C, Winter PD. Fetal and infant growth and impaired glucose tolerance at age 64. *BMJ* 1991;303: 1019–22.

Harding, J. Nutritional basis for the fetal origins of adult disease. In: Langley-Evans SC, editor. Fetal nutrition and adult disease. Wallingford: Cabi, 2004: 21–54.

Harrison M, Langley-Evans SC. Intergenerational programming of impaired nephrogenesis and hypertension in rats following maternal protein restriction during pregnancy. *Br J Nutr* 2008;101: 1020–30.

Hughson MD, Douglas-Denton R, Bertram JF, Hoy WE. Hypertension, glomerular number, and birth weight in African Americans and white subjects in the southeastern United States. *Kidney Int* 2006;69: 671–8.

Joles JA, Sculley DV, Langley-Evans SC. Proteinuria in aging rats due to low-protein diet during mid-gestation. *J DOHAD* 2010;1: 75–83.

Kind KL, Simonetta G, Clifton PM, Robinson JS, Owens JA. Effect of maternal feed restriction on blood pressure in the adult guinea pig. *Exp Physiol* 2002;87: 469–77.

Kwong WY, Wild AE, Roberts P, Willis AC, Fleming TP. Maternal undernutrition during the pre-implantation period of rat development causes blastocyst abnormalities and programming of postnatal hypertension. *Development* 2000;127: 4195–4202.

Langley-Evans SC. Nutrition: A lifespan approach. Oxford: Wiley-Blackwell, 2009.

Langley SC, Jackson AA. Increased systolic blood pressure in adult rats induced by fetal exposure to maternal low protein diets. *Clin Sci* 1994;86: 217–22.

Langley-Evans SC, Welham SJ, Sherman RC, Jackson AA. Weanling rats exposed to maternal low-protein diets during discrete periods of gestation exhibit differing severity of hypertension. *Clin Sci* 1996a;91: 607–15.

Langley-Evans SC, Gardner DS, Jackson AA. Association of disproportionate growth of fetal rats in late gestation with raised systolic blood pressure in later life. *J Reprod Fert* 1996b;106: 307–12.

Langley-Evans SC, Gardner DS, Jackson AA. Evidence of programming of the hypothalamic-pituitary-adrenal axis by maternal protein restriction during pregnancy. *J Nutr* 1996c;126: 1578–85.

Langley-Evans S, Phillips G, Benediktsson R, Gardner DS, Edwards CRW, Jackson AA, Seckl JR. Protein intake in pregnancy, placental glucocorticoid metabolism and the programming of hypertension in the rat. *Placenta* 1996d; 17: 169–72.

Langley-Evans SC. Maternal carbenoxolone treatment lowers birthweight and induces hypertension in the offspring of rats fed a low protein diet. *Clin Sci* 1997;93: 423–9.

Langley-Evans SC, Welham SJM, Jackson AA. Fetal exposure to a maternal low protein diet impairs nephrogenesis and promotes hypertension in the rat. *Life Sci* 1999;64: 965–74.

Langley-Evans AJ, Langley-Evans SC. Relationship between maternal nutrient intakes in early and late pregnancy and infants weight and proportions at birth: prospective cohort study. *J R Soc Health* 2003;123: 210–6.

Lillycrop KA, Phillips ES, Jackson AA, Hanson MA, Burdge GC. Dietary protein restriction of pregnant rats induces and folic acid supplementation prevents epigenetic modification of hepatic gene expression in the offspring. *J Nutr* 2005;135: 1382–6.

Lillycrop KA, Slater-Jefferies JL, Hanson MA, Godfrey KM, Jackson AA, Burdge GC. Induction of altered epigenetic regulation of the hepatic glucocorticoid receptor in the offspring of rats fed a protein-restricted diet during pregnancy suggests that reduced DNA methyltransferase-1 expression is involved in impaired DNA methylation and changes in histone modifications. *Br J Nutr* 2007;97: 1064–73.

Lindsay RS, Lindsay RM, Edwards CR, Seckl JR. Inhibition of 11-beta-hydroxysteroid dehydrogenase in pregnant rats and the programming of blood pressure in the offspring. *Hypertension* 1996;27: 1200–4.

Lucas A. Early Diet and Later Consequences. London: British Nutrition Foundation, 1991.

Mallinson J, Sculley DV, Craigon J, Plant R, Langley-Evans SC, Brameld JM. Fetal exposure to a maternal low protein diet during mid gestation results in muscle-specific effects on fibre type composition in young rats. *Br J Nutr* 2007; 98: 292–9.

Mathews F, Yudkin P, Neil A. Influence of maternal nutrition on outcome of pregnancy: prospective cohort study. *BMJ* 1999;319: 339–43.

McMullen S, Gardner DS, Langley-Evans SC. Prenatal programming of angiotensin II type 2 receptor expression in the rat. *Br J Nutr* 2004;91: 133–40.

Mehta G, Roach HI, Langley-Evans SC, Reading I, Oreffo ROC, Aihie-Sayer A, Clarke NMP, Cooper C. Intrauterine exposure to a maternal low protein diet reduces adult bone mass and alters growth plate morphology. *Calc Tiss Intl* 2002;79: 493–8.

Owens JA, Thavaneswaran P, De Blasio MJ, McMillen IC, Robinson JS, Gatford KL. Specific effects of placental restriction on components of the metabolic syndrome in young adult sheep. *Am J Physiol Endocrinol Metab* 2007;292: E1879–89.

Persson E, Jansson T. Low-birth-weight is associated with elevated adult blood pressure in the chronically catheterized guinea-pig. *Acta Physiol Scand* 1992;145: 195–6.

Plagemann A, Harder T, Rake A, Melchior K, Rohde W, Dörner G. Hypothalamic nuclei are malformed in weanling offspring of low protein malnourished rat dams. *J Nutr* 2000;130: 2582–9.

Seckl JR. Prenatal glucocorticoids and long-term programming. *Eur J Endocrinol* 2004;151 Suppl 3: U49–62.

Shams M, Kilby MD, Somerset DA, Howie AJ, Gupta A, Wood PJ, Afnan M, Stewart PM. 11Beta-hydroxysteroid dehydrogenase type 2 in human pregnancy and reduced expression in intrauterine growth restriction. *Hum Reprod* 1998;13: 799–804.

Sinclair KD, Allegrucci C, Singh R, Gardner DS, Sebastian S, Bispham J, Thurston A, Huntley JF, Rees WD, Maloney CA, Lea RG, Craigon J, McEvoy TG, Young LE. DNA methylation, insulin resistance, and blood pressure in offspring determined by maternal periconceptional b vitamin and methionine status. *Proc Natl Acad Sci U S A* 2007;104: 19351–6.

Snoeck A, Remacle C, Reusens B, Hoet JJ. Effect of a low protein diet during pregnancy on the fetal rat endocrine pancreas. *Biol Neonate* 1990;57: 107–18.

Torrens C, Brawley L, Anthony FW, Dance CS, Dunn R, Jackson AA, Poston L, Hanson MA. Folate supplementation during pregnancy improves offspring cardiovascular dysfunction induced by protein restriction. *Hypertension* 2006;47: 982–7.

Vehaskari VM, Aviles DH, Manning J. Prenatal programming of adult hypertension in the rat. *Kidney Int* 2001;59: 238–45.

Vickers MH, Breier BH, McCarthy D, Gluckman PD. Sedentary behavior during postnatal life is determined by the prenatal environment and exacerbated by postnatal hypercaloric nutrition. *Am J Physiol Regul Integr Comp Physiol* 2003;285: R271–3.

Watkins AJ, Wilkins A, Cunningham C, Perry VH, Seet MJ, Osmond C, Eckert JJ, Torrens C, Cagampang FR, Cleal J, Gray WP, Hanson MA, Fleming TP. Low protein diet fed exclusively during mouse oocyte maturation leads to behavioural and cardiovascular abnormalities in offspring. *J Physiol* 2008;586: 2231–44.

Woodall SM, Johnston BM, Breier BH, Gluckman PD. Chronic maternal undernutrition in the rat leads to delayed postnatal growth and elevated blood pressure of offspring. *Pediatr Res* 1996;40: 438–43.

Yates Z, Tarling EJ, Langley-Evans SC, Salter AM. Maternal undernutrition programmes atherosclerosis in the Apo E*3 Leiden mouse. *Br J Nutr* 2008;101: 1185–94.

5 Fetal programming of endocrine function in IUGR offspring depends on the cause of low birth weight: Evidence from animal models and the human FIPS-study

Eva Nüsken, Anja Tzschoppe, Jörg Dötsch, and Kai-Dietrich Nüsken

Low birth weight and intrauterine growth restriction (IUGR) can be caused by a number of different conditions, which are not accounted for in many experimental settings. Therefore, the objective of our present studies is to analyze the impact of different causes of low birth weight on fetal programming of endocrine function using the example of two key candidate molecules: IGF-1 and leptin.

Methodologically, we have established two different models of intrauterine growth restriction in the rat – the model of bilateral uterine artery ligation (UAL) and the model of low protein nutrition (LPN). In humans, we have established a prospective multicenter study ("FIPS") studying placental tissue and umbilical cord blood from growth-restricted neonates with anomalous placental Doppler velocimetry (IUGR), small for gestational age neonates with normal placental Doppler (small for gestational age [SGA]) and healthy controls (appropriate for gestational age [AGA]).

Our results indicate that fetal programming of leptin and IGF-1 depends on the cause of low birth weight rather than birth weight itself. UAL and LPN both induce IUGR but have opposing impacts on placental as well as fetal hepatic leptin and IGF-1 gene expressions at birth. In addition to differing windows of exposure, we speculate that availability of nutrients and occurrence of hypoxia, respectively, might be the pivotal differences leading to distinct programming. In humans, the underlying cause for fetal programming of metabolic disease via reduced neonatal free leptin might be prenatal unfavorable placental environment (IUGR, as evidenced by reduced placental perfusion), not low birth weight (SGA). In conclusion, morbidity after low birth weight should be analyzed referring to the underlying pathophysiological cause rather than referring to low birth weight itself.

5.1 Introduction

Intrauterine growth restriction is known to be associated with disease in later life (Varvarigou, 2010). Consequently, the importance of early human development on the predisposition for disease in later life has become an important topic of research, and various models have been developed to study the effect of low birth weight on later morbidity. In humans, low birth weight and intrauterine growth restriction are caused by a number of different conditions. In many experimental settings, however, these different causes are not accounted for. Therefore, the objective of our present clinical and experimental studies is to analyze the impact of different causes of low birth weight on fetal programming of endocrine function.

5.2 Leptin and IGF-1, two key candidate molecules of endocrine programming

More than a decade ago it was demonstrated that uterine artery ligation (UAL) results in decreased serum levels of IGF-1 and elevated serum concentrations of IGFBP-1 in the fetus (Unterman et al., 1993). Offspring of UAL dams develop impaired glucose tolerance as well as altered lipid metabolism and global adiposity in later life (Nüsken et al., 2008; Simmons, Templeton, and Gertz, 2001). Similarly to rodent data, IGF-1 is decreased and IGFBP-1 is elevated in cord blood from human SGA neonates (Verhaeghe et al., 1993) who are at higher risk to develop a disturbed glucose tolerance and diabetes mellitus, respectively (Hales et al., 1991). Altered IGF-1 (Brugts et al., 2010; Dunger, Yuen, and Ong, 2004; Rajpathak et al., 2009) and IGFBP-1 (Heald et al., 2001; Lewitt et al., 2008) levels are associated with disturbed glucose tolerance in adults. Likewise, decreased IGF-1 serum concentrations as well as IGF-1 hepatic gene expression, respectively, and elevated IGFBP-1 serum concentrations and elevated IGFBP-1 hepatic gene expression were measured in rats with streptozotocin-induced diabetes mellitus (Han, Kang, and Park, 2006). Thus, IGF-1 and IGFBP-1 might play a pivotal role in fetal programming of later metabolic disease and are of high interest when comparing different models of IUGR.

Leptin was discovered in 1994 and plays an essential role in the regulation of energy homeostasis, food intake, body composition, and reproductive function (Ahima and Flier, 2000). It is known to reduce food intake by regulating the activity of neurons in the hypothalamus (Bouret, Draper, and Simerly, 2004). In this context, Bouret and colleagues were able to show that leptin deficiency during a critical period of brain development in neonatal mice induced permanent disruption of neural projection pathways from the arcuate nucleus of the hypothalamus, leading to the development of adiposity later on (Bouret et al., 2004). Because a dysregulation of appetite might be responsible for the development of adiposity in SGA infants, leptin is a key candidate of metabolic programming. Additionally, leptin is of interest in IUGR as it seems to be related to intrauterine growth (Koistinen et al., 1997) and insulin sensitivity (Miras et al., 2010). However, leptin data from IUGR studies is conflicting. Leptin gene expression in perirenal visceral fat from male IUGR lambs was significantly decreased compared to controls (Duffield et al., 2009). In humans, some authors report increased leptin cord blood levels in IUGR infants (Shekhawat et al., 1998) whereas most others found decreased umbilical leptin concentrations (Jaquet et al., 1998; Pighetti et al., 2003; Yildiz, Avci, and Ingeç, 2002). These conflicting results might be explained by the fact that the underlying pathophysiological cause is not accounted for in most IUGR studies.

5.3 Animal models of IUGR

Worldwide, various animal models have been used to study the impact of intrauterine growth restriction. In our group, we have established two different, widely used models of IUGR in the rat. The model of bilateral UAL is used to induce IUGR by placental insufficiency (Nüsken et al., 2008), whereas the model of low protein (LP) nutrition simulates the situation of mothers who suffer from malnutrition (Plank et al., 2006).

In UAL dams, we perform the ligation on day 19 of pregnancy. Both uterine horns are carefully pulled out of the abdomen and both uterine arteries and veins are ligated at the most caudal point accessible. After the ligation, blood flow to the fetuses is only supplied from cranially via the ovarian artery. Therefore, the phenotype of intrauterine growth restriction is most severe in caudal fetuses. Fetuses from ligated dams (LIG) are compared to both fetuses of sham-operated dams ([SOP] in whom the suture material was not fixed but removed after identical anesthetic and surgical procedures) and to fetuses of unoperated controls (C). In the LPN model, dams are fed a low protein diet (LP; 8% casein) throughout pregnancy. The control dams are fed an isocaloric normal protein (NP) diet (17% casein).

In studies using the UAL model, there are several methodological aspects to be considered. As to the fetal position in the uterine horn, we found that caudal fetuses from ligated dams were most severely growth-restricted and that placental gene expression of insulin-like growth factor binding protein 1 (IGFBP-1) measured by RNA protection assay at birth was increased only in fetuses near the ligation site (caudal) but not in fetuses far from the ligation (Nüsken et al., 2007; ▶Tab. 5.1). It is also important to note that the UAL model requires untreated controls because sham operation alone induces not only IUGR but also alterations of gene expression at birth as well as long-term pathogenic programming of adiposity and disturbed lipid metabolism (Nüsken et al., 2008).

Comparing the UAL model with the LPN model, there are three main methodological differences. First, the cause of low birth weight is different (low blood flow vs. malnutrition). Secondly, the window of exposure varies (last 4 days of pregnancy vs. complete pregnancy). Thirdly, birth weight in fetuses of ligated dams (LIG) and of sham-operated dams (SOP) depends on the fetal position in relation to the ligation site (Nüsken et al., 2007; ▶Tab. 5.1), whereas all fetuses of LP dams are born too small irrespective of their position in the uterine horn. Analysis of gene expression at birth demonstrated that leptin expression in the placentas of LIG and SOP fetuses was significantly down-regulated compared to control fetuses. Conversely, leptin in placentas of LP fetuses

Tab. 5.1: Dependence of birth weight and placental IGFBP-1 expression on the fetal position in the uterine horn. Data are shown as mean ± SD.

Fetal position in the uterine horn	No. of fetuses investigated	Body weight at cesarean delivery (g)	IGFBP-1 expression (mean percentage relative to control fetuses)
Close to ligation site (1st and 2nd fetus)	8	3.86 ± 0.8	404 ± 734
Intermediate position	5	4.22 ± 0.4	106 ± 136
Far from ligation site (last and 2nd last fetus)	8	4.75 ± 0.5	152 ± 212

(derived from Nüsken et al., 2007)

was significantly upregulated compared to NP. Similarly, IGF-1 gene expression in the placenta was reduced in group LIG but increased in group LP. In fetal liver, IGF-1 expression was significantly downregulated in LIG fetuses but unaltered in LP fetuses (Nüsken et al., 2011).

In conclusion, comparison of the UAL model with the LPN model provides strong evidence that the *cause* of low birth weight, not low birth weight itself, is crucial when studying IUGR-associated fetal programming. In addition to differing windows of exposure, we speculate that availability of nutrients and occurrence of hypoxia, respectively, might be the pivotal differences leading to distinct programming.

5.4 Human IUGR study (FIPS)

In humans, we have established a prospective multicenter study (Fetal programming – IUGR – Placental markers – Study; FIPS) to identify placental genes with predictive value for the development of obesity and metabolic disorders after intrauterine growth restriction based on the hypothesis of an alteration of gene expression by fetal programming. As we define IUGR by a birth weight Z-score < 10th percentile *and* anomalous placental Doppler velocimetry during pregnancy, all of the IUGR pregnancies in this study experience placental insufficiency. Further inclusion and exclusion criteria are listed in detail by Tzschoppe et al. (2010a).

In the present study (Tzschoppe et al., 2010a, 2010b) we primarily aimed to compare placental leptin synthesis and leptin binding capability in venous cord blood between IUGR newborns and neonates born AGA. Secondly, these parameters were analyzed in an additional group of neonates with low birth weight but normal uterine and umbilical artery Doppler velocimetry (SGA, defined by a birth weight Z-score < 10th percentile) and also compared to IUGR newborns. We enrolled 21 newborns with prenatal ultrasound-proven IUGR (9 males, 12 females), 33 healthy AGA neonates (19 males, 14 females), and 14 SGA newborns without IUGR (7 males, 7 females). 62% of the IUGR, none of the SGA, and 45% of the AGA infants were premature. Further clinical characteristics of the three groups at birth are listed in ▶Tab. 5.2. In all neonates, we determined the concentration of leptin and soluble leptin receptor (sOB-R) in venous cord blood at birth. Moreover, placental gene and protein expression of leptin were measured. For statistical analysis, measurements were log-transformed to normalize the data.

Comparing IUGR to AGA neonates, plasma log-leptin concentration in venous cord blood did not differ significantly. However, the concentration of log-sOB-R was significantly elevated in IUGR newborns ($p = 0.01$, ▶Fig. 5.1).

On the placental level, log-leptin mRNA was significantly higher in IUGR than in AGA neonates (relative gene expression, $p = 0.01$). Ligand blotting analysis revealed that the increase in leptin mRNA levels was accompanied by increased leptin protein expression in placentas of IUGR infants (▶Fig. 5.2).

To investigate the effect of prenatal placental environment on potential pathological fetal programming in lean human neonates, we compared IUGR newborns with the additional group of SGA neonates. Whereas no significant difference was found for plasma log-leptin concentration in venous cord blood ($p = 0.70$, ▶Fig. 5.3), the concentration of log-sOB-R was elevated in IUGR ($p = 0.01$, ▶Fig. 5.3) compared to SGA neonates.

Tab. 5.2: Birth characteristics of IUGR, AGA, and SGA neonates. Data are shown as mean ± SEM and median (minimum–maximum).

	IUGR (n = 21)	AGA (n = 33)	SGA (n = 14)	Significance
Gestational age (weeks)	35.1 ± 0.6 35.3 (30–40)	36.4 ± 0.4 37.1 (30–41)	39.3 ± 0.2 39.2 (38–41)	[1]p = 0.08 [2]p < 0.001 [3]p = 0.001
Spontaneous delivery; cesarean section (n; n)	2; 19	12; 21	10; 4	[1]p = 0.054 [2]p < 0.001 [3]p = 0.053
Maternal age (years)	30.0 ± 1.2 30.5 (19–39)	31.3 ± 1.0 32.0 (20–38)	27.3 ± 1.3 27.5 (20–36)	[1]p = 0.39 [2]p = 0.16 [3]p = 0.02
Maternal BMI before pregnancy (kg/m²)	21.6 ± 0.7 21.4 (17.0–27.8)	22.9 ± 0.6 22.7 (18.3–29.1)	20.7 ± 0.6 20.3 (17.6–23.3)	[1]p = 0.16 [2]p = 0.40 [3]p = 0.04
Maternal BMI at term (kg/m²)	26.3 ± 1.1 26.1 (18.8–39.3)	27.8 ± 0.8 27.9 (19.1–36.7)	25.6 ± 1.2 24.0 (21.7–32.4)	[1]p = 0.28 [2]p = 0.72 [3]p = 0.18
Maternal smoking (n/n recorded)	2/19	2/31	4/10	[1]p = 0.64 [2]p = 0.19 [3]p = 0.06
Placental weight (g)	360 ± 23 350 (190–540)	503 ± 21 515 (320–780)	458 ± 29 470 (315–690)	[1]p < 0.001 [2]p = 0.01 [3]p = 0.22
Birth weight SDS	−2.3 ± 0.1 −2.2 (−3.5 − −1.1)	−0.4 ± 0.1 −0.4 (−1.1–0.2)	−2.0 ± 0.1 −2.0 (−2.5 − −1.4)	[1]p < 0.001 [2]p = 0.11 [3]p < 0.001

[1] IUGR-AGA, [2] IUGR-SGA, [3] AGA-SGA

(derived from Tzschoppe et al., 2010b)

Considering placental gene expression, log-leptin mRNA was significantly higher in IUGR than in SGA newborns (relative gene expression, $p < 0.001$, ▶Fig. 5.4).

Ligand blotting analysis showed that leptin protein expression was reduced in SGA compared to IUGR neonates (▶Fig. 5.2).

Thus, not low birth weight (SGA), but prenatal unfavorable placental environment as evidenced by reduced placental perfusion (IUGR) might be the underlying cause for fetal programming of metabolic disease via reduced neonatal free leptin. In analogy to rodent models (Bouret et al., 2004), we speculate that leptin deficiency after IUGR might induce a dysregulation of appetite and energy expenditure due to insufficient formation of specific hypothalamic circuits. In conclusion, morbidity after low birth weight should be analyzed referring to the underlying pathophysiological cause rather than referring to low birth weight itself.

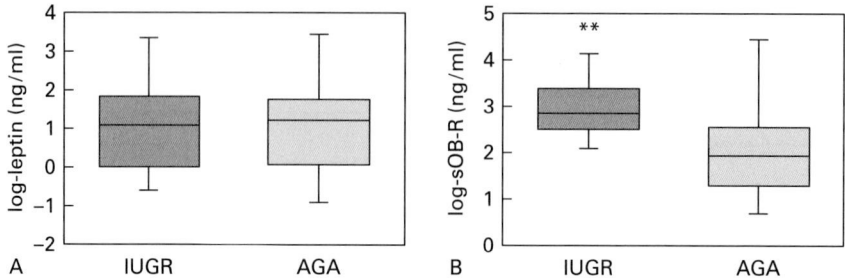

Fig. 5.1: Concentration of log-transformed leptin (A) and log-transformed sOB-R (B) in the umbilical vein of IUGR ($n = 21$) and AGA ($n = 33$) neonates after birth. There is a significant difference in the concentration of log-transformed sOB-R between IUGR and AGA newborns (**$p = 0.01$). Data are shown as boxplots.

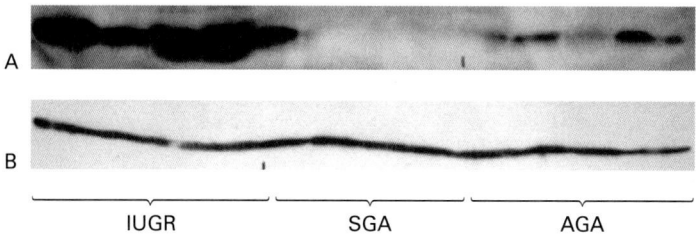

Fig. 5.2: Illustration of leptin in placental tissue of IUGR, SGA, and AGA neonates as evaluated by Western Blot analysis. Leptin (16kDa) showed higher protein expression in IUGR samples compared to SGA and AGA samples (A). ß-actin detection (43kDa) served as loading control (B).

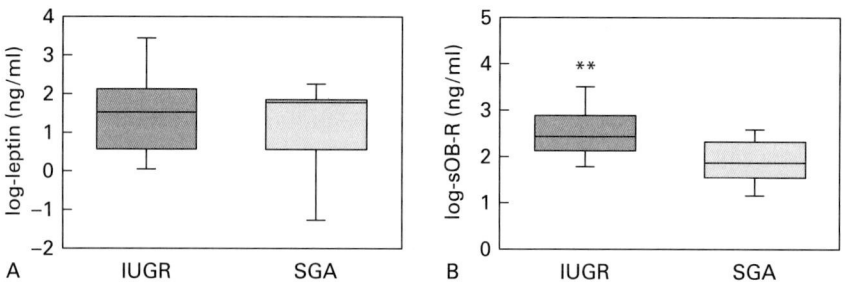

Fig. 5.3: Concentration of log-transformed leptin (A) and log-transformed sOB-R (B) in the umbilical vein of IUGR ($n = 21$) and SGA ($n = 14$) neonates after birth. There is a significant difference in the concentration of log-transformed sOB-R between IUGR and SGA newborns (**$p = 0.01$). Data are shown as boxplots.

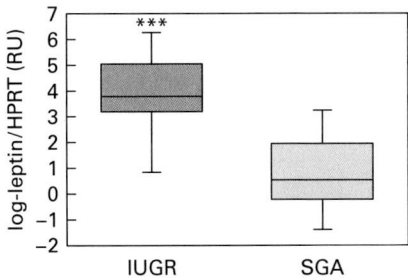

Fig. 5.4: Placental leptin gene expression in IUGR (*n* = 21) and SGA (*n* = 14) neonates. There is a significant difference between IUGR and SGA newborns (***p < 0.001). Gene expression data are log-transformed and are related to the housekeeping gene hypoxanthine guanine phosphoribosyl transferase (HPRT). Data are shown as boxplots. (RU = relative units.)

5.5 Summary

Following the first publications by, for example, Dörner (Dörner and Mohnike, 1973) and Barker (Barker and Osmond, 1986) on the association between early human development and morbidity in later life, numerous clinical and experimental studies have focused on the implications of low birth weight. However, in many of these studies, it is unclear whether intrauterine growth restriction (IUGR) is present, and the underlying pathophysiological cause of low birth weight is not accounted for. Looking at leptin and IGF-1, which are both key molecules of endocrine programming, our present studies in animals and humans demonstrate that fetal programming of endocrine systems does not depend on low birth weight itself, but on the cause of low birth weight.

In rats, uterine artery ligation (UAL) on day 19 of pregnancy, as well as low protein nutrition (LPN) throughout pregnancy, are established models for the induction of low birth weight subsequent to IUGR. The experimental setting of both models clearly varies in the window of exposure (last 4 days of pregnancy vs. complete pregnancy) and in the underlying pathophysiological cause of low birth weight (low blood flow vs. malnutrition). Although both models induce IUGR, they have opposing impact on placental as well as fetal hepatic leptin and IGF-1 gene expressions at birth (Nüsken et al., 2011). This is reflected by the distinct long-term outcome of the two animal models. Offspring of ligated dams develop disturbed glucose tolerance, altered lipid metabolism, and global adiposity in later life (Nüsken et al., 2008; Simmons et al., 2001). In contrast, our specific low protein nutrition results in only minor metabolic changes in the offspring (Plank et al., 2008). Additionally, LPN seems to induce arterial hypertension and kidney disease much earlier in life than UAL (Langley-Evans, Langley-Evans, and Marchand, 2003; Vehaskari, Aviles, and Manning, 2001; Wlodek et al., 2008). Thus, these models provide strong evidence that the cause of low birth weight is crucial when studying IUGR-models.

Because the relevance of observations in animals for humans is limited, we have initiated a prospective controlled multicenter study in humans named "FIPS" (Fetal programming – IUGR – Placental markers – Study), aiming at predicting later disease by analyzing the placenta and venous cord blood right after birth (Dötsch, Schild, and

Struwe, 2008). In the afterbirth of infants suffering from intrauterine deprivation resulting in IUGR (proved by pathological Doppler velocimetry of the umbilical and/or uterine arteries during pregnancy), important regulating systems for cell growth and transport through the placenta are studied. During the following 6 years, the patients are examined annually with regard to growth, overweight, blood pressure, kidney function, and glucose tolerance.

As to leptin, data from the FIPS study indicates that increased leptin binding capacity results in reduced biologically active circulating leptin concentrations in IUGR neonates, but not in neonates with low birth weight and normal Doppler (SGA). Furthermore, current preliminary data demonstrates that IUGR neonates only, but not SGA neonates, show a significant decrease of circulating IGF-1 (Tzschoppe et al., 2010a, 2010b). Therefore, human data also demonstrates that the cause of low birth weight is a key factor for fetal programming of endocrine systems.

In conclusion, morbidity after low birth weight should be analyzed referring to the underlying pathophysiological cause rather than referring to low birth weight itself.

References

Ahima RS, Flier JS. Leptin. *Annu Rev Physiol* 2000;62: 413–37.

Barker DJ, Osmond C. Infant mortality, childhood nutrition, and ischaemic heart disease in England and Wales. *Lancet* 1986;1: 1077–81.

Bouret SG, Draper SJ, Simerly RB. Trophic action of leptin on hypothalamic neurons that regulate feeding. *Science* 2004;304: 108–10.

Brugts MP, van Duijn CM, Hofland LJ, Witteman JC, Lamberts SW, Janssen JA. Igf-I bioactivity in an elderly population: relation to insulin sensitivity, insulin levels, and the metabolic syndrome. *Diabetes* 2010;59: 505–8.

Dörner G, Mohnike A. [Possible importance of pre- and-or early postnatal nutrition in the pathogenesis of diabetes mellitus]. *Acta Biol Med Ger* 1973;31: K7–10.

Dötsch J, Schild RL, Struwe E. Can the afterbirth play a role after birth? *Hum Ontogenet* 2008;2: 25–8.

Duffield JA, Vuocolo T, Tellam R, et al. Intrauterine growth restriction and the sex specific programming of leptin and peroxisome proliferator-activated receptor gamma (PPARgamma) mRNA expression in visceral fat in the lamb. *Pediatr Res* 2009;66: 59–65.

Dunger D, Yuen K, Ong K. Insulin-like growth factor I and impaired glucose tolerance. *Horm Res* 2004;62: 101–7.

Hales CN, Barker DJ, Clark PM, Cox LJ, Fall C, Osmond C, Winter PD. Fetal and infant growth and impaired glucose tolerance at age 64. *BMJ* 1991;303: 1019–22.

Han HJ, Kang CW, Park SH. Tissue-specific regulation of insulin-like growth factors and insulin-like growth factor binding proteins in male diabetic rats in vivo and in vitro. *Clin Exp Pharmacol Physiol* 2006;33: 1172–9.

Heald AH, Cruickshank JK, Riste LK, et al. Close relation of fasting insulin-like growth factor binding protein-1 (IGFBP-1) with glucose tolerance and cardiovascular risk in two populations. *Diabetologia* 2001;44: 333–9.

Jaquet D, Leger J, Levy-Marchal C, Oury JF, Czernichow P. Ontogeny of leptin in human fetuses and newborns: effect of intrauterine growth retardation on serum leptin concentrations. *J Clin Endocrinol Metab* 1998;83: 1243–6.

Koistinen HA, Koivisto VA, Andersson S, et al. Leptin concentration in cord blood correlates with intrauterine growth. *J Clin Endocrinol Metab* 1997;82: 3328–30.

Langley-Evans SC, Langley-Evans AJ, Marchand MC. Nutritional programming of blood pressure and renal morphology. *Arch Physiol Biochem* 2003;111: 8–16.

Lewitt MS, Hilding A, Ostenson CG, Efendic S, Brismar K, Hall K. Insulin-like growth factor-binding protein-1 in the prediction and development of type 2 diabetes in middle-aged Swedish men. *Diabetologia* 2008;51: 1135–45.

Miras M, Ochetti M, Martín S, et al. Serum levels of adiponectin and leptin in children born small for gestational age: relation to insulin sensitivity parameters. *J Pediatr Endocrinol Metab* 2010;23: 463–71.

Nüsken KD, Dötsch J, Rauh M, Rascher W, Schneider H. Uteroplacental insufficiency after bilateral uterine artery ligation in the rat: impact on postnatal glucose and lipid metabolism and evidence for metabolic programming of the offspring by sham operation. *Endocrinology* 2008;149: 1056–63.

Nüsken KD, Warnecke C, Hilgers KF, Schneider H. Intrauterine growth after uterine artery ligation in rats: dependence on the fetal position in the uterine horn and need for prenatal marking of the animals. *J Hypertens* 2007;25: 247–8.

Nüsken KD, Schneider H, Plank C, et al. Fetal programming of gene expression in growth-restricted rats depends on the cause of low birth weight. *Endocrinology* 2011,152: 1327–35.

Pighetti M, Tommaselli GA, D'Elia A, et al. Maternal serum and umbilical cord blood leptin concentrations with fetal growth restriction. *Obstet Gynecol* 2003;102: 535–43.

Plank C, Grillhösl C, Ostreicher I, et al. Transient growth hormone therapy to rats with low protein-inflicted intrauterine growth restriction does not prevent elevated blood pressure in later life. *Growth Factors* 2008;26: 355–64.

Plank C, Ostreicher I, Hartner A, et al. Intrauterine growth retardation aggravates the course of acute mesangioproliferative glomerulonephritis in the rat. *Kidney Int* 2006;70: 1974–82.

Rajpathak SN, Gunter MJ, Wylie-Rosett J, et al. The role of insulin-like growth factor-I and its binding proteins in glucose homeostasis and type 2 diabetes. *Diabetes Metab Res Rev* 2009;25: 3–12.

Shekhawat PS, Garland JS, Shivpuri C, et al. Neonatal cord blood leptin: its relationship to birth weight, body mass index, maternal diabetes, and steroids. *Pediatr Res* 1998;43: 338–43.

Simmons RA, Templeton LJ, Gertz SJ. Intrauterine growth retardation leads to the development of type 2 diabetes in the rat. *Diabetes* 2001;50: 2279–86.

Tzschoppe AA, Struwe E, Dörr HG, et al. Differences in gene expression dependent on sampling site in placental tissue of fetuses with intrauterine growth restriction. *Placenta* 2010a;31: 178–85.

Tzschoppe A, Struwe E, Rascher W, et al. Intrauterine growth restriction (IUGR) is associated with increased leptin synthesis and binding capability in neonates. *Clin Endocrinol* 2010b; ahead of print. doi: 10.1111/j.1365–2265.2010.03943.x.

Unterman TG, Simmons RA, Glick RP, Ogata ES. Circulating levels of insulin, insulin-like growth factor-I (IGF-I), IGF-II, and IGF-binding proteins in the small for gestational age fetal rat. *Endocrinology* 1993;132: 327–36.

Varvarigou AA. Intrauterine growth restriction as a potential risk factor for disease onset in adulthood. *J Pediatr Endocrinol Metab* 2010;23: 215–24.

Vehaskari VM, Aviles DH, Manning J. Prenatal programming of adult hypertension in the rat. *Kidney Int* 2001;59: 238–45.

Verhaeghe J, Van Bree R, Van Herck E, Laureys J, Bouillon R, Van Assche FA. C-peptide, insulin-like growth factors I and II, and insulin-like growth factor binding protein-1 in umbilical cord serum: correlations with birth weight. *Am J Obstet Gynecol* 1993;169: 89–97.

Wlodek ME, Westcott K, Siebel AL, Owens JA, Moritz KM. Growth restriction before or after birth reduces nephron number and increases blood pressure in male rats. *Kidney Int* 2008;74: 187–95.

Yildiz L, Avci B, Ingeç M. Umbilical cord and maternal blood leptin concentrations in intrauterine growth retardation. *Clin Chem Lab Med* 2002;40: 1114–7.

6 Intrauterine corticosteroids for lung maturation: Observations of HPA axis function and cardiac autonomic balance in the neonate

Leonhard Schäffer, Tilo Burkhardt, Maren Tomaske, Manfred Rauh, and Ernst Beinder

The putative long-term effects of antenatal glucocorticoid treatment for accelerating lung maturation in pregnancies at risk for preterm birth is still a matter of debate. Different animal models have shown that antenatal glucocorticoid exposure has a persistent impact on the hypothalamus-pituitary-adrenal (HPA) – axis regulation and that the developing cardiac autonomic system is sensitive toward antenatal glucocorticoids. In the human, the situation is less clear. Long-term observations in adolescents and young adults have rather focused on classic signs of disease manifestation such as blood pressure. Risk-factors for cardiovascular and metabolic disease, however, may transform into apparent clinical manifestation at a more advanced age when stability of these systems can be less compensated by the organism. Our studies analyzed whether a single course of antenatal betamethasone treatment has a direct and continuous effect on the developing HPA axis and the cardiac autonomic system. To this end, resting- and stress-induced salivary levels for cortisol, cortisone, and α-amylase as well as heart rate variability parameters as early signs of system alteration were analyzed. These studies were conducted in healthy newborns born late preterm or at term. Our studies show that a single course of antenatal betamethasone treatment induces a significant suppression of HPA-axis reactivity in healthy infants that is present several weeks later in early postnatal life. In contrast, the cardiac autonomic balance appears not to be primarily affected. Antenatal betamethasone treatment may therefore alter the HPA axis in a manner that predisposes these individuals toward a development of diseases in later life.

6.1 Introduction

Antenatal glucocorticoid administration is an established procedure in pregnancies with an imminent risk for preterm delivery. Before 34 weeks of gestation, maternal administration of synthetic glucocorticoids, such as betamethasone or dexamethasone, significantly reduces perinatal mortality and morbidity by maturational effects on the immature fetal lungs and decreases the risk for necrotizing enterocolitis and severe cerebral hemorrhage (Roberts and Dalziel, 2006).

Evidence from animal models, however, suggests that excess glucocorticoid exposure during intrauterine development may entail long-term alterations in the functionality and balance of homeostasis regulating systems. Indeed, major physiologic systems involved in the development of hypertension and the metabolic syndrome are glucocorticoid sensitive targets during intrauterine development (Drake, Tang, and Nyirenda, 2007; Seckl, 2004). In the rat, maternal antenatal dexamethasone treatment results in elevated blood pressure in the offspring (Benediktsson et al., 1993; Woods and Weeks, 2005). Likewise, the maternal administration of dexamethasone in the sheep induces hypertension during adulthood (Dodic et al., 1998, 2002). Glucocorticoids are likewise involved in programming of glucose tolerance and metabolism. Again, in the rat as well as in the sheep, persistent alterations in glucose and insulin levels have been found in adult offspring after intrauterine glucocorticoid exposure (Moss et al., 2001; Nyirenda et al., 1998).

6.2 Vulnerability of the hypothalamic-pituitary-adrenal (HPA) axis

The hypothalamic-pituitary-adrenal (HPA) axis represents the organism's central organ of stress regulation and is involved in preservation of cardiovascular and metabolic stability, and elevated cortisol levels have been linked to arteriosclerosis and diabetes (Sapolsky, Romero, and Munck, 2000). The HPA axis and its key limbic regulator, the hippocampus, are especially sensitive to glucocorticoids because this system is tightly regulated through a feedback mechanism involving glucocorticoid (GR) and mineralocorticoid receptors (MR) at the level of the hippocampus, hypothalamus, and pituitary gland to inhibit HPA activity (Jacobson and Sapolsky, 1991). The HPA axis has been shown to be vulnerable to excess glucocorticoid exposure during its maturational stage (Kapoor, Petropoulos, and Matthews, 2008; Owen, Andrews, and Matthews, 2005). As such, overexposure to glucocorticoids results in attenuated hippocampal GR and MR expression. The resulting permanently increased cortisol levels and hypertension in the adult rats suggest an impaired negative feedback sensitivity of the HPA axis (Levitt et al., 1996). Further alterations at different levels of the HPA axis are likewise targets of glucocorticoid receptor alterations (Dean et al., 2001). Thus, glucocorticoid induced permanent alterations of these receptors may induce a resetting of the balance and reactivity of the HPA axis in later life.

6.3 Vulnerability of the sympathetic nervous system

The sympathetic nervous system (SNS) development has been shown to be sensitive toward antenatal glucocorticoids as well. In fact, the SNS is closely interconnected with the HPA axis as glucocorticoids provide direct signals for noradrenergic system maturation in the brainstem and thus on central noradrenergic activity (Slotkin et al., 1992). Furthermore, cardiac noradrenergic innervation is directly affected by glucocorticoids (Bian, Seidler, and Slotkin, 1993). Adrenergic cardiovascular drive and noradrenergic influences play a key role in the development or progression of hypertension and the metabolic syndrome in the adult (Grassi et al., 2009), making this system another key candidate for glucocorticoid induced long-term alterations in system balance. This notion is supported by experiments showing a sustained elevation of blood pressure and altered baroreceptor heart rate response in fetal sheep and the baboon and increased central and peripheral vascular resistance after glucocorticoid administration (Derks et al., 1997; Fletcher et al., 2002; Koenen et al., 2002; Schwab et al., 2000).

6.4 Findings in humans

Findings of putative alterations of HPA-axis activity and SNS balance in the human after intrauterine glucocorticoid exposure are less clear. Premature neonates failed to increase cortisol levels in response to a stressor after intrauterine exposure to gluco-corticoids for lung maturation (Davis et al., 2004, 2006). In the neonate as well as in a cohort of preterm born children at the age of 14 years, blood pressure was significantly increased after prenatal glucocorticoid treatment (Doyle et al., 2000; Kari et al., 1994). In contrast, a large prospective follow-up study did not find significant alterations in blood pressure and resting cortisol levels in 30-year-old adults after a single course of antenatal betamethasone treatment for lung maturation. Physiological functional-ity when challenging these systems was not available. Nevertheless, during a glucose challenge, clear indicators for the presence of insulin resistance were present in these individuals (Dalziel et al., 2005). In fact, studies have mainly focused on classical signs of disease manifestation; however, these signs may not become apparent until a later age when compensatory mechanisms fail after a certain threshold is reached.

If indeed the HPA axis and the SNS experience permanent alterations after intrauter-ine glucocorticoid exposure, these alterations should be detectable after birth. Consider-ing the fact that these alterations may be mild and clinically not apparent during early life due to a high compensatory reserve being only "exhausted" over many years, we aimed to not only analyze HPA and SNS balance under resting conditions but also to challenge these systems.

A further rationale to analyze these systems in neonates was that in a normal postna-tal period, temporarily challenged systems normalize in response to a normal postnatal environment, while permanently altered systems may become apparent, but postnatal compensatory system reactions may not have had the time to develop.

6.5 HPA axis functionality in neonates after intrauterine betamethasone treatment

To analyze the functionality of the HPA axis, we applied a simple noninvasive method by measuring cortisol and cortisone levels in salivary samples. Salivary cortisol reflects the unbound, active fraction of cortisol and is highly correlated with plasma cortisol levels (Calixto et al., 2002; Gunnar, 1989), making this method especially valuable for infants where blood sampling is less desired by parents. Likewise, to analyze for functionality under challenge, we made use of the routinely conducted heel-prick test 72–96 h after delivery, which has been shown to be an adequate stimulus for HPA-axis activation (Gunnar, 1992). Resting cortisol levels and cortisol levels after this challenge were measured. While resting levels of cortisol were comparable between the infants with antenatal betamethasone treatment and controls, we found that the neonatal HPA axis was significantly suppressed in infants with betamethasone treatment after the stimulus as these infants failed to adequately increase cortisol release (Schäffer et al., 2009; ▶Fig. 6.1). Because these infants were born near or at term and the mean interval between glucocorticoid treatment and delivery was more than 8 weeks, it is rather unlikely that these effects may only be a transient short-term effect consider-ing that short-term effects of antenatal glucocorticoid exposure have been described to last for about 1 week after administration (Ballard et al., 1980; Parker et al., 1996).

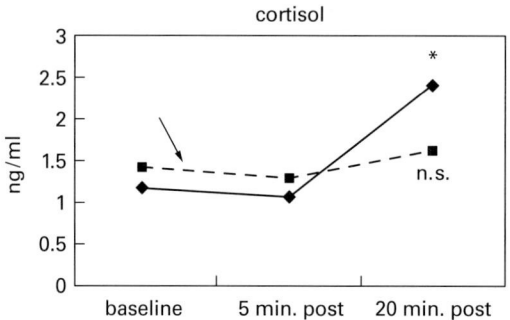

Fig. 6.1: Median cortisol levels during resting- (baseline) and post-stress induction (5 min. post, 20 min. post) phases in betamethasone exposed neonates (- - -) and controls (—). Arrow indicates stress induction. $*p < 0.05$, n.s.: not significant.

The possibility that the decreased cortisol response in the study group would be the result of an increased conversion of cortisol to cortisone by an altered activity of the 11ß-hydroxysteroid dehydrogenase could also be excluded because cortisol and cortisone levels were strongly correlated in the study group, thus excluding this possibility. Therefore, it appears that a single course of antenatal betamethasone treatment for imminent preterm delivery has a suppressive effect on HPA-axis reactivity that persists at least for more than a mean of 8 weeks when these pregnancies continue and infants are delivered near or at term.

6.6 The cardiac autonomic system after intrauterine betamethasone treatment

A sensitive parameter to analyze early alterations in the cardiac sympathetic – parasympathetic balance is heart rate variability (HRV), which is a well-established noninvasive measure of cardiac autonomic control that has been shown to be related to hypertension (Guzzetti et al., 1991; Langewitz, Ruddel, and Schachinger, 1994) and to predict future adverse cardiovascular events in adults (Algra et al., 1993). Analyses of HRV have been suggested for putative prognostic use in children as well (Stewart, 2000). Analysis from 24 h Holter electrocardiogram (ECG) tracings calculating various parameters for short- and long-term analyses during active and resting states did not reveal any significant difference between betamethasone exposed infants and controls (Schäffer et al., 2010).

To further support our conclusion, we supplemented our electrophysiological studies by measuring salivary α-amylase levels during resting conditions and after a stressful stimulus (heel-prick test). Salivary α-amylase is secreted by acinar cells in the salivary glands that are richly innervated by both sympathetic and parasympathetic nerve fibers, influencing the release of α-amylase by classic neurotransmitters (Turner and Sugiya, 2002). Studies in humans and animals have suggested that the activation of the autonomic nervous system leads to a high activity of salivary α-amylase (Asking and Gjorstrup, 1987; Chatterton et al., 1996; Schneyer and Hall, 1991; Steerenberg et al., 1997). Furthermore, α-amylase levels have been found to be associated with cardiovascular physiology and are suggested to be a surrogate for cardiovascular autonomic system balance (Granger et al., 2007), thereby making this parameter a promising indicator for cardiac autonomic function.

Interestingly, α-amylase levels rather decreased in betamethasone-exposed neonates in response to the stress event as compared to controls (Schäffer et al., 2010). We speculate that the slightly attenuated α-amylase response might be explained by the altered HPA-system sensitivity rather than by direct effects of steroid exposure on the sympathetic system as these systems are closely interconnected. Thus, it appears that the neonatal cardiac autonomic system is primarily unaffected by a single course of betamethasone treatment for lung maturation.

6.7 Summary

To our best knowledge, the presented studies are the first to analyze stress physiology in healthy term or near term delivered infants after a single course of betamethasone administration at a much earlier time in pregnancy. These early signs for alterations in the balance and activity of the HPA axis and the cardiac autonomic system may further contribute to the understanding of origins of disease development.

According to our results, a single course of antenatal betamethasone treatment for imminent preterm delivery entails alterations in HPA-axis responsiveness that persist into postnatal life. If this alteration of the HPA-axis balance really persists during life, it may represent a significant risk factor for the development of diseases in later life. In contrast, according to our results, cardiac autonomic balance appears to be preserved after exogenous glucocorticoid treatment at least in the neonate. However, due to the mutual interaction between the HPA axis and the SNS, this system may be subject to later alterations as the organism further matures.

Considering the beneficial effects of antenatal glucocorticoids to significantly reduce infant morbidity and mortality in pregnancies at risk for preterm delivery before 34 weeks of gestation, it is clear that these measures outweigh putative long-term risks according to current knowledge. Nevertheless, thorough evaluation in these cases is mandatory to ensure a clear indication for antenatal glucocorticoids. Prophylactic treatment in low-risk situations for preterm delivery should be avoided.

References

Algra A, Tijssen JG, Roelandt JR, Pool J, Lubsen J. Heart rate variability from 24-hour electrocardiography and the 2-year risk for sudden death. *Circulation* 1993;88: 180–5.

Asking B, Gjorstrup P. Synthesis and secretion of amylase in the rat parotid gland following autonomic nerve stimulation in vivo. *Acta Physiol Scand* 1987;130: 439–45.

Ballard PL, Gluckman PD, Liggins GC, Kaplan SL, Grumbach MM. Steroid and growth hormone levels in premature infants after prenatal betamethasone therapy to prevent respiratory distress syndrome. *Pediatr Res* 1980;14: 122–7.

Benediktsson R, Lindsay RS, Noble J, Seckl JR, Edwards CR. Glucocorticoid exposure in utero: new model for adult hypertension. *Lancet* 1993;341: 339–41.

Bian X, Seidler FJ, Slotkin TA. Fetal dexamethasone exposure interferes with establishment of cardiac noradrenergic innervation and sympathetic activity. *Teratology* 1993;47: 109–17.

Calixto C, Martinez FE, Jorge SM, Moreira AC, Martinelli CE Jr. Correlation between plasma and salivary cortisol levels in preterm infants. *J Pediatr* 2002;140: 116–8.

Chatterton RT, Jr, Vogelsong KM, Lu YC, Ellman AB, Hudgens GA. Salivary alpha-amylase as a measure of endogenous adrenergic activity. *Clin Physiol* 1996;16: 433–48.

Dalziel SR, Walker NK, Parag V, et al. Cardiovascular risk factors after antenatal exposure to beta-methasone: 30-year follow-up of a randomised controlled trial. *Lancet* 2005;365: 1856–62.

Davis EP, Townsend EL, Gunnar MR, et al. Effects of prenatal betamethasone exposure on regulation of stress physiology in healthy premature infants. *Psychoneuroendocrinology* 2004;29: 1028–36.

Davis EP, Townsend EL, Gunnar MR, et al. Antenatal betamethasone treatment has a persisting influence on infant HPA axis regulation. *J Perinatol* 2006;26: 147–53.

Dean F, Yu C, Lingas RI, Matthews SG. Prenatal glucocorticoid modifies hypothalamo-pituitary-adrenal regulation in prepubertal guinea pigs. *Neuroendocrinology* 2001;73: 194–202.

Derks JB, Giussani DA, Jenkins SL, et al. A comparative study of cardiovascular, endocrine and behavioural effects of betamethasone and dexamethasone administration to fetal sheep. *J Physiol* 1997;499: 217–26.

Dodic M, Hantzis V, Duncan J, et al. Programming effects of short prenatal exposure to cortisol. *FASEB J* 2002;16: 1017–26.

Dodic M, May CN, Wintour EM, Coghlan JP. An early prenatal exposure to excess glucocorticoid leads to hypertensive offspring in sheep. *Clin Sci* (Lond) 1998;94: 149–55.

Doyle LW, Ford GW, Davis NM, Callanan C. Antenatal corticosteroid therapy and blood pressure at 14 years of age in preterm children. *Clin Sci* (Lond) 2000;98: 137–42.

Drake AJ, Tang JI, Nyirenda MJ. Mechanisms underlying the role of glucocorticoids in the early life programming of adult disease. *Clin Sci* (Lond) 2007;113: 219–32.

Fletcher AJ, McGarrigle HH, Edwards CM, Fowden AL, Giussani DA. Effects of low dose dexamethasone treatment on basal cardiovascular and endocrine function in fetal sheep during late gestation. *J Physiol* 2002;545: 649–60.

Granger DA, Kivlighan KT, el-Sheikh M, Gordis EB, Stroud LR. Salivary alpha-amylase in biobehavioral research: recent developments and applications. *Ann NY Acad Sci* 2007;1098: 122–44.

Grassi G, Arenare F, Quarti-Trevano F, Seravalle G, Mancia G. Heart rate, sympathetic cardiovascular influences, and the metabolic syndrome. *Prog Cardiovasc Dis* 2009;52: 31–7.

Gunnar MR. Studies of the human infant's adrenocortical response to potentially stressful events. *New Dir Child Dev* 1989;45: 3–18.

Gunnar MR. Reactivity of the hypothalamic-pituitary-adrenocortical system to stressors in normal infants and children. *Pediatrics* 1992;90: 491–7.

Guzzetti S, Dassi S, Pecis M, et al. Altered pattern of circadian neural control of heart period in mild hypertension. *J Hypertens* 1991;9: 831–8.

Jacobson L, Sapolsky R. The role of the hippocampus in feedback regulation of the hypothalamic-pituitary-adrenocortical axis. *Endocr Rev* 1991;12: 118–34.

Kapoor A, Petropoulos S, Matthews SG. Fetal programming of hypothalamic-pituitary-adrenal (HPA) axis function and behavior by synthetic glucocorticoids. *Brain Res Rev* 2008;57: 586–95.

Kari MA, Hallman M, Eronen M, et al. Prenatal dexamethasone treatment in conjunction with rescue therapy of human surfactant: a randomized placebo-controlled multicenter study. *Pediatrics* 1994;93: 730–6.

Koenen SV, Mecenas CA, Smith GS, Jenkins S, Nathanielsz PW. Effects of maternal betamethasone administration on fetal and maternal blood pressure and heart rate in the baboon at 0.7 of gestation. *Am J Obstet Gynecol* 2002;186: 812–7.

Langewitz W, Ruddel H, Schachinger H. Reduced parasympathetic cardiac control in patients with hypertension at rest and under mental stress. *Am Heart J* 1994;127: 122–8.

Levitt NS, Lindsay RS, Holmes MC, Seckl JR. Dexamethasone in the last week of pregnancy attenuates hippocampal glucocorticoid receptor gene expression and elevates blood pressure in the adult offspring in the rat. *Neuroendocrinology* 1996;64: 412–8.

Moss TJ, Sloboda DM, Gurrin LC, Harding R, Challis JR, Newnham JP. Programming effects in sheep of prenatal growth restriction and glucocorticoid exposure. *Am J Physiol Regul Integr Comp Physiol* 2001;281: R960–70.

Nyirenda MJ, Lindsay RS, Kenyon CJ, Burchell A, Seckl JR. Glucocorticoid exposure in late gestation permanently programs rat hepatic phosphoenolpyruvate carboxykinase and glucocorticoid receptor expression and causes glucose intolerance in adult offspring. *J Clin Invest* 1998;101: 2174–81.

Owen D, Andrews MH, Matthews SG. Maternal adversity, glucocorticoids and programming of neuroendocrine function and behaviour. *Neurosci Biobehav Rev* 2005;29: 209–26.

Parker CR Jr, Atkinson MW, Owen J, Andrews WW. Dynamics of the fetal adrenal, cholesterol, and apolipoprotein B responses to antenatal betamethasone therapy. *Am J Obstet Gynecol* 1996;174: 562–5.

Roberts D, Dalziel S. Antenatal corticosteroids for accelerating fetal lung maturation for women at risk of preterm birth. *Cochrane database of systematic reviews* (Online) 2006;3, CD004454.

Sapolsky RM, Romero LM, Munck AU. How do glucocorticoids influence stress responses? Integrating permissive, suppressive, stimulatory, and preparative actions. *Endocr Rev* 2000;21: 55–89.

Schäffer L, Burkhardt T, Tomaske M, et al. Effect of antenatal betamethasone administration on neonatal cardiac autonomic balance. *Pediatr Res* 2010;68: 286–91.

Schäffer L, Luzi F, Burkhardt T, Rauh M, Beinder E. Antenatal betamethasone administration alters stress physiology in healthy neonates. *Obstet Gynecol* 2009;113: 1082–8.

Schneyer CA, Hall HD. Effects of varying frequency of sympathetic stimulation on chloride and amylase levels of saliva elicited from rat parotid gland with electrical stimulation of both autonomic nerves. *Proc Soc Exp Biol Med* 1991;196: 333–7.

Schwab M, Roedel M, Anwar MA, et al. Effects of betamethasone administration to the fetal sheep in late gestation on fetal cerebral blood flow. *J Physiol* 2000;528: 619–32.

Seckl JR. Prenatal glucocorticoids and long-term programming. *Eur J Endocrinol* 2004;151: U49–62.

Slotkin TA, Lappi SE, McCook EC, Tayyeb MI, Eylers JP, Seidler FJ. Glucocorticoids and the development of neuronal function: effects of prenatal dexamethasone exposure on central noradrenergic activity. *Biol Neonate* 1992;61: 326–36.

Steerenberg PA, van Asperen IA, van Nieuw Amerongen A, Biewenga A, Mol D, Medema GJ. Salivary levels of immunoglobulin A in triathletes. *Eur J Oral Sci* 1997;105: 305–9.

Stewart JM. Does heart rate variability explain increased blood pressure in adolescents? *J Pediatr* 2000;137: 6–8.

Turner RJ, Sugiya H. Understanding salivary fluid and protein secretion. *Oral Dis* 2002;8: 3–11.

Woods LL, Weeks DA. Prenatal programming of adult blood pressure: role of maternal corticosteroids. *Am J Physiol Regul Integr Comp Physiol* 2005;289: R955–62.

7 Feast or Famine: In the fast lane to puberty

Deborah M. Sloboda, Angelica B. Bernal, Graham J. Howie,
Mark B. Hampton, and Mark H. Vickers

Early life adversity, particularly inadequate nutrition, has been shown to induce long-term adverse metabolic and cardiovascular consequences in offspring. Research into the developmental programming of disease has now incorporated aspects of reproductive physiology, suggesting that reproductive function may similarly have a developmental origin. Although evidence for early life nutritional influences on reproductive function is mounting, a clear understanding of the link between maternal nutrition and offspring ovarian maturation has not been established. We have shown that maternal undernutrition, and in some circumstances, maternal high fat feeding, before or during pregnancy or during early postnatal life, can alter the reproductive function of the offspring. This early nutritional imbalance may exert its effects on reproductive factors such as timing of puberty, gonadal development and pituitary-gonadal activity. Very few studies have investigated the effects of maternal undernutrition on ovarian function/development. Nevertheless, it is clear that the developing gonad is sensitive to its immediate environment and nutritional perturbations can have long-term consequences on adult reproductive function.

7.1 Introduction

There is now considerable epidemiological and experimental evidence indicating that early life environmental signals, including nutrition, affect subsequent development leading to patho-physiologies including obesity and insulin resistance. These signals induce highly integrated responses in endocrine-related homeostasis, resulting in persistent changes to the developmental trajectory producing an altered adult phenotype (Hanson and Gluckman, 2008). However where the intrauterine and postnatal environments differ markedly, such modifications to the developmental trajectory may prove maladaptive (Gluckman et al., 2008). Evidence that reproductive maturation and function is similarly influenced by early life events is now emerging from animal studies and selected human populations. As the reproductive system and its hormonal control mechanisms are largely established during fetal life, adverse environmental influences such as inadequate maternal nutrition can exert deleterious effects on the structure and function of reproductive organs.

Over the past century, the average age at menarche has advanced considerably: in Europe, menarcheal age has fallen from 17 to ~12.5 years of age, although the rate of decline is slowing (Kaplowitz, 2006; Parent et al., 2003). Historically, the onset of menarche was proposed to be dependent upon a critical level of body fat (Frisch 1987), but evidence now exists across populations for the role of prenatal nutritional influences and the age at menarche (Cooper et al.; 1996, Cox et al., 2009a; Garn, 1987). Over a decade ago, Cooper et al. first demonstrated that low birth weight predicted altered female reproductive function (Cooper et al., 1996). Since then, early life events have been associated with ovarian and breast cancer (Elias et al., 2004), the timing of onset of menarche (Sloboda et al., 2007) and menopause (Elias et al., 2003) and factors likely to negatively impact on reproductive function (Elias et al., 2007; Ibanez and de Zegher, 2006; de Zegher and Ibanez, 2009).

Studies of selected human populations have provided insight into the mechanisms that might underpin associations between early life events and reproductive function. Girls born at a low birth weight (LBW) showed a marked reduction in ovarian and uterine size both during neonatal life and in adolescence (Ibanez et al., 2000; Ibanez et al., 2003) and demonstrated concentrations of gonadotrophins that were persistently elevated by almost 50% at 18 years of age (Ibanez et al., 2003). It has been reported that growth restricted girls demonstrated a reduction in primordial follicle number compared to gestationally matched appropriately grown infants (de Bruin et al., 1998; de Bruin et al., 2001), suggestive of reduced ovarian follicular reserve (Broekmans et al., 2006).

In large Caucasian cohorts, LBW and greater weight gain in childhood acted independently to reduce the age at menarche (Adair, 2001; Cooper et al., 1996; Sloboda et al., 2007). Similar effects are seen in central fat distribution and insulin sensitivity at age 8 years (Garnett et al., 2001; Ibanez et al., 2008). We have recently shown in a normal population of adolescent girls that birth weight and postnatal BMI predicted age at menarche (Sloboda et al., 2007). The earliest age at menarche was seen in girls with lower than the median estimated birth weight and higher than the median BMI at 8 years of age. Our data, together with those previously reported, suggest that the association between intrauterine and postnatal growth patterns and age at menarche can be extended to encompass the entire birth weight range, and not simply selected growth-restricted populations (Sloboda et al., 2007).

Alterations in reproductive function have clear impacts on future generations and investigations of the transgenerational effects of early life events on reproductive function have increased in number. In women whose early menarche was associated with increased adult weight and shorter height, their offspring were more likely to be taller and fatter (Ong et al., 2007), pointing towards a feed forward cycle of obesity and early reproductive maturation. Children of overweight and obese mothers are more likely to become obese and overweight putting them at risk of early pubertal maturation. The need to break this cycle of early maturation and obesity is essential, a cycle that likely results in subsequent re-programming of the next generation for the same fate.

Ovarian function is exquisitely sensitive to nutritional status and clinical and experimental studies have demonstrated that a decline in ovarian follicular reserve, changes in ovulation rates and altered age at onset of menarche are all vulnerable to early life influences (Gardner et al., 2009; Sloboda et al., 2009). Recently, reports suggest that nutritional quality as well as the source of macronutrients has been associated with pubertal onset. Children with lower diet quality pre-puberty experienced pubertal growth spurt at an earlier age than children with a higher diet quality (Cheng et al., 2010). Further, protein intake from dairy but not animal meat particularly at age 5–6 years in childhood, was associated with earlier indices of puberty (pubertal growth spurt, menarche, voice break; Gunther et al., 2010). Intriguingly, these associations were independent of body mass index. Early life cues influence development during critical periods that extend prior to childhood and infancy right to conception and including the early embryonic or fetal period. Follow-up studies of survivors of the Dutch Hunger Winter have attributed altered reproductive function in the offspring of mothers who experienced famine, to contrasting prenatal and postnatal nutritional status; although no significant effect on long term fertility was observed in this cohort (Lumey, 1998). However menstrual irregularity (Elias et al., 2007), decreased age at natural menopause (Elias et al., 2003), and increased risk of breast cancer (Elias et al., 2004) were observed.

When considering present day social and cultural conditions however, the globalization of agriculture and food processing has changed worldwide food availability and the last thirty years have seen a 10-fold increase in the number of people with access to high caloric diets (Seidell, 1999; Seidell, 2000). Many studies of populations undergoing transition from relatively poor nutrition to a "Westernized" high fat and high carbohydrate diet have demonstrated that this transition may alter key health indices in adult life and lead to lifelong adverse effects, which may include impacts on reproductive function (Victora et al., 2008). Together, with changes in the physical demands of work and increased mechanization (Seidell, 2000) a significant increase in the global incidence of obesity now exists. In developed countries, 15–20% of women between the ages of 25 and 55 years are obese (Seidell, 2000), and therefore have increased risks of infertility and cardiovascular and metabolic disease. Increasing numbers of women in developed countries are starting pregnancy overweight and gaining excess weight during pregnancy. In developed societies caloric and/or fat consumption are generally excessive and, maternal obesity is now a common pregnancy complication (Catalano, 2007). Importantly, these effects may be self-perpetuating, as offspring of obese mothers are themselves prone to obesity, giving rise to transgenerational effects (Armitage et al. 2008; Shankar et al., 2008). The effects of maternal obesity on reproductive function in the offspring are unclear, although childhood obesity and insulin resistance is associated with early menarche, suggesting that reproductive and metabolic complications of offspring born to obese mothers are likely to go hand in hand (Armitage et al., 2005; Kaplowitz, 2008).

7.2 Animal studies

Much of what we know regarding nutrition and reproductive outcomes is derived from experimental studies in animals. Maternal protein restriction throughout pregnancy in the rat had either no effect on pubertal age in male and female offspring, but significantly reduced both long-term fertility (Zambrano et al., 2005) and longevity in adult females (Guzman et al., 2006) or delayed pubertal onset and reduced Kiss1 mRNA levels in the hypothalamus (Iwasa et al., 2010). Experimental fetal growth restriction in the rat using uterine artery ligation late in pregnancy delayed puberty in the offspring, as did late gestational and postnatal caloric restriction (Engelbregt et al., 2001; Leonhardt et al., 2003). Altered follicular development, reflected by an increased number of antral follicles of small size and reduced number of large sized antral/Graafian follicles has been reported following a maternal global dietary restriction of 50%; this is consistent with increased circulating FSH levels observed at weaning. The reduced number of mature antral follicles implies that factors involved in later stage of follicular development may be disturbed by perinatal maternal undernutrition (Leonhardt et al., 2003).

Maternal protein restriction during pregnancy or lactation resulted in delayed puberty and increased reproductive cycle length (Guzman et al., 2006). Similar results are also evident for maternal malnutrition occurring during lactation, via protein and energy restriction, with disrupted folliculogenesis (reduction in primordial, large antral follicles and corpora lutea), altered levels of steroid hormone receptor isoforms and factors required for ovarian angiogenesis (Veiga Ferreira et al., 2010). Furthermore, decreased mRNA expression of key factors regulating ovarian function, namely aromatase, leptin and FSH, LH and leptin receptors are also observed in the ovaries of adult rat offspring (da Silva Faria et al., 2009).

Hilakivi-Clarke and colleagues demonstrated that consumption of a high-fat diet throughout pregnancy resulted in an early pubertal onset in the offspring independent of either changes in total body weight or caloric intake before puberty (Hilakivi-Clarke et al., 1997). It has been suggested that pubertal onset was accelerated in offspring of undernourished mothers to maintain the ability to reproduce in a high-risk environment and in offspring of high-fat fed mothers, advanced pubertal onset was to opportunistically enhance reproductive fitness (Sloboda et al., 2009). Although maternal nutritional adversity assigns effects on pubertal onset in offspring, the mechanisms underpinning these changes are largely unknown.

We have recently investigated both 'feast' and 'famine' conditions early in life effects on reproduction. We have shown that nutritional deficits and excesses during intrauterine, lactational and post-weaning periods resulted in the acceleration of pubertal onset and subsequent changes in ovarian function (Sloboda et al., 2009).

In our studies, depending on the offspring's nutritional history during the prenatal and lactational periods, subsequent nutrition and body weight gain did not further influence offspring reproductive tempo and was rather dominated by prenatal nutrition (▶Figs. 7.1 and 7.2). These results suggest that nutrition during early critical developmental windows sets the tempo of reproductive development.

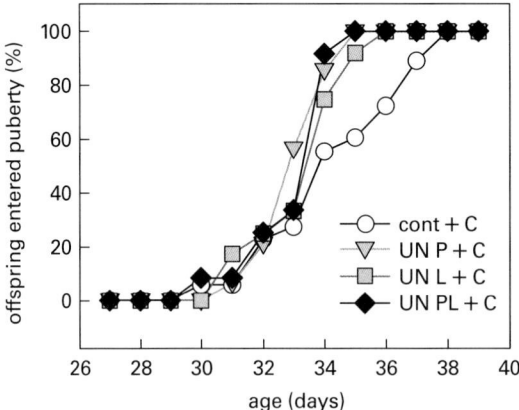

Fig. 7.1: Percentage of offspring entering puberty over time whose mothers received 50% of normal ad-libitum nutrition. Cont – control pregnancies; UN P – mothers undernourished during pregnancy only; UN L – mothers undernourished during lactation only; UN PL – mothers undernourished during pregnancy and lactation. C-postnatal chow diet. Data represent at least six litters per maternal dietary group. Maternal diet effect $p < 0.001$.

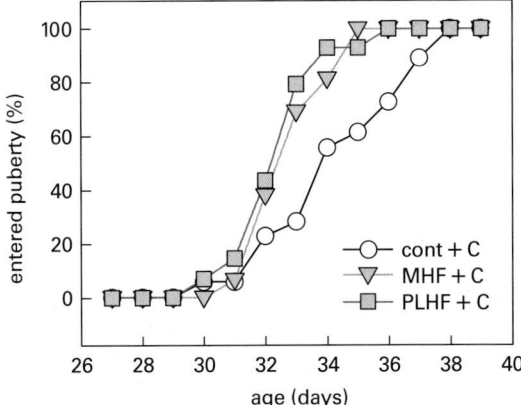

Fig. 7.2: Percentage of offspring entering puberty over time whose mothers received a high fat diet. Cont – control pregnancies; MHF – mothers fed a HF diet pre-conceptionally and throughout pregnancy and lactation; PLHF – dams fed a chow diet pre-conceptionally and a HF diet through pregnancy and lactation only. C – postnatal chow diet. Data represent at least six litters per maternal dietary group. Maternal diet effect $p < 0.001$.

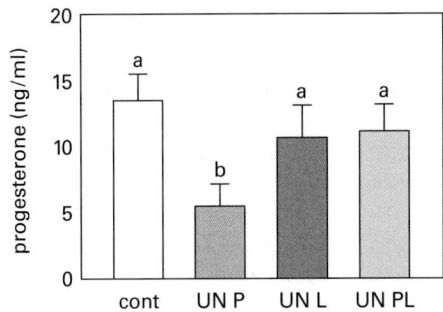

Fig. 7.3: Circulating adult female progesterone concentrations at proestrous in offspring whose mothers received 50% of normal nutrition or control diet throughout pregnancy and/or lactation. Cont – control pregnancies; UN P – mothers undernourished during pregnancy only; UN L – mothers undernourished during lactation only; UN PL – mothers undernourished during pregnancy and lactation. Data are expressed as group means ± SEM. Groups marked by different letters are significantly different at $p < 0.05$.

We also demonstrated that whereas maternal calorie restriction led to early pubertal onset, it also resulted in a reduction in progesterone concentrations in offspring later in life (▶Fig. 7.3).

In contrast, we found that maternal high fat feeding induced early maturation but was associated with elevated progesterone concentrations in adult offspring, although this reached statistical significance in the PLHF offspring only (▶Fig. 7.4). We suggest that two different developmental pathways in our study led to the acceleration of pubertal timing but with different consequences for ovarian function (Sloboda et al., 2009).

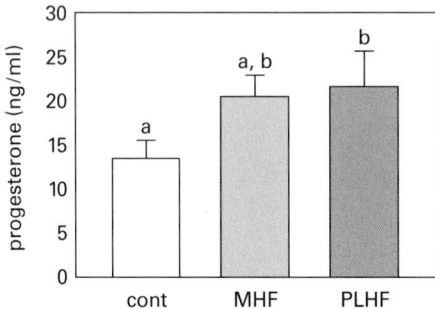

Fig. 7.4: Circulating adult female progesterone concentrations at proestrous in offspring whose mothers received a high fat diet or control diet. Cont – control pregnancies; MHF – mothers fed a high fat diet pre-conceptionally and throughout pregnancy and lactation; PLHF – mothers fed a chow diet pre-conceptionally and a high fat diet through pregnancy and lactation only. Data are expressed as group means ± SEM. Groups denoted by different letters are significantly different at $p < 0.05$.

The mechanisms underlying these changes are unclear. Altered oxidative stress conditions may underpin many of the known associations between early life nutritional adversity and altered later life physiologic function (Loui et al., 2009; Theys et al., 2009). Oxidative stress plays an important role in normal reproductive processes and has been implicated in reproductive pathologies (Agarwal et al., 2006). It is possible that oxidative stress may be the common link between early life nutritional insults and altered reproductive function. Although relatively little is known about the role of oxidative stress during intrauterine fetal development, experimental studies have documented the role of redox balance in the modification of gene expression and the deleterious effects of oxidized proteins contributing to cell toxicity, inflammation, apoptosis and endothelial dysfunction (Luo et al., 2006). Mitochondrial function was altered in embryos and oocytes of mothers that were nutritionally challenged (Igosheva et al., 2010). It is well recognized that disruption of redox homeostasis alters gene expression and that the accumulation of oxidized proteins has a deleterious effect on cell function (Chakravarti and Chakravarti, 2007). Although the accumulation of carbonylated proteins is a general marker of oxidative stress in damaged and aging tissue, the monitoring of specific protein modifications can provide additional insight into the nature and site of oxidative stress. The peroxiredoxin family of antioxidant thiol proteins, which includes the mitochondrial protein peroxiredoxin 3 (Prx 3), is responsible for breaking down endogenous hydroperoxides (Cox et al., 2010). Excess hydrogen peroxide can also hyperoxidize the active site cysteine of Prxs, thereby inactivating the protein (Cox et al., 2009b; Musicco et al., 2009).

In our studies of maternal nutrient manipulation, we have observed that maternal undernutrition significantly reduced primordial, secondary and antral follicle number in adult offspring in a manner that was dependent upon the timing of nutrient restriction. Specifically, a reduction in early stage follicle populations was observed in offspring born to mothers undernourished throughout both pregnancy and lactation, whereas antral follicles were reduced in offspring born to all mothers that were undernutrition regardless of whether the period of undernutrition was restricted to pregnancy or lactation or both (unpublished observations). These reductions were associated with decreased mRNA levels of genes critical for follicle maturation and ovulation. We also demonstrated increased ovarian oxidative stress in offspring born to undernourished mothers regardless of the timing of the undernutrition. However, only those mothers whose undernutrition included the period of pregnancy produced offspring with reduced ovarian peroxidoxin 3 mRNA levels (unpublished observations). We hypothesize that this reduction may be suggestive of an inability to cope with increased oxidative stress conditions. Taken together, we propose that these data support the possibility that maternal undernutrition, especially during the period of pregnancy, results in accelerated ovarian ageing in offspring.

7.3 Conclusions

Our findings specifically highlight the importance of the prenatal environment and further contribute to the mounting evidence for the influence of early life factors, in particular maternal nutrition, on reproductive function in later life. Disorders of reproductive health are increasingly common and are of major public health importance in both developed and developing societies. Further studies will provide better insight into the mechanisms underlying these processes and may have significant implications not only for the current understanding of reproductive pathologies but also for future generations' reproductive ability.

References

Adair LS. Size at birth predicts age at menarche. *Pediatrics* 2001;107: e59.

Agarwal A, Gupta S, Sikka S. The role of free radicals and antioxidants in reproduction. *Curr Opin Obstet Gynecol* 2006;18: 325–32.

Armitage JA, Poston L, Taylor PD. Developmental origins of obesity and the metabolic syndrome: The role of maternal obesity. *Front Horm Res* 2008;36: 73–84.

Armitage JA, Taylor PD, Poston, L. Experimental models of developmental programming: Consequences of exposure to an energy rich diet during development. *J Physiol* 2005;565: 3–8.

Broekmans FJ, Kwee J, Hendriks DJ, Mol BW, Lambalk CB. A systematic review of tests predicting ovarian reserve and ivf outcome. *Hum Reprod Update* 2006;12: 685–718.

Catalano PM. Increasing maternal obesity and weight gain during pregnancy: The obstetric problems of plentitude. *Obstet Gynecol* 2007;110: 743–4.

Chakravarti B, Chakravarti DN. Oxidative modification of proteins: Age-related changes. *Gerontology* 2007;53: 128–39.

Cheng G, Gerlach S, Libuda L, Kranz S, Gunther ALB, Karaolis-Danckert N, Kroke A, Buyken AE. Diet quality in childhood is prospectively associated with the timing of puberty but not with body composition at puberty onset. *J Nutr* 2010;140: 95–102.

Cooper C, Kuh D, Egger P, Wadsworth M, Barker D. Childhood growth and age at menarche. *Br J Obstet Gynaecol* 1996;103: 814–7.

Cox AG, Pearson AG, Pullar JM, Jonsson TJ, Lowther WT, Winterbourn CC, Hampton MB. Mitochondrial peroxiredoxin 3 is more resilient to hyperoxidation than cytoplasmic peroxiredoxins. *Biochem J* 2009a;421: 51–8.

Cox AG, Peskin AV, Paton LN, Winterbourn CC, Hampton MB. Redox potential and peroxide reactivity of human peroxiredoxin 3. *Biochemistry* 2009b;48: 6495–501.

Cox AG, Winterbourn CC, Hampton MB. Mitochondrial peroxiredoxin involvement in antioxidant defence and redox signalling. *Biochem J* 2010;425: 313–25.

Da Silva Faria T, De Bittencourt Brasil F, Sampaio FJ, Da Fonte Ramos C. Maternal malnutrition during lactation affects folliculogenesis, gonadotropins, and leptin receptors in adult rats. *Nutrition* 2010;26: 1000–7.

De Bruin JP, Dorland M, Bruinse HW, Spliet W, Nikkels PG, Te Velde ER. Fetal growth retardation as a cause of impaired ovarian development. *Early Hum Dev* 1998;51: 39–46.

De Bruin JP, Nikkels PG, Bruinse HW, Van Haaften M, Looman CW, Te Velde ER. Morphometry of human ovaries in normal and growth-restricted fetuses. *Early Hum Dev* 2001;60: 179–92.

De Zegher F, Ibanez L. Early origins of polycystic ovary syndrome: Hypotheses may change without notice. *J Clin Endocrinol Metab* 2009;94: 3682–5.

Elias SG, Peeters PH, Grobbee DE, Van Noord PA. Breast cancer risk after caloric restriction during the 1944–1945 dutch famine. *J Natl Cancer Inst* 2004;96: 539–46.

Elias SG, Van Noord PA, Peeters PH, Den Tonkelaar I, Grobbee DE. Caloric restriction reduces age at menopause: The effect of the 1944–1945 dutch famine. *Menopause* 2003;10: 399–405.

Elias SG, Van Noord PAH, Peeters PHM, Den Tonkelaar I, Kaaks R, Grobbee DE. Menstruation during and after caloric restriction: The 1944–1945 dutch famine. *Fertility and Sterility* 2007;88: 1101–7.

Engelbregt MJ, Van Weissenbruch MM, Popp-Snijders C, Lips P, Delemarre-Van De Waal HA. Body mass index, body composition, and leptin at onset of puberty in male and female rats after intrauterine growth retardation and after early postnatal food restriction. *Pediatr Res* 2001;50: 474–8.

Frisch RE. Body fat, menarche, fitness and fertility. *Hum Reprod* 1987;2: 521–33.

Gardner DS, Ozanne SE, Sinclair KD. Effect of the early-life nutritional environment on fecundity and fertility of mammals. Philosophical Transactions of the Royal Society B: *Biological Sciences* 2009;364: 3419–27.

Garn SM. The secular trend in size and maturational timing and its implications for nutritional assessment. *J Nutr* 1987;117: 817–23.

Garnett SP, Cowell CT, Baur LA, Fay RA, Lee J, Coakley J, Peat JK, Boulton TJ. Abdominal fat and birth size in healthy prepubertal children. *Int J Obes Relat Metab Disord* 2001;25: 1667–73.

Gluckman PD, Hanson MA, Beedle AS, Spencer HG. Predictive adaptive responses in perspective. *Trends in Endocrinology & Metabolism* 2008;19: 109–10.

Gunther ALB, Karaolis-Danckert N, Kroke A, Remer T, Buyken AE. Dietary protein intake throughout childhood is associated with the timing of puberty. *J Nutr* 2010;140: 565–71.

Guzman C, Cabrera R, Cardenas M, Larrea F, Nathanielsz PW, Zambrano E. Protein restriction during fetal and neonatal development in the rat alters reproductive function and accelerates reproductive ageing in female progeny. *J Physiol* 2006;572: 97–108.

Hanson MA, Gluckman PD. Developmental origins of health and disease: New insights. *Basic & Clinical Pharmacology & Toxicology* 2008;102: 90–3.

Hilakivi-Clarke L, Clarke R, Onojafe I, Raygada M, Cho E, Lippman M. A maternal diet high in n-6 polyunsaturated fats alters mammary gland development, puberty onset, and breast cancer risk among female rat offspring. *Proc Natl Acad Sci U S A* 1997;94: 9372–7.

Ibanez L, De Zegher F. Puberty after prenatal growth restraint. *Horm Res* 2006;65: 112–5.

Ibanez L, Potau N, Enriquez G, De Zegher F. Reduced uterine and ovarian size in adolescent girls born small for gestational age. *Pediatr Res* 2000;47: 575–7.

Ibanez L, Potau N, Enriquez G, Marcos MV, Zegher FD. Hypergonadotrophinaemia with reduced uterine and ovarian size in women born small-for-gestational-age. *Hum Reprod* 2003;18: 1565–9.

Ibanez L, Suarez L, Lopez-Bermejo A, Diaz M, Valls C, De Zegher F. Early development of visceral fat excess after spontaneous catch-up growth in children with low birth weight. *J Clin Endocrinol Metab* 2008;93: 925–8.

Igosheva N, Abramov AY, Poston L, Eckert JJ, Fleming TP, Duchen MR, Mcconnell J. Maternal diet-induced obesity alters mitochondrial activity and redox status in mouse oocytes and zygotes. *PLoS ONE* 2010;5: e10074.

Iwasa T, Matsuzaki T, Murakami M, Fujisawa S, Kinouchi R, Gereltsetseg G, Kuwahara A, Yasui T, Irahara M. Effects of intrauterine undernutrition on hypothalamic kiss1 expression and the timing of puberty in female rats. *J Physiol* 2010;588: 821–9.

Kaplowitz P. Pubertal development in girls: Secular trends. *Curr Opin Obstet Gynecol* 2006;18: 487–91.

Kaplowitz PB. Link between body fat and the timing of puberty. *Pediatrics* 2008;121: S208–17.

Leonhardt M, Lesage J, Croix D, Dutriez-Casteloot I, Beauvillain JC, Dupouy JP. Effects of perinatal maternal food restriction on pituitary-gonadal axis and plasma leptin level in rat pup at birth and weaning and on timing of puberty. *Biol Reprod* 2003;68: 390–400.

Loui A, Raab A, Maier RF, Bratter P, Obladen M. Trace elements and antioxidant enzymes in extremely low birthweight infants. *J Trace Elem Med Biol* 2009;24: 111–8.

Lumey LH. Reproductive outcomes in women prenatally exposed to undernutrition: A review of findings from the dutch famine birth cohort. *Proc Nutr Soc* 1998;57: 129–35.

Luo ZC, Fraser WD, Julien P, Deal CL, Audibert F, Smith GN, Xiong X, Walker M. Tracing the origins of "Fetal origins" of adult diseases: Programming by oxidative stress? *Med Hypotheses* 2006;66: 38–44.

Musicco C, Capelli V, Pesce V, Timperio AM, Calvani M, Mosconi L, Zolla L, Cantatore P, Gadaleta MN. Accumulation of overoxidized peroxiredoxin iii in aged rat liver mitochondria. *Biochim Biophys Acta* 2009;1787: 890–6.

Ong KK, Northstone K, Wells JC, Rubin C, Ness AR, Golding J, Dunger DB. Earlier mother's age at menarche predicts rapid infancy growth and childhood obesity. *PLoS Med* 2007;4: e132.

Parent AS, Teilmann G, Juul A, Skakkebaek NE, Toppari J, Bourguignon JP. The timing of normal puberty and the age limits of sexual precocity: Variations around the world, secular trends, and changes after migration. *Endocr Rev* 2003;24: 668–93.

Seidell JC. Prevention of obesity: The role of the food industry. *Nutr Metab Cardiovasc Dis* 1999;9: 45–50.

Seidell JC. Obesity, insulin resistance and diabetes – a worldwide epidemic. *Br J Nutr* 2000;83: S5–8.

Shankar K, Harrell A, Liu X, Gilchrist JM, Ronis MJ, Badger TM. Maternal obesity at conception programs obesity in the offspring. *Am J Physiol Regul Integr Comp Physiol* 2008;294: R528–38.

Sloboda DM, Hart R, Doherty DA, Pennell CE, Hickey M. Age at menarche: Influences of prenatal and postnatal growth. *J Clin Endocrinol Metab* 2007;92: 46–50.

Sloboda DM, Howie GJ, Pleasants A, Gluckman PD, Vickers MH. Pre- and postnatal nutritional histories influence reproductive maturation and ovarian function in the rat. *PLoS ONE* 2009;4: e6744.

Theys N, Clippe A, Bouckenooghe T, Reusens B, Remacle C. Early low protein diet aggravates unbalance between antioxidant enzymes leading to islet dysfunction. *PLoS One* 2009;4: e6110.

Veiga Ferreira R, Meireles Gombar F, Da Silva Faria T, Silva Costa W, Barcellos Sampaio FJ, Da Fonte Ramos C. Metabolic programming of ovarian angiogenesis and folliculogenesis by maternal malnutrition during lactation. *Fertil Steril* 2010;93: 2572–80.

Victora CG, Adair L, Fall C, Hallal PC, Martorell R, Richter L, Sachdev HS. Maternal and child undernutrition: Consequences for adult health and human capital. *The Lancet* 2008;371: 340–57.

Zambrano E, Rodriguez-Gonzalez GL, Guzman C, Garcia-Becerra R, Boeck L, Diaz L, Menjivar M, Larrea F, Nathanielsz PW. A maternal low protein diet during pregnancy and lactation in the rat impairs male reproductive development. *J Physiol* 2005;563: 275–84.

8 Early life origins of diabetes and obesity: General aspects and the thin – fat baby paradigm

Chittaranjan S. Yajnik, Urmila S. Deshmukh

The increasing realization that obesity and type 2 diabetes are best prevented has focused researchers' attention on the influence of early life factors. The environment in utero has been shown to program the body composition and metabolic-endocrine axes, which determine the individual's adaptability to later-life exposures. Accumulating evidence suggests that epigenetic mechanisms contribute to this programming. Thus, maternal factors (nutrition and metabolism) that influence the in utero milieu have a large role to play in the primordial prevention of chronic diseases. Optimizing adolescent health rather than focusing only on adult lifestyle modifications would be much more beneficial and cost effective in preventing obesity and diabetes.

8.1 Introduction

The escalating burden of chronic noncommunicable diseases (NCDs) such as obesity, diabetes, cardiovascular disease (CVD), and cancer is well recognized, although these do not appear in the millennium development goals. Obesity and diabetes are now epidemic in many economically developing and newly industrialized nations (low and middle income countries [LMIC]), and are considered to be the most challenging health problems in the 21st century. These conditions affect a very large number of people; more than 1 billion adults are overweight in the world (World Health Organization, 2010), and 285 million people are diabetic (International Diabetes Federation, 2009). Together, the two are major contributors to the global burden of chronic diseases and disability.

The current dogma proposes that obesity, diabetes, and other related disorders have a genetic susceptibility and are precipitated by adult lifestyle factors, including poor diet and lack of physical activity. Recent diabetes prevention trials have therefore targeted the middle-aged, obese, and glucose-intolerant subjects for *primary* prevention of diabetes. We consider these as attempts to fix the problem after the horse has bolted.

There is increasing interest in the newly established field of developmental origins of health and disease (International Society for Developmental Origins of Health and Disease, 2010). Recent discoveries have highlighted that intrauterine factors influence susceptibility to NCDs by nongenetic mechanisms. This has led to a growing belief in the possibility of primordial prevention of diabetes and related disorders.

This review focuses on the impact of the intrauterine environment on the risk of diabetes and obesity in later life.

8.2 Nutrition and diabetes

It is interesting to see the evolution of ideas in this field. In 1965, a WHO Expert Committee on diabetes commented, "evidence that malnutrition protects adult populations from diabetes seems unassailable" (World Health Organization, 1965). In 1980, another WHO Expert Committee wrote, "malnutrition is probably a major determinant of diabetes" (World Health Organization, 1980). They introduced a new category: malnutrition-related diabetes mellitus (MRDM). However, in 1997 the Expert Committee dropped the entity of MRDM from their classification (The Expert Committee Report, 1997). Even though there can be no doubt that overnutrition precipitates type 2 diabetes (T2D), it is relevant that India, the world's capital of diabetes, also figures prominently in the world hunger map. In addition to holding more than 50 million diabetic patients in 2010, India also holds the largest number of low birth weight (LBW) babies and more than 8 million severely undernourished children. These statistics point toward contribution of both early life undernutrition and later life overnutrition in the etiology of T2D. Our research focused attention on these factors by describing the thin – fat Indian diabetic patient (Yajnik et al., 2002), which refers to poor lean mass and a relative excess of fat mass, especially deposited in and around the abdomen. More excitingly, we described that the small and thin Indian baby was adipose (Yajnik et al., 2003), thus focusing the attention on intrauterine life as an important determinant of the epidemic of diabetes and CVD.

Our findings were stimulated by the research of Hales and Barker, who caused a sensation in the 1980s by describing an association between birth weight and risk of diabetes (Hales and Barker, 1992). They proposed that fetal undernutrition disturbed the development of fetal pancreas and also promoted insulin resistance (IR) in various organs. Thus, low birth weight predicted diabetes, which they called the "thrifty phenotype" hypothesis. This idea was variously expressed as "fetal origins of adult diseases," "small baby syndrome," etc. During this period considerable stress was given on *low* birth weight, though Barker and his colleagues had described a continuous and graded association of the birth weight (Barker, 1997).

One of the difficulties for the scientists to appreciate the association of lower birth weight with diabetes was the previously described association between macrosomia and future risk of diabetes in babies born to diabetic mothers. These two ideas have stimulated a considerable amount of research in the link between intrauterine growth and future risk of diabetes. This chapter discusses some aspects of this association.

8.3 Maternal nutrition, fetal growth, and future health

More than 50 years ago, McCance wrote, 'The size attained in utero depends on the services which the mother is able to supply; these are mainly food and accommodation' (McCance, 1962). Thus, maternal size and the nutrients transferred through placenta determine the size of the fetus.

Pedersen and Freinkel were the first to highlight the role of maternal diabetes in influencing the long-term health of the offspring. Pedersen proposed that maternal glucose and other fuels cross the placenta and cause fetal islet hyperplasia and hyperinsulinism, which causes overgrowth in *insulin sensitive* organs (Pedersen, 1977).

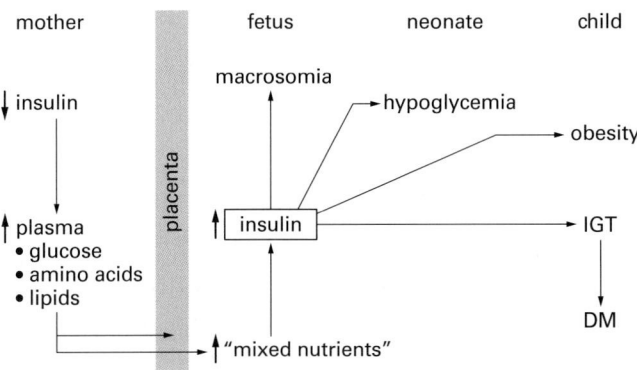

Fig. 8.1: Fuel-mediated teratogenesis of Pedersen and Freinkel. Maternal fuels cross the placenta and influence islet development and fetal insulin secretion. In diabetic pregnancies there is islet hyperplasia, hyperinsulinism, and excess growth of insulin responsive tissues and organs. This leads to macrosomia, perinatal metabolic problems, and early onset obesity and type 2 diabetes (modified from Freinkel, 1980).

Freinkel expanded the use of the term *teratogenesis* from the conventional reference to fetal malformation to include fetal macrosomia and future obesity and diabetes (fuel-mediated teratogenesis) (Freinkel, 1980) (▶Fig. 8.1).

During development, different organs and systems are susceptible to the maternal metabolic changes at different times based on the developmental schedule. Freinkel (1980) suggested that pregestational diabetes, which affects the fetus until conception, would have more wide-ranging effects than *gestational* diabetes (GDM), which begins later. Severity of maternal metabolic disturbance will determine the size of the effect.

Data from Pima Indians in Arizona, US, showed that the risk of obesity and diabetes was higher in offspring who were born to mothers who were diabetic during the pregnancy, compared with those born to nondiabetic mothers and mothers with pre-diabetes (Pettitt et al., 1988). This finding indicates a stronger role for intrauterine hyperglycemia in the etiology of obesity and diabetes compared to genetics. However, it is possible that mothers who are diagnosed with diabetes at a younger age might transmit an excess of genetic risk. A subsequent study of siblings in the same population showed that those born after the mother was diagnosed with diabetes were heavier and more likely to have diabesity (diabetes and obesity) compared with those who were born before mother was diagnosed with diabetes (Dabelea, Hanson, and Lindsay, 2000). There was no corresponding paternal influence. These findings confirm a role for pregnancy hyperglycemia rather than genetics or postnatal environment in the risk of childhood obesity. Studies in Chicago (Silverman et al., 1995) showed similar findings in the offspring of diabetic mothers and also showed an association between amniotic fluid insulin concentration and risk of obesity-hyperglycemia in the offspring.

On the other hand, a follow-up study of people born in Hertfordshire, UK, demonstrated that lower birth weight increased the risk of diabetes and associated disorders (Barker, 1997). Interesting findings were reported in children of Dutch women who were exposed to Hunger Winter, providing a more direct proof of association between intrauterine undernutrition and risk of NCDs (Roseboom, de Rooij, and Painter, 2006). One of the first studies involving these offspring showed that if the exposure to famine was in the third trimester of pregnancy, offspring were less likely to be obese in adult life, but exposure to famine during the first and second trimesters was associated with higher risk of obesity (Ravelli, Stein, and Susser, 1976).

Subsequent to the demonstration of the association of birth weight and type 2 diabetes, Lucas defined fetal programming as "a process whereby a stimulus applied in utero establishes a permanent response in the fetus leading to enhanced susceptibility to later disease" (Lucas, 1991). There is now ample evidence that maternal nutritional imbalance involving both macro- and micronutrients has a *programming* effect on the fetus. Data on the role of specific nutrients is now accumulating from animal and human studies. We have coined the term *nutrient-mediated teratogenesis* to describe this phenomenon (Yajnik, 2009).

Maternal obesity without hyperglycemia can also have substantial effect on the risk of obesity in the child (Catalano et al., 2009). This raises the possibility that nonglucose fuels (e.g., lipids) might also be important. In clinical practice we have been too glucocentric and have forgotten about the original concept of *mixed nutrients* in the teratogenic process.

8.4 Developmental plasticity, programming, teratogenesis, and predictive adaptive response

The ability of the growing fetus to respond to the environmental cues and assume different sizes and functional characteristics is called *developmental plasticity* (Bateson, Barker, and Clutton-Brock, 2004). It describes the ability of the fetus to achieve different phenotypes with a given genotype. An intrauterine challenge puts constraint on the structural and functional development of the fetus, limiting its ability to respond effectively to a changing environment. It is thought that the fetus perceives these environmental cues as indicative of the postnatal environment, and the adaptations are appropriate for such an environment (predictive adaptive response) (Gluckman, Hanson, and Spencer, 2005). If the postnatal environment is different, the adaptations may become inappropriate, and the individual has an increased susceptibility to disease.

The concept of *nutrient-mediated teratogenesis* and *fuel-mediated teratogenesis* refers to different ends of the spectrum of the effects of nutritional and metabolic challenges in utero, and can be looked upon as the two sides of the same coin. We have used the term *dual teratogenesis* to describe the situation in rapidly transiting populations (▶Fig. 8.2) (Yajnik, 2009).

Intrauterine undernutrition produces small, thin, and adipose babies who are insulin resistant and remain so (small, thin, and insulin resistant) if postnatal nutrition is not excessive. These individuals have low rates of NCD, as seen in rural populations in India. Postnatal overnutrition promotes obesity and hyperglycemia, frequently without correction of the micronutrient deficiencies. For example, in a study in Mysore, India, GDM was associated with low circulating vitamin B_{12} concentrations (Krishnaveni et al., 2009). In such a condition, the fetus is exposed to multiple adverse programming influences, resulting in a phenotype of excess adiposity, pancreatic islet dysfunction, and a tendency toward diabetes and CVD at a young age. Such a dual teratogenesis

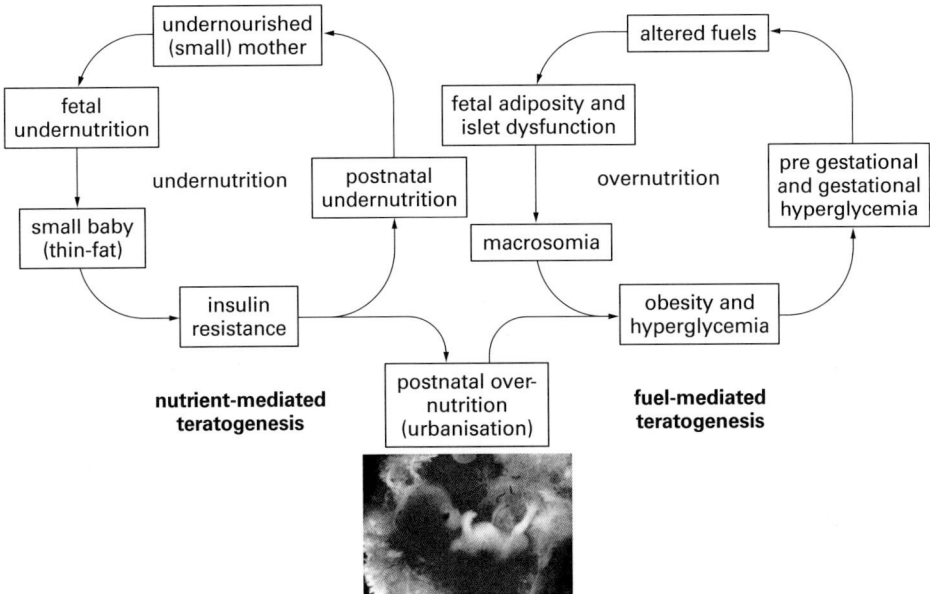

Fig. 8.2: The figure shows the interrelationship of two major maternal factors (undernutrition and overnutrition) in fetal programming. An undernourished mother produces a small (thin-fat), insulin resistant baby. If this baby remains undernourished in postnatal life, the cycle is propagated. If the thin-fat insulin-resistant baby is overnourished it becomes obese and hyperglycemic. An obese and hyperglycemic mother produces a *macrosomic* baby at higher risk of obesity and hyperglycemia. Thus, the intergenerational insulin resistance – diabetes cycle is propagated through a girl child. Rapid transition shifts the balance from undernutrition to overnutrition and contributes to escalation of the diabetes epidemic. Improving health of a girl child is of paramount importance in controlling the diabetes epidemic (Yajnik, 2009).

is proposed to contribute to the rapidly rising epidemic of obesity – diabetes in modern India (Yajnik, 2009).

8.5 Birth weight: An exposure, an intermediate variable, or only a marker?

It is important to note that the biological association between birth weight and diabetes is U-shaped, that is, both low and high birth weight are associated with higher risk of diabetes. The risk associated with large birth weight is mostly ascribed to the effect of maternal hyperglycemia, but risk of maternal obesity also is increasingly recognized.

A recently published systematic review (Whincup et al., 2008) covering data from 31 populations examined the association of birth weight and type 2 diabetes in 152,084 individuals, including 6,090 diabetes cases. The association between birth weight and type 2 diabetes was inverse in 23 populations (statistically significant in 9) and positive in 8 (statistically significant in 2 native North American populations). Overall,

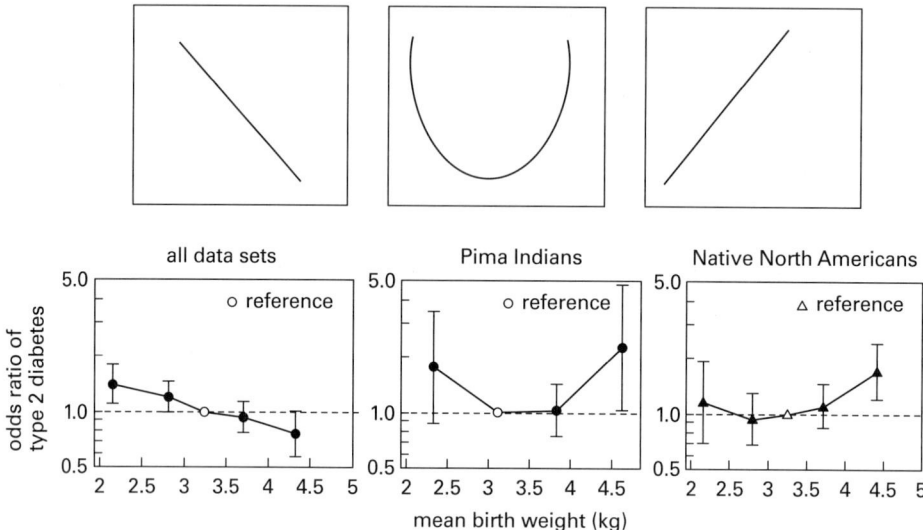

Fig. 8.3: Associations of birth weight with type 2 diabetes. The biological association appears to be U-shaped, that is, both low and high birth weight are associated with the risk of diabetes. Depending on the relative role of maternal undernutrition (nutrient-mediated teratogenesis) and overnutrition (fuel-mediated teratogenesis), the shape of the graph varies as shown from the systematic review by Whincup et al. (Compiled from Yajnik, 2004 and Whincup et al., 2008).

1 kg increase in birth weight reduced type 2 diabetes risk by 25%, and by 30% after adjusting for adult BMI. The association was strongly graded and continuous (▶Fig. 8.3).

It is important to understand that the story is not about birth weight but about fetal programming and that intergenerational prevention of type 2 diabetes and obesity will need to target maternal nutrition and metabolism.

8.6 Role of postnatal growth

Longitudinal follow up in birth cohorts from both developing and developed populations has helped our understanding of the interactions between intrauterine and postnatal growth and risk of type 2 diabetes and CVD.

In the Pune Children's Study (PCS) at the King Edward Memorial Hospital, Pune, we followed up more than 400 children whose birth weights were available from the labor-room record. At 4 years of age we studied their anthropometry, glucose tolerance, and circulating insulin concentrations. We demonstrated that after oral glucose load, 30 min plasma glucose and insulin concentrations were inversely related to the birth weight (Yajnik et al., 1995). This provided the first proof for Barker's hypothesis in a developing country. We followed up these children at 8 years of age to study their metabolic characteristics. In addition to confirming the association of low birth weight with increased insulin resistance, we observed that the levels of risk factors for diabetes and CVD (glucose, insulin resistance, lipids, blood pressure, leptin concentrations, etc.) were highest in children who were born the lightest but were heaviest at 8 years of age

(Bavdekar et al., 1999). The offspring from New Delhi Birth Cohort who are followed from birth were studied at 28 years of age (Bhargava et al., 2004). Those who were diabetic were born lighter, had grown slower during infancy but had grown progressively faster from 3 years of age, and had an earlier adiposity rebound compared to those who were normal glucose tolerant.

Glucose tolerance was tested in adults participating in the Helsinki Birth Cohort Study (1934–1944) (Eriksson et al., 2006). Both, impaired glucose tolerance and type 2 diabetes, were associated with low birthweight ($p < 0.0001$, adjusting for current BMI), and low weight gain between birth and 2 years increased the risk. A one standard deviation (*SD*) increase in weight at 2 years protected against hyperglycemia (odds ratio [OR] 0.76, 95% confidence interval [CI] 0.69–0.84); the effect was greatest in those with low birth weight. Thus, this study defined intrauterine life, infancy, and childhood as critical periods for future risk of insulin resistance and hyperglycemia.

8.7 Contributions of the Pune Maternal Nutrition Study

The Pune Maternal Nutrition Study (PMNS) cohort was established between 1992 and 1996 in six villages near Pune, India, to investigate the influence of maternal body size and nutrition during pregnancy on fetal growth and future metabolic risks in the offspring (Rao et al., 2001). More than 800 pregnancies were studied. The average mother in the PMNS was aged 21 years, weighed 42 kg (BMI 18.1 kg/m²), and had a dietary intake of 1700 kcal/day and 45 g proteins/day during pregnancy. The newborns weighed

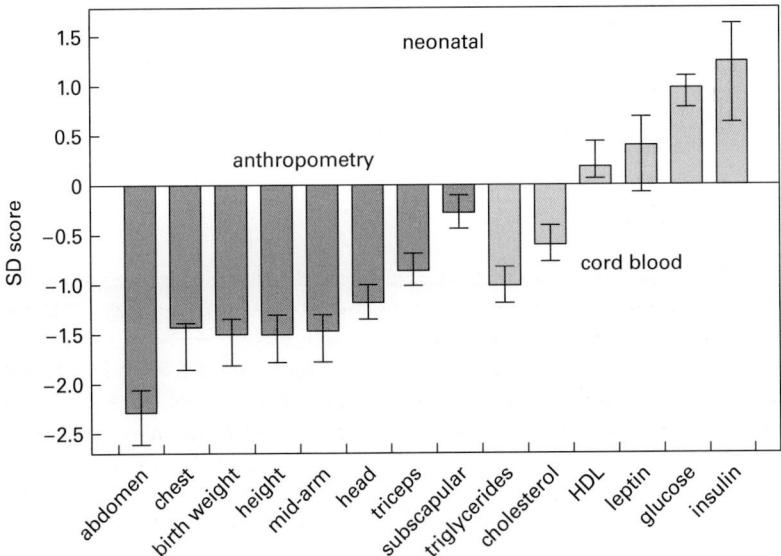

Fig. 8.4: Comparison of Indian and UK babies. UK measurements are used as a reference (0). The Indian babies were smaller than the British babies in all measurements of size. Cord plasma leptin concentration was similar, and cord plasma glucose and insulin concentrations were higher in the Indian babies. (Yajnik et al., 2002).

on average 2700 g with a ponderal index of 24.1 kg/cm³; 28% were LBW (<2500g). In comparison with babies born in the UK (3500 g, ponderal index 27.3 kg/cm³), Indian babies were lighter, shorter (47.3 cm vs. 50.2 cm), and thinner, but the sub-scapular skin-fold measurements were relatively well preserved (z score −0.53; 95% CI −0.61, −0.46) (▶Fig. 8.4) (Yajnik et al., 2002, 2003). Thus, the Indian babies were short and thin but fat, corroborating our description of Indian adults.

Recently, we compared whole body magnetic resonance imaging (MRI) measurements of adipose tissue and its distribution in healthy full-term Indian babies (Pune) with those in white European newborns (London, UK) (Modi et al., 2009). Though smaller in weight (95% CI for difference −0.757 to −0.385 kg, $p < 0.001$), head circumference (−2.15 to −0.9 cm, $p < 0.001$) and length (−2.9 to −1.1 cm $p < 0.001$), the Indian babies had similar whole body adipose tissue content (−0.175 to 0.034 l, $p = 0.2$) (▶Fig. 8.5).

Adipose tissue distribution was distinctly different. Indian babies had significantly greater absolute adiposity in all three abdominal compartments, internal (visceral) (0.012 to 0.023 l, $p < 0.001$), deep subcutaneous (0.003 to 0.017 l, $p = 0.006$), and superficial subcutaneous (0.006 to 0.043 l, $p = 0.011$) but a significant reduction in non-abdominal superficial subcutaneous adipose tissue (−0.184 to −0.029 l, $p = 0.008$). Thus, this study confirmed that differences in adipose tissue distribution exist at birth, which could be an important risk factor for diabetes and related disorders. Conventional measurements of birth size are not sensitive to these vital differences. Further research must focus on periconceptional, intrauterine, and early postnatal exposures that modify the tissue deposition pattern. In yet another study we demonstrated higher insulin and leptin concentrations but lower adiponectin concentrations in the cord blood of Indian babies compared to the European babies (▶Fig. 8.4) (Yajnik et al., 2002).

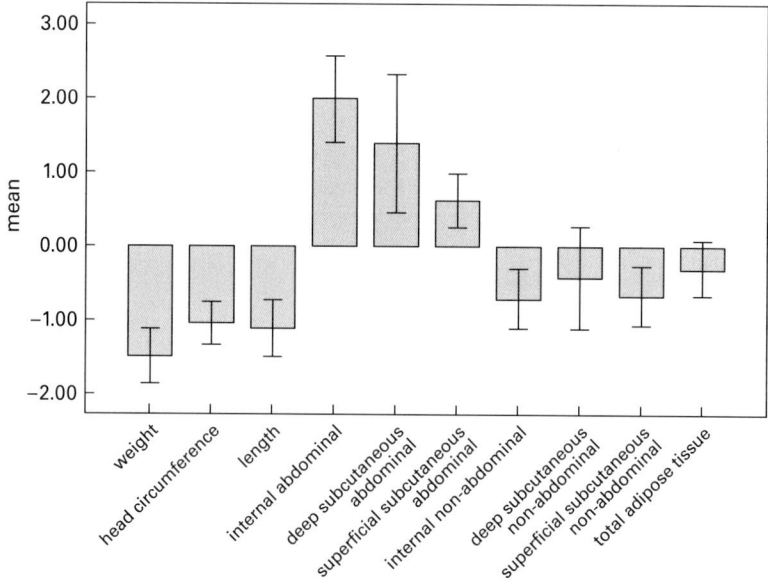

Fig. 8.5: Anthropometry and adipose tissue compartments: Z scores (mean ± 95% CI) for Indian babies with white European babies as baseline (Modi et al., 2009). (Error bars: 95% CI).

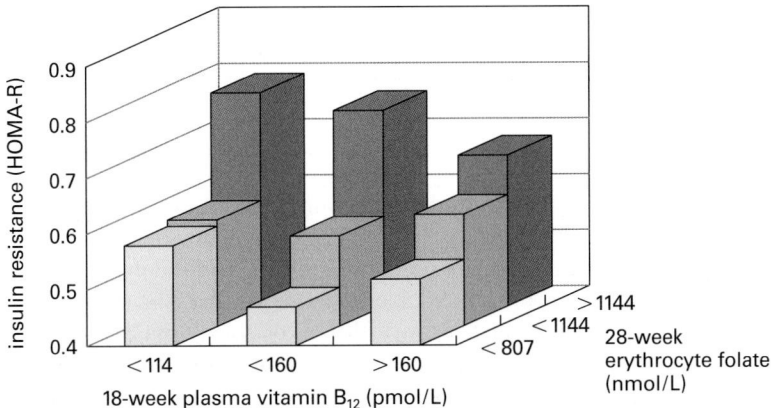

Fig. 8.6: Pune Maternal Nutrition Study: Insulin resistance (HOMA-R) in the children at 6 y in relation to maternal plasma vitamin B_{12} (at 18 wk) and erythrocyte folate (at 28 wk) concentrations. Maternal folate concentrations in pregnancy directly predict insulin resistance in the child. The most insulin-resistant children were born to mothers who had the lowest vitamin B_{12} and highest folate concentrations (Yajnik et al., 2008).

The PMNS also improved our knowledge of maternal determinants of fetal growth. More frequent intake of green leafy vegetables, fruit, and milk (foods rich in micronutrients) by mother predicted larger newborn size, whereas macronutrient intake (calories and proteins) did not, highlighting the importance of micronutrients in fetal growth (Rao et al., 2001). About two-thirds of women had low vitamin B_{12} concentrations; hardly anyone was folate deficient. About one-third had high total homocysteine (tHcy) concentrations, and more than 90% had high methyl malonic acid (MMA) concentrations, attributable to the deficiency of vitamin B_{12} (Yajnik et al., 2008).

High maternal tHcy concentration predicted intrauterine growth restriction (Yajnik et al., 2005). Higher maternal frequency of consumption of green leafy vegetables and milk and higher erythrocyte folate concentrations during pregnancy predicted higher offspring adiposity at 6 years. The effect of maternal folate was exaggerated by vitamin B_{12} deficiency; the offspring of mothers who had lowest vitamin B_{12} and highest folate concentrations were the most insulin resistant (▶Fig. 8.6) (Yajnik et al., 2008).

Thus, attention was focused on the importance of maternal one-carbon metabolism for fetal growth and programming of diabetes and related disorders. One-carbon metabolism is important for nucleic acid and protein synthesis and epigenetic methylation of DNA. This regulates cellular growth and differentiation.

8.8 Genetics and epigenetics of fetal growth and diabetes-obesity

Do genetic factors have a role in fetal growth and programming of NCDs? One obvious pathway to investigate was insulin mediated fetal growth, which was proposed as an important mechanism for fuel-mediated teratogenesis. Hattersley et al. (1998) investigated the possibility that genetic determinants of insulin secretion and activity could explain the association between fetal size and future risk of diabetes (fetal insulin hypothesis).

They investigated the influence of the glucokinase gene (GCK) on fetal growth, and showed an important interaction between maternal genotype (GCK mutation) and phenotype (hyperglycemia) with fetal genotype in influencing offspring birth weight (Hattersley et al., 1998). After the discovery of many type 2 diabetes predisposing polymorphisms in the genome wide association studies (GWAS), they have demonstrated that some of these markers are also associated with birth weight (e.g., fat mass and obesity-associated gene [FTO]). Additionally, in GWAS of birth weight (Freathy et al., 2009), they found that some of the polymorphisms predicting birth weight are also type 2 diabetes genes. These findings will no doubt improve our understanding of regulation of fetal growth and etiology of type 2 diabetes. However, the effect of maternal nutrition and metabolism is crucial for fetal growth. This is obvious from the variability of birth weight between and within populations, between the first and later pregnancies, and from the description of a reduction in offspring birth weight after maternal bariatric surgery (Smith et al., 2009).

Animal data also highlights the role of maternal rather than paternal influence on fetal growth. It is interesting, however, that skeletal growth of the fetus seems to be more influenced by paternal factors (presumably genetic) (Knight et al., 2005).

One recent exciting development is the discovery of the factors regulating gene expression. These factors have improved our understanding of the interactions between the environment and genes. Developmental plasticity is largely a function of regulation of gene function. Waddington called these processes *epigenetic* (Van Spebroeck, 2002). Current understanding is that the methylation of DNA bases, acetylation of histones, and noncoding RNAs (iRNA) are important mechanisms that regulate the gene expression. Methylation of cytosine residues in the cytosine-phosphatidyl-guanosine (CpG) islands is regulated by methyl donors in the diet, including folate, vitamin B_{12}, betaine, and choline (Waterland and Jirtle, 2003). Our demonstration of the role of folate and vitamin B_{12} in regulation of fetal growth, body composition, and programming of insulin resistance therefore assumes a special significance (Yajnik et al., 2008).

Waterland and Jirtle (2003) fed agouti mice with a methylating cocktail during pregnancy. The progeny had varying coat color and were less obese compared to controls, despite inheriting the same genotype. This was related to methylation of the promoter region of the agouti gene, which is responsible for determining coat color. Such epigenetic changes are heritable for many generations and potentially may be involved in fetal programming.

This idea is also supported by experiments in sheep. Ewes were made methionine deficient, their ova were fertilized in vitro, and the blastocysts were transferred to surrogate mothers with normal methionine status (Sinclair et al., 2007). The offspring (especially males) were obese and insulin resistant and had alterations in DNA methylation at a number of sites within the genome. Epigenetic regulation of glucocorticoid receptor and peroxisome proliferator activator alpha (PPAR-α) genes have been shown to be involved in fetal programming due to a low protein diet in rodents (Lillycrop et al., 2005). The first evidence in humans supporting the hypothesis that early-life environmental conditions can cause epigenetic changes in humans that persist throughout life has been provided in the Dutch Hunger Winter Families Study (Heijmans et al., 2008). They showed that individuals who were prenatally exposed to famine during the Dutch Hunger Winter in 1944–45 had, 6 decades later, less DNA methylation of the imprinted

IGF2 gene compared with their unexposed, same-sex siblings. The association was specific for periconceptional exposure.

The GWAS polymorphisms associated with birth weight, obesity, and type 2 diabetes are the obvious candidates for future epigenetic studies to inform on the important environmental regulators.

8.9 Conclusion

We suggest a modification to the conventional gene-lifestyle dogma of type 2 diabetes. The susceptibility to diabetes and other NCDs is also influenced by epigenetic processes and fetal programming. Maternal nutrition and metabolism are major determinants of these processes. Prevention of obesity, type 2 diabetes, and other NCDs should start with improvement of the health of young girls who would be mothers tomorrow. The current models of diabetes prevention in postreproductive, obese, glucose intolerant women are unlikely to reduce the escalating epidemic in the young. Along with efforts to control hyperglycemia in the elderly, there is an urgent need to plan intergenerational prevention by improving nutrition and metabolism of young girls before conception. This could provide a multigenerational benefit and should be the focus of future research.

References

Barker DJP. Fetal nutrition and cardiovascular disease in later life. *Br Med Bul* 1997;53: 96–108.

Bateson P, Barker D, Clutton-Brock T. Developmental plasticity and human health. *Nature* 2004;430: 419–21.

Bavdekar A, Yajnik CS, Fall CH, et al. Insulin resistance syndrome in 8-year-old Indian children: small at birth, big at 8 years, or both? *Diabetes* 1999;48: 2422–9.

Bhargava SK, Sachdev HS, Fall CHD, et al. Relation of serial changes in childhood body-mass index to impaired glucose tolerance in young adulthood. *N Engl J Med* 2004;350: 865–75.

Catalano PM, Presley L, Minium J, Hauguel-de Mouzon S. Fetuses of obese mothers develop insulin resistance in utero. *Diabetes Care* 2009;32: 1076–80.

Dabelea D, Hanson RL, Lindsay RS. Intrauterine exposure to diabetes conveys risks for type 2 diabetes and obesity: a study of discordant sibships. *Diabetes* 2000;49: 2208–11.

Eriksson JG, Osmond C, Kajantie E, Forsén TJ, Barker DJ. Patterns of growth among children who later develop type 2 diabetes or its risk factors. *Diabetologia* 2006;49: 2853–8.

The Expert Committee on the Diagnosis and Classification of Diabetes Mellitus: Report of the expert committee on the diagnosis and classification of diabetes mellitus. *Diabetes Care* 1997;20: 1183–97.

Freathy RM, Bennett AJ, Ring SM, et al. Type 2 diabetes risk alleles are associated with reduced size at birth. *Diabetes* 2009;58: 1428–33.

Freinkel N. Banting Lecture 1980. Of pregnancy and progeny. *Diabetes* 1980;29: 1023–35.

Gluckman PD, Hanson MA, Spencer HG. Predictive adaptive responses and human evolution. *Trends Ecol Evol* 2005;20: 527–33.

Hales CN, Barker DJP. Type 2 (non-insulin dependent) diabetes mellitus: the thrifty phenotype hypothesis. *Diabetologia* 1992;35: 595–601.

Hattersley AT, Beards F, Ballantyne E, Appleton M, Harvey R, Ellard S. Mutations in the glucokinase gene of the fetus result in reduced birth weight. *Nat Genet* 1998;19: 268–70.

Heijmans BT, Tobi EW, Stein AD, et al. Persistent epigenetic differences associated with prenatal exposure to famine in humans. *Proc Natl Acad Sci USA* 2008;105: 17046–9.

International Diabetes Federation 2009. http://www.diabetesatlas.org/content/diabetes-and-impaired-glucose-tolerance. Accessed September 30, 2010.

International Society for Developmental Origins of Health and Disease (DOHaD). http://www.mrc.soton.ac.uk/dohad/. Accessed September 30, 2010.

Knight B, Shields BM, Turner M, Powell RJ, Yajnik CS, Hattersley AT. Evidence of genetic regulation of fetal longitudinal growth. *Early Hum Dev* 2005;81: 823–31.

Krishnaveni GV, Hill JC, Veena SR, et al. Low plasma vitamin B(12) in pregnancy is associated with gestational "diabesity" and later diabetes. *Diabetologia* 2009;52: 2350–8.

Lillycrop KA, Phillips ES, Jackson AA, Hanson MA, Burdge GC. Dietary protein restriction of pregnant rats induces and folic acid supplementation prevents epigenetic modification of hepatic gene expression in the offspring. *J Nutr* 2005;135: 1382–6.

Lucas A. Programming by early nutrition in man. In: Bock GR, Whelan J, editors. *The Childhood Environment and Adult Disease*. CIBA Foundation Symposium 156. Chichester: Wiley; 1991: 38–55.

McCance RA. Food, growth, and time. *Lancet* 1962;2: 621–6.

Modi N, Thomas EL, Uthaya SN, Umranikar S, Bell JD, Yajnik CS. Whole body magnetic resonance imaging of healthy newborn infants demonstrates increased central adiposity in Asian Indians. *Pediatr Res* 2009;65: 584–7.

Pedersen J. Hyperglycaemia-hyperinsulinism theory and birthweight. In: *The Pregnant Diabetic and Her Newborn: Problems and Management*. Baltimore: Williams & Wilkins; 1977: 211–20.

Pettitt DJ, Aleck KA, Baird HR, Carraher MJ, Bennett PH, Knowler WC. Congenital susceptibility to NIDDM: role of intrauterine environment. *Diabetes* 1988;37: 622–8.

Rao S, Yajnik CS, Kanade A, et al. Intake of micronutrient-rich foods in rural Indian mothers is associated with the size of their babies at birth: Pune Maternal Nutrition Study. *J Nutr* 2001;131: 1217–24.

Ravelli GP, Stein ZA, Susser MW. Obesity in young men after famine exposure in utero and early infancy. *N Engl J Med* 1976;295: 349–53.

Roseboom T, de Rooij S, Painter R. The Dutch famine and its long-term consequences for adult health. *Early Hum Dev* 2006;82: 485–91.

Silverman BL, Metzger BE, Cho NH, Loeb CA. Impaired glucose tolerance in adolescent offspring of diabetic mothers. Relationship to fetal hyperinsulinism. *Diabetes Care* 1995;18: 611–7.

Sinclair KD, Allegrucci C, Singh R, et al. DNA methylation, insulin resistance, and blood pressure in offspring determined by maternal periconceptional B vitamin and methionine status. *Proc Natl Acad Sci USA* 2007;104: 19351–6.

Smith J, Cianflone K, Biron S, et al. Effects of maternal surgical weight loss in mothers on intergenerational transmission of obesity. *J Clin Endocrinol Metab* 2009;94: 4275–83.

Waterland RA, Jirtle RL. Transposable elements: targets for early nutritional effects on epigenetic gene regulation. *Mol Cell Biol* 2003;23: 5293–300.

Whincup PH, Kaye SJ, Owen CG, et al. Birth weight and risk of type 2 diabetes: a systematic review. *JAMA* 2008;300: 2886–97.

World Health Organization. Diabetes Mellitus: Report of a WHO Expert Committee. Tech. Rep. Ser., no. 310, Geneva, 1965.

World Health Organization. Expert Committee on Diabetes Mellitus. Tech. Rep. Ser., no. 646, Geneva, 1980.

World Health Organization. http://www.who.int/dietphysicalactivity/media/en/gsfs_obesity. Accessed September 30, 2010.

Yajnik CS, Fall CHD, Vaidya U, et al. Fetal growth and glucose and insulin metabolism in four year old Indian children. *Diabetic Medicine* 1995;12: 330–6.

Yajnik CS, Lubree HG, Rege SS, et al. Adiposity and hyperinsulinemia in Indians are present at birth. *J Clin Endocrinol Metab* 2002;87: 5575–80.

Yajnik CS, Fall CHD, Coyaji KJ, et al. Neonatal anthropometry: the thin-fat Indian baby: The Pune Maternal Nutrition Study. *Int J Obes* 2003;26: 173–80.

Yajnik CS. Obesity epidemic in India: intrauterine origin? *Proc Nutr Soc* 2004;63: 387–96.

Yajnik CS, Deshpande SS, Panchanadikar AV, et al. Maternal total homocysteine concentration and neonatal size in India. *Asia Pacific J of Clin Nutr* 2005;14: 179–81.

Yajnik CS, Deshpande SS, Jackson AA, et al. Vitamin B_{12} and folate concentrations during pregnancy and insulin resistance in the offspring: The Pune Maternal Nutrition Study. *Diabetologia* 2008;51: 29–38.

Yajnik CS. Nutrient-mediated teratogenesis and fuel-mediated teratogenesis: two pathways of intrauterine programming of diabetes. *Int J Gynaecol Obstet* 2009;104: S27–31.

9 The outcome in offspring of obese mothers: Clinical and experimental aspects

Lucilla Poston

Obesity amongst pregnant women has increased in recent decades and has become a major concern for health care providers because of the associated risk of morbidity and mortality for mother and child. Increasingly it is recognized that there may be longer term consequences for the infant, with evidence supporting a role for an independent association between exposure to maternal obesity *in utero* and the risk of later obesity. Observational and prospective mother-child cohort studies provide an increasing evidence base for this 'transgenerational transfer' of obesity risk but causality is difficult to establish. Animal models have provided strong and consistent supportive data and also have shed light on mechanistic pathways, notably the likelihood that maternal humoral factors adversely influence development of the hypothalamus leading to irreversible changes in energy balance. These and other recent studies highlighting the presence of hypertension in young offspring of obese rodents are beginning to influence protocol design in human – child cohorts and have considerable potential to inform intervention studies in obese women to reduce the incidence of childhood obesity.

9.1 Introduction

The number of obese adults is predicted to rise to over 700 million by 2015 (World Health Organization, 2006). More than 42 million children under 5 are estimated as overweight and childhood obesity tracks strongly to adolescence and adulthood (Reilly et al., 2003; Wardle et al., 2006). Because of associated morbidity and mortality, this world wide epidemic of obesity is likely to lead to a reversal in the trend of longer life expectancy (Franks et al., 2010; Olshansky et al., 2005).

Amongst the many complications of obesity are those which influence reproductive health. Inevitably, in recent years, the numbers of obese pregnant women have increased in parallel with the incidence of obesity in the general population. Few countries have nationally available statistics but cohort studies in the UK show upward trajectories in pregnant women (Heslehurst et al., 2010), and in the United States, approximately 20% of Americans are obese when they become pregnant (Chu et al., 2009; Kim et al., 2007). Obesity in pregnancy presents a substantial increase in risk for the health of the mother and her unborn child. Obese women have a higher than average risk of early pregnancy loss, gestational diabetes and pre-eclampsia and are more likely to suffer from complications in labor and post partum haemorrhage. Their infants are at greater risk of congenital anomalies, macrosomia, still birth and of complications in early post natal life (Nelson et al., 2010). These and a wide range of other maternal and infant complications are likely to arise from the profoundly altered maternal metabolic state associated with obesity. Obese pregnant women demonstrate marked peripheral and hepatic insulin resistance (Sivan et al., 1997) and in the post-prandial state, the circulatory increase in metabolic fuels; glucose, lipids and amino acids facilitate transfer of excess nutrients to the fetus (Nelson et al., 2010). Whilst the immediate consequences of this are apparent in the demonstration of increased birthweight and adiposity infants of obese women (Hull et al., 2008; Sewell et al., 2006), there may be longer term consequences of pre-natal exposure to maternal obesity for the health of the child, notably an increased risk of obesity in later life.

9.2 Associations between obesity in mother and child

Parental obesity is a strong risk factor for childhood obesity, with many reports identifying associations between paternal or maternal obesity and offspring BMI (Lake et al., 1997). With regard to the influence of obesity in pregnancy on the developing child, numerous observational studies have reported independent associations between maternal BMI as measured in pregnancy and the BMI of the offspring in childhood and adulthood (Koupil and Toivanen, 2008; Laitinen et al., 2001; Li et al., 2005; Li et al., 2007; Reilly et al., 2005; Salsberry and Reagan, 2005; Whitaker, 2004). However, BMI provides a poor index of fat mass, and interpretation is confounded by the lack of accurate body compositional analysis in either the mother or the child, or both. Nonetheless, in the few reports where associations between maternal BMI/adiposity in pregnancy and offspring adiposity have been addressed, an independent and positive association has also been reported (Blair et al., 2007; Burdette et al., 2006; Gale et al., 2007; Mingrone et al., 2008). Importantly, if there were to be a specific added risk of obesity to the child from an *in utero* influence, a stronger association of the child's BMI or adiposity with maternal obesity than with paternal obesity would be expected. Relatively few studies have both maternal and paternal weight data available at the time of the index pregnancy but several have shown a stronger association of maternal than paternal BMI with offspring BMI (Catalano et al., 2009; Lawlor et al., 2007; Lawlor et al., 2008; Pirkola et al., 2010; Salsberry and Reagan, 2005). In one investigation from the UK ALSPAC cohort, the predominant maternal effect was reported to be explicable by inheritance of the variant of the FTO gene association with obesity (Lawlor et al., 2008). However, most of the larger studies have relied upon self-reported parental weights and heights, and some may have inherent bias when paternal height and weight is supplied by the mother, as in the ALSPAC cohort (Davey Smith et al., 2007). In a recent study using data pooled from the Annual Health Surveys for England in which parental BMI was directly measured (but not during pregnancy), a strong and graded association was found between parental weight status and risk of childhood obesity, which was significantly stronger for maternal weight (Whitaker et al., 2010). This was interpreted as possibly supporting a role for a direct influence of the maternal environment but, as recognized by the authors, this association may have alternative explanations such as the role played by the mother in determining the diet of the child, specifically because of the recognized lower degree of control of familial diets among families with obese mothers (Wardle et al., 2002).

9.2.1 Gestational weight gain and childhood obesity

Excessive gestational weight gain (GWG) is associated with adverse pregnancy outcome (Rasmussen and Yaktine, 2009) and an association between GWG and offspring BMI has been reported by some (Kleiser et al., 2009; Mamun et al., 2009; Moreira et al., 2007; Oken et al., 2007; Oken et al., 2008), but not all investigations (Catalano et al., 1995; Koupil and Toivanen, 2008). Two recent studies have addressed relationships between gestational weight gain and childhood fat mass, as directly measured, and both of these have reported positive associations (Crozier et al., 2010; Fraser et al., 2010).

9.2.2 Association or causality?

In light of current evidence it is not possible to attribute causality to relationships between maternal obesity or gestational weight gain and the risk of obesity in the child. To date no prospective randomised trial in obese pregnant women has determined whether or not an intervention can reduce adiposity in the child which, if proven, would provide strong support for causality. Several small studies have attempted to improve pregnancy outcome through lifestyle interventions in obese women but although a few have shown a reduction in gestational weight gain, none was powered to address neonatal outcome or for relevant outcomes in the children beyond infancy (Nelson et al., 2009; Ronnberg and Nilsson, 2010). In the absence of interventional trials, several observational cohort studies have addressed the role of potential modifiers of the relationship between obesity in mother and child, including shared dietary and physical activities, and some have shown little modification effect. However few cohorts have the capability to address the potential confounding influence of all the recognized early life determinants of childhood obesity, including duration of breast-feeding, maternal smoking, short duration of childhood hours of sleep and a rapid post natal growth trajectory (Gillman et al., 2008; Monasta et al., 2010). Furthermore only one attempt has been made to address the role of shared genetic susceptibility in defining the more pronounced maternal BMI *versus* paternal BMI association with childhood obesity (Lawlor et al., 2008). Several large intervention studies currently underway in obese pregnant women have the potential to directly address the validity of the hypothesis of maternal-child 'transmission' of obesity, and by determination of obesity related genetic traits, identify the role of gene-environment interactions (Nelson et al., 2010). According to the hypothesis, a reduction of pre-pregnancy BMI would also have the potential to reduce offspring adiposity, but hitherto no RCT has recruited women to a weight loss regime or normal care prior to pregnancy and followed the children to assess the effect on childhood adiposity. One report indicates that pre-pregnancy weight loss reduces the risk of obesity in the child; increasing numbers of morbidly obese women are undergoing surgical intervention to promote weight loss and this observational study has shown that children born to women after biliopancreatic diversion bariatric surgery have a lower risk of obesity than siblings born before their mother had surgery (Smith et al., 2009). This certainly infers, but does not prove, an influence of the maternal *in utero* environment on offspring obesity risk.

9.3 Experimental models of maternal obesity

Whilst observational studies from human cohorts have provided a strong rationale for pursuit of the hypothesis of transgenerational 'transmission of obesity', the current evidence base is less than adequate to inform public health strategy. Because of the rapid expansion of supporting evidence, national and international public health recommendations and guidelines have highlighted the immediate need for intervention studies in obese women to confirm or refute the hypothesis (National Institute for Health and Clinical Excellence, 2010; Poston et al., 2011), and several are underway. However, the optimal intervention should be developed from a sound understanding of the underlying mechanistic pathways, and in this regard animal models have the potential to provide important insight.

Several laboratories, including our own, have addressed the hypothesis that maternal obesity predisposes the progeny to obesity in later life. We have investigated the offspring of obese dams in an experimental design in which female rats and mice are fed a sugar and fat rich highly palatable diet before pregnancy and during pregnancy and lactation (Nivoit et al., 2009; Samuelsson et al., 2008). Adult offspring develop an increase in fat mass with age (Samuelsson et al., 2008). As these observations parallel many from other laboratories, the transgenerational transmission of obesity in rodents is reproducible and occurs in different strains of mice and rats, despite diverse dietary protocols used for generation of maternal obesity (Bayol et al., 2007; Chang et al., 2008; Dunn and Bale, 2009; Ferezou-Viala et al., 2007; Levin and Govek, 1998; Sen and Simmons, 2010; Shankar et al., 2008; Srinivasan et al., 2006). The variety of maternal diets might suggest that obesity *per se* rather than elements of the diet are responsible for the 'programming' of offspring obesity. However, distinction between the relative influence of maternal obesity and diet represents a practical challenge in study design, although one elegantly designed investigation in which the weight of rats dams fed an obesogenic diet was maintained at the control level by pair feeding to controls suggested that maternal fat mass was the critical determinant, since the offspring as the pair fed animals maintained the same weight as controls (White et al., 2009). Other investigators consider that the increased saturated fat content of an obesogenic diet alone is adequate for development of offspring obesity (Carmody et al., 2010). Also, in a recent study of non-human primates in which Japanese macaque monkeys were fed a high fat diet during pregnancy the offspring developed increased adiposity at 6 months of age (McCurdy et al., 2009), which was independent of maternal weight and therefore considered to be induced by an element of the diet. Several studies in which rodents have been fed purified diets with differing fat composition during pregnancy have demonstrated widely differing effects on the offspring phenotype depending on the fatty acid composition (Amusquivar et al., 2000; Korotkova et al., 2005). For example, a recent report demonstrated that a maternal diet rich in medium chain fatty acids can offer protection against the development of obesity in offspring when they are challenged with a fat rich diet (Dong et al., 2011). This literature at present does not present a clear message as to which dietary fats are to be avoided or which may afford protection against offspring obesity, most likely due to the variety of dietary protocols and feeding regimes used and differing methods of assessment of offspring adiposity. Nonetheless, with improved standardization of methods between laboratories, these studies could play an important role in understanding of the relative influences of maternal dietary fatty acids and fat mass *per se* on the risk of obesity in the offspring, and thereby translate to dietary advice for obese pregnant women.

Whilst it is clear that obesity and/or diets rich in saturated fat increase the risk of obesity in the offspring, few laboratories have attempted dietary intervention studies in obese dams to investigate the potential for reversal of increased offspring adiposity, although these would be necessary to inform interventions in pregnant women. An interesting addition to the recent literature is the observation that antioxidant supplementation in obese pregnant rats prevents the development of obesity in the offspring. Supplementing rat dams' fat rich 'western diet' with vitamins A, E and C led to reversal of adiposity in 2 week old and in 2 month old offspring (Sen and Simmons, 2010). Whilst vitamin A is contraindicated in human pregnancy, an intervention with antioxidant supplements could be feasible in pregnant women, although we have previously reported adverse pregnancy outcomes of high dose antioxidants (vitamins C and E) when administered to pregnant women at increased risk of pre-eclampsia, which included a large sub group of obese women (Poston et al., 2006).

9.3.1 Pathways contributing to development of offspring obesity

Recent developments provide important insight into the mechanisms which underlie the association between maternal obesity and offspring obesity in the various animal models. Some investigators, including ourselves, have suggested that adipocyte function may be permanently affected. We reported an increase in adipocyte size and increased mRNA expression of genes involved in adipocyte differentiation in offspring of obese mice (beta-adrenoceptor 2 and 3, 11 beta HSD-1, and PPAR-γ 2) (Samuelsson et al., 2008). In addition, Sen and Simmons observed that the antioxidant supplement regime led to reversal of altered offspring fat tissue expression of proadipogenic and lipogenic genes (PPARγ, Pref-1,Wisp 2, SREBP1, AcCoA, FAS, FAT) (Sen and Simmons, 2010); the gene expression profile in the offspring prenatally exposed to maternal obesity could infer that the exposure leads to continued expansion beyond neonatal life of the adipocyte pre-cursor pool which would contribute to the development of obesity. This profile may also indicate that obesity related oxidative stress may contribute to an increase in adipocyte differentiation and fat tissue expansion.

Changes in adipocyte development and differentiation may play a permissive role in the generation of offspring obesity, but ultimately increase in fat mass must result from a change in energy balance in which expenditure is less than intake. Persistently altered mitochondrial function acquired early in life could influence energy balance (Symonds et al., 2009) and we have reported abnormalities in mitochondrial function in skeletal muscle from offspring of obese dams which may have widespread implications for energy homeostasis (Shelley et al., 2009). Further investigations are required to interrogate the role of mitochondrial function in the different models, especially in adipocytes and from the different fat depots. This is a pertinent area of research which is relatively underexplored.

The most remarkable and consistent phenotypic feature of the animal models is the observation from our laboratory and others that the offspring of obese or fat fed dams are hyperphagic, with the suggestion that 'programming' of enhanced appetite plays a major role in increasing fat tissue mass in the offspring (Chang et al., 2008; Nivoit et al., 2009; Samuelsson et al., 2008; Walker et al., 2008). Associations between obesity in mothers and satiety in their children has never been formally studied in mother-child cohorts but there are validated methods by which satiety can be addressed and these animal studies have already influenced ongoing studies, now addressing the effects of maternal obesity on childhood appetite.

Several plausible mechanisms for the increase in offspring appetite in the animal models have been proposed; firstly the potential role of fetal hyperinsulinemia. Obesity in pregnant women is associated with increased risk of GDM and we have shown that diet induced obesity in pregnant rats is associated with maternal insulin resistance (Holemans et al., 2004), and associated maternal post prandial hyperglycemia would be expected to lead to fetal hyperinsulinemia. Plagemann and colleagues propose that fetal hyperinsulinemia leads to dysfunction of critical pathways of development in the neuronal hypothalamic networks central to appetite regulation, thus permanently increasing food intake leading to adulthood obesity and insulin resistance (Plagemann, 2005; Plagemann et al., 1999a; Plagemann et al., 1999b; Plagemann et al., 1998). Although not specifically investigated in models of maternal diet induced obesity, fetal hyperinsulinemia could play an important role in development of the hyperphagia observed.

A second mechanism, the focus of recent investigations in our laboratory, is the potential role of hyperleptinemia and its influence on hypothalamic development of appetite regulatory pathways. Rodents demonstrate a post natal leptin 'surge' which is unrelated to appetite regulation or growth and is considered to play a physiological role in development of the hypothalamic appetite regulatory pathways (Bouret, 2010). In rat pups from obese dams we measured the post natal leptin profile from birth to weaning and showed an exaggerated surge compared to controls. In weanling pups we also reported evidence for altered development of neural projections between the arcuate and paraventricular nuclei of the hypothalamus. This was associated with markers of central leptin resistance, as demonstrated by measurement of pSTAT3 expression in the arcuate nucleus in response to exogenous leptin administration; pSTAT3 expression normally increases in response to leptin but this was blunted in the offspring of the obese dams compared to the controls. In addition, leptin administration did not lead to the anticipated reduction in food intake observed in control animals. Thus the young offspring of obese dams demonstrated central leptin resistance (Kirk et al., 2009), leading to the hypothesis that the exaggerated leptin surge promotes central leptin resistance which in turn prevents normal development of the hypothalamic appetite regulatory pathways, thereby leading to persistent hyperphagia and increased adiposity. Others have similarly shown that offspring from dams fed a high fat diet have reduced sensitivity to the anorectic effects of leptin (Walker et al., 2008). The relationship of these observations to the human situation is unknown, although maternal visceral fat mass is the major determinant of plasma leptin in pregnant from the first trimester and obese pregnant women demonstrate hyperleptinemia (Fattah et al., 2011). In human pregnancy fetal hypothalamic development is almost complete by birth, therefore the period of hypothalamic vulnerability to leptin, should leptin similarly be a neurotrophic hormone in man, is more likely to be in the antenatal, rather than the postnatal period (Grayson et al., 2010a).

Obesity, as well as consumption of a high fat diet, is associated with a marked inflammatory profile, and prenatal exposure to inflammatory mediators may influence fetal brain development. Grayson et al have reported that fetuses of Japanese macaques

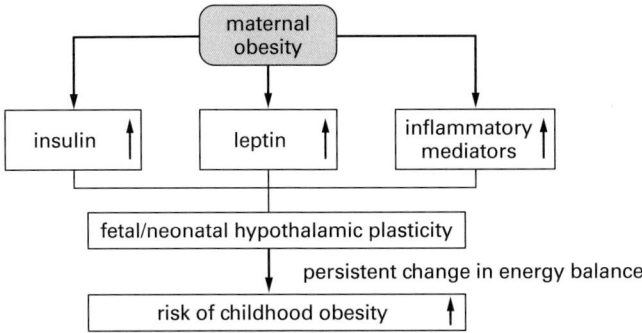

Fig. 9.1: Relationship between maternal and offspring obesity; proposed mechanistic pathways inferred from studies in experimental animals.

consuming a high fat diet demonstrate increased circulating and hypothalamic cytokines, and have postulated that these contribute to the perturbations in the central melanocortin (proopiomelanocortin, POMC) and serotonin systems observed in the fetal brain which may affect energy homeostasis and cardiovascular function, as well as offspring behaviour (Grayson et al., 2010b; Sullivan et al., 2010). Notably, reversal of the maternal diet after four years of a high fat dietary intake was associated with normal fetal proopiomelanocortin mRNA expression. The inflammatory state of obesity is also associated with oxidative stress and it would be interesting to determine whether antioxidant supplementation in these non-human primate achieves reversal of offspring adiposity as reported in obese rat dams and their offspring (Sen and Simmons, 2010) (▶Fig. 9.1).

Should any or all of these proposed pathways be proven to contribute to the development of obesity in offspring of obese/fat fed animals, then different approaches to intervention could be developed for obese pregnant women. In relation to hyperinsulinemia, strategies which improve insulin resistance should be considered; indeed several ongoing randomized controlled trials are relevant e.g. the UPBEAT trial in the UK, which aims to improve pregnancy outcome in obese women by recommending a low glycemic index diet and/or increased physical activity. Follow up of children from trial participants will be invaluable in establishing whether improved control of maternal glucose homeostasis may reduce childhood adiposity. Current strategies for reducing gestational weight gain to improve pregnancy outcome, which focus more on calorie restriction may however be more apposite should hyperleptinemia and inflammatory responses be greater determinants of offspring adiposity. In addition, the fat composition of the diet may be all important. Whilst further corroborative studies are needed, especially in non-human primates, animal models have considerable potential to inform future interventions in pregnancy which may contribute to curtailment of childhood obesity.

9.3.2 Cardiovascular function in the offspring of obese animals

There are many examples of developmental programming of cardiovascular dysfunction by states of maternal undernutrition, recently reviewed (Ojeda et al., 2008) but few investigators have addressed whether exposure to maternal obesity in animals is associated with cardiovascular dysfunction in the offspring. The hypothalamus plays a critical role in blood pressure control through the melanocortin system, and in circadian variation of blood pressure via the suprachiasmatic nucleus. Since developmental plasticity of the hypothalamus appears to be central in determining abnormal energy balance in the offspring of obese dams, investigation of cardiovascular function is also of obvious interest. Furthermore, several studies have reported an association between maternal BMI or gestational weight gain in human pregnancy and offspring blood pressure (Lawlor et al., 2004; Mamun et al., 2009; Oken, 2009; West et al., 2010). However, because of the established relationship between obesity and blood pressure, it is important to determine whether the development of childhood obesity underpins this relationship or whether there is an independent risk of hypertension in the child of an obese mother; indeed in a recent study of 99 diabetic women and their children an association between maternal BMI and offspring systolic blood pressure, which was independent of maternal diabetes status, was attenuated towards null after adjustment for child attained BMI. However correction for offspring BMI did not impact upon an association between maternal BMI and offspring E-selectin, a cardiovascular risk marker (West et al., 2010).

Animal studies offer the opportunity to delineate 'cause and effect relationships'. We have shown that adult offspring of diet-induced obese mice and rats develop hypertension (Samuelsson et al., 2008; Samuelsson et al., 2010) using protocols in which blood pressure was measured by the method of remote telemetry, enabling continuous measurement of blood pressure in conscious unrestrained animals. By assessment in young male and female rat offspring (30 days) with prior exposure to maternal obesity we were able to demonstrate elevation of blood pressure before development of increased fat mass. The blood pressure was also higher than controls at 90 days of age, and by 180 days the increase in blood pressure in male offspring was associated with loss of diurnal variation. The 30 day and 90 day old offspring dams also showed an enhanced response to restraint stress, and supranormal renal noradrenaline content and renin mRNA expression. Spectral analysis of the blood pressure tracings revealed increased low frequency oscillations in 30 and 90 day old offspring compared to controls, and at 90 days investigation of blood pressure responses to noradrenaline and sodium nitroprusside identified reduced baroreflex sensitivity. Taken together, these observations strongly suggested the hypertension is of sympathetic origin. We also investigated the blood pressure response to exogenous leptin. Leptin increases blood pressure through an increase in hypothalamic and nucleus tractus solitarius efferent sympathetic tone via the renal nerve (Mark et al., 2009). The offspring of the obese dams demonstrated an enhanced pressor response to leptin injection. Although in apparently contrast to the leptin resistance observed in relation to food intake, it is recognized that cardiovascular and appetite regulatory actions of leptin are attributed to different regions of the hypothalamus. Indeed, the young lean offspring presented a very similar phenotype of 'selective leptin resistance' to that observed in adult obese rodents (Rahmouni et al., 2005). Future research will focus on defining the central mechanisms responsible, particularly the role of the POMC system and the melanocortin receptor types 3 and 4 (MC3/4R) since these are implicated in leptin induced elevation of blood pressure (Tallam et al., 2006). Importantly, these observations have provided a rationale for investigation of blood pressure and blood pressure variability in the children of obese mothers in ongoing mother-child cohort studies. Indeed, there is already some limited evidence to suggest that children of obese mothers may be prone to hypertension through altered autonomic control including a report of an association between maternal BMI and fetal cardiac sympathovagal activation (Ojala et al., 2009).

9.4 Summary

In summary, the evidence for an independent association between maternal obesity and offspring obesity is strong, although causality remains to be proven. Animal studies have shown unequivocal support for the transgenerational influence of maternal obesity on the developing offspring and, importantly have provided mechanistic insight at a depth practically not possible in human studies. These have already informed ongoing mother-child cohort studies and, inevitably, will play an important role in development of intervention studies in obese women with the aim of preventing childhood obesity.

References

Amusquivar E, Ruperez FJ, Barbas C, Herrera E. Low arachidonic acid rather than alpha-tocopherol is responsible for the delayed postnatal development in offspring of rats fed fish oil instead of olive oil during pregnancy and lactation. *J Nutr* 2000;130: 2855–65.

Bayol SA, Farrington SJ, Stickland NC. A maternal 'junk food' diet in pregnancy and lactation promotes an exacerbated taste for 'junk food' and a greater propensity for obesity in rat offspring. *Br J Nutr* 2007;98: 843–51.

Blair NJ, Thompson JM, Black PN, Becroft DM, Clark PM, Han DY, Robinson E, Waldie KE, Wild CJ, Mitchell EA. Risk factors for obesity in 7-year-old European children: the Auckland Birthweight Collaborative Study. *Arch Dis Child* 2007;92: 866–71.

Bouret SG. Development of hypothalamic neural networks controlling appetite. *Forum Nutr* 2010;63: 84–93.

Burdette HL, Whitaker RC, Hall WC, Daniels SR. Maternal infant-feeding style and children's adiposity at 5 years of age. *Arch Pediatr Adolesc Med* 2006;160: 513–20.

Carmody JS, Wan P, Accili D, Zeltser LM, Leibel RL. Respective contributions of maternal insulin resistance and diet to metabolic and hypothalamic phenotypes of progeny. *Obesity* 2010; October 14, ahead of print.

Catalano PM, Drago NM, Amini SB. Maternal carbohydrate metabolism and its relationship to fetal growth and body composition. *Am J Obstet Gynecol* 1995;172: 1464–70.

Catalano PM, Farrell K, Thomas A, Huston-Presley L, Mencin P, De Mouzon SH, Amini SB. Perinatal risk factors for childhood obesity and metabolic dysregulation. *Am J Clin Nutr* 2009;90: 1303–13.

Chang GQ, Gaysinskaya V, Karatayev O, Leibowitz SF. Maternal high-fat diet and fetal programming: increased proliferation of hypothalamic peptide-producing neurons that increase risk for overeating and obesity. *J Neurosci* 2008;28: 12107–19.

Chu SY, Kim SY, Bish CL. Prepregnancy obesity prevalence in the United States 2004–2005. *Matern Child Health J* 2009;13: 614–20.

Crozier SR, Inskip HM, Godfrey KM, Cooper C, Harvey NC, Cole ZA, Robinson SM. Weight gain in pregnancy and childhood body composition: findings from the Southampton Women's Survey. *Am J Clin Nutr* 2010;91: 1745–51.

Davey Smith G, Steer C, Leary S, Ness A. Is there an intrauterine influence on obesity? Evidence from parent child associations in the Avon Longitudinal Study of Parents and Children (ALSPAC). *Arch Dis Child* 2007;92: 876–80.

Dong YM, Li Y, Ning H, Wang C, Liu JR, Sun CH. High dietary intake of medium-chain fatty acids during pregnancy in rats prevents later-life obesity in their offspring. *J Nutr Biochem* 2011;22: 791–7.

Dunn GA, Bale TL. Maternal high-fat diet promotes body length increases and insulin insensitivity in second-generation mice. *Endocrinology* 2009;150: 4999–5009.

Fattah C, Barry S, O'connor N, Farah N, Stuart B, Turner MJ. Maternal leptin and body composition in the first trimester of pregnancy. *Gynecol Endocrinol* 2011;27: 263–6.

Ferezou-Viala J, Roy AF, Serougne C, Gripois D, Parquet M, Bailleux V, Gertler A, Delplanque B, Djiane J, Riottot M, Taouis M. Long-term consequences of maternal high-fat feeding on hypothalamic leptin sensitivity and diet-induced obesity in the offspring. *Am J Physiol Regul Integr Comp Physiol* 2007;293: R1056–62.

Franks PW, Hanson RL, Knowler WC, Sievers ML, Bennett PH, Looker HC. Childhood obesity other cardiovascular risk factors and premature death. *N Engl J Med* 2010;362: 485–93.

Fraser A, Tilling K, Macdonald-Wallis C, Sattar N, Brion MJ, Benfield L, Ness A, Deanfield J, Hingorani A, Nelson SM, Smith GD, Lawlor DA. Association of maternal weight gain in pregnancy with offspring obesity and metabolic and vascular traits in childhood. *Circulation* 2010;121: 2557–64.

Gale CR, Javaid MK, Robinson SM, Law CM, Godfrey KM, Cooper C. Maternal size in pregnancy and body composition in children. *J Clin Endocrinol Metab* 2007;92: 3904–11.

Gillman MW, Rifas-Shiman SL, Kleinman K, Oken E, Rich-Edwards JW, Taveras EM. Developmental origins of childhood overweight: potential public health impact. *Obesity (Silver Spring)* 2008;16: 1651–6.

Grayson BE, Kievit P, Smith MS, Grove KL. Critical determinants of hypothalamic appetitive neuropeptide development and expression: species considerations. *Front Neuroendocrinol* 2010a;31: 16–31.

Grayson BE, Levasseur PR, Williams SM, Smith MS, Marks DL, Grove KL. Changes in melanocortin expression and inflammatory pathways in fetal offspring of nonhuman primates fed a high-fat diet. *Endocrinology* 2010b;151: 1622–32.

Heslehurst N, Rankin J, Wilkinson JR, Summerbell CD. A nationally representative study of maternal obesity in England UK: trends in incidence and demographic inequalities in 619 323 births 1989–2007. *Int J Obes* 2010;34: 420–8.

Holemans K, Caluwaerts S, Poston L, Van Assche FA. Diet-induced obesity in the rat: a model for gestational diabetes mellitus. *Am J Obstet Gynecol* 2004;190: 858–65.

Hull HR, Dinger MK, Knehans AW, Thompson DM, Fields DA. Impact of maternal body mass index on neonate birthweight and body composition. *Am J Obstet Gynecol* 2008;198: 416 e1–6.

Kim SY, Dietz PM, England L, Morrow B, Callaghan WM. Trends in pre-pregnancy obesity in nine states 1993–2003. *Obesity* 2007;15: 986–93.

Kirk SL, Samuelsson AM, Argenton M, Dhonye H, Kalamatianos T, Poston L, Taylor PD, Coen CW. Maternal obesity induced by diet in rats permanently influences central processes regulating food intake in offspring. *PLoS One* 2009;4: e5870.

Kleiser C, Schaffrath Rosario A, Mensink GB, Prinz-Langenohl R, Kurth BM. Potential determinants of obesity among children and adolescents in Germany: results from the cross-sectional KiGGS Study. *BMC Public Health* 2009;9: 46.

Korotkova M, Gabrielsson BG, Holmang A, Larsson BM, Hanson LA, Strandvik B. Gender-related long-term effects in adult rats by perinatal dietary ratio of n-6/n-3 fatty acids. *Am J Physiol Regul Integr Comp Physiol* 2005;288: R575–9.

Koupil I, Toivanen P. Social and early-life determinants of overweight and obesity in 18-year-old Swedish men. *Int J Obes* 2008;32: 73–81.

Laitinen J, Power C, Jarvelin MR. Family social class maternal body mass index childhood body mass index and age at menarche as predictors of adult obesity. *Am J Clin Nutr* 2001;74: 287–94.

Lake JK, Power C, Cole TJ. Child to adult body mass index in the 1958 British birth cohort: associations with parental obesity. *Arch Dis Child* 1997;77: 376–81.

Lawlor DA, Najman JM, Sterne J, Williams GM, Ebrahim S, Davey Smith G. Associations of parental birth and early life characteristics with systolic blood pressure at 5 years of age: findings from the Mater-University study of pregnancy and its outcomes. *Circulation* 2004;110: 2417–23.

Lawlor DA, Smith GD, O'callaghan M, Alati R, Mamun AA, Williams GM, Najman JM. Epidemiologic evidence for the fetal overnutrition hypothesis: findings from the mater-university study of pregnancy and its outcomes. *Am J Epidemiol* 2007;165: 418–24.

Lawlor DA, Timpson NJ, Harbord RM, Leary S, Ness A, Mccarthy MI, Frayling TM, Hattersley AT, Smith GD. Exploring the developmental overnutrition hypothesis using parental-offspring associations and FTO as an instrumental variable. *PLoS Med* 2008;5: e33.

Levin BE, Govek E. Gestational obesity accentuates obesity in obesity-prone progeny. *Am J Physiol* 1998;275: R1374–9.

Li C, Goran MI, Kaur H, Nollen N, Ahluwalia JS. Developmental trajectories of overweight during childhood: role of early life factors. *Obesity* 2007;15: 760–71.

Li C, Kaur H, Choi WS, Huang TT, Lee RE, Ahluwalia JS. Additive interactions of maternal prepregnancy BMI and breast-feeding on childhood overweight. *Obes Res* 2005;13: 362–71.

Mamun AA, O'callaghan M, Callaway L, Williams G, Najman J, Lawlor DA. Associations of gestational weight gain with offspring body mass index and blood pressure at 21 years of age: evidence from a birth cohort study. *Circulation* 2009;119: 1720–7.

Mark AL, Agassandian K, Morgan DA, Liu X, Cassell MD, Rahmouni K. Leptin signaling in the nucleus tractus solitarii increases sympathetic nerve activity to the kidney. *Hypertension* 2009;53: 375–80.

Mccurdy CE, Bishop JM, Williams SM, Grayson BE, Smith MS, Friedman JE, Grove KL. Maternal high-fat diet triggers lipotoxicity in the fetal livers of nonhuman primates. *J Clin Invest* 2009;119: 323–35.

Mingrone G, Manco M, Mora ME, Guidone C, Iaconelli A, Gniuli D, Leccesi L, Chiellini C, Ghirlanda G. Influence of maternal obesity on insulin sensitivity and secretion in offspring. *Diabetes Care* 2008;31: 1872–6.

Monasta L, Batty GD, Cattaneo A, Lutje V, Ronfani L, Van Lenthe FJ, Brug J. Early-life determinants of overweight and obesity: a review of systematic reviews. *Obes Rev* 2010;11: 695–708.

Moreira P, Padez C, Mourao-Carvalhal I, Rosado V. Maternal weight gain during pregnancy and overweight in Portuguese children. *Int J Obes* 2007;31: 608–14.

National Institute for Health and Clinical Excellence (Nice). Weight Management Guidelines. 2010. http://guidance.nice.org.uk/PH27, accessed January 18, 2011.

Nelson SM, Matthews P, Poston L. Maternal metabolism and obesity: modifiable determinants of pregnancy outcome. *Hum Reprod Update* 2010;16: 255–75.

Nivoit P, Morens C, Van Assche FA, Jansen E, Poston L, Remacle C, Reusens B. Established diet-induced obesity in female rats leads to offspring hyperphagia adiposity and insulin resistance. *Diabetologia* 2009;52: 1133–42.

Ojala T, Aaltonen J, Siira S, Jalonen J, Ekholm E, Ekblad U, Laitinen K. Fetal cardiac sympathetic activation is linked with maternal body mass index. *Early Hum Dev* 2009;85: 557–60.

Ojeda NB, Grigore D, Alexander BT. Role of fetal programming in the development of hypertension. *Future Cardiol* 2008;4: 163–74.

Oken E. Maternal and child obesity: the causal link. *Obstet Gynecol Clin North Am* 2009;36: 361–77.

Oken E, Rifas-Shiman SL, Field AE, Frazier AL, Gillman MW. Maternal gestational weight gain and offspring weight in adolescence. *Obstet Gynecol* 2008;112: 999–1006.

Oken E, Taveras EM, Kleinman KP, Rich-Edwards JW, Gillman MW. Gestational weight gain and child adiposity at age 3 years. *Am J Obstet Gynecol* 2007;196: 322 e1–8.

Olshansky SJ, Passaro DJ, Hershow RC, Layden J, Carnes BA, Brody J, Hayflick L, Butler RN, Allison DB, Ludwig DS. A potential decline in life expectancy in the United States in the 21st century. *N Engl J Med* 2005;352: 1138–45.

Pirkola J, Pouta A, Bloigu A, Hartikainen AL, Laitinen J, Jarvelin MR, Vaarasmaki M. Risks of overweight and abdominal obesity at age 16 years associated with prenatal exposures to maternal prepregnancy overweight and gestational diabetes mellitus. *Diabetes Care* 2010;33: 1115–21.

Plagemann A. Perinatal programming and functional teratogenesis: impact on body weight regulation and obesity. *Physiol Behav* 2005;86: 661–8.

Plagemann A, Harder T, Janert U, Rake A, Rittel F, Rohde W, Dörner G. Malformations of hypothalamic nuclei in hyperinsulinemic offspring of rats with gestational diabetes. *Dev Neurosci* 1999a;21: 58–67.

Plagemann A, Harder T, Melchior K, Rake A, Rohde W, Dörner G. Elevation of hypothalamic neuropeptide Y-neurons in adult offspring of diabetic mother rats. *Neuroreport* 1999b;10: 3211–6.

Plagemann A, Harder T, Rake A, Melchior K, Rittel F, Rohde W, Dörner G. Hypothalamic insulin and neuropeptide Y in the offspring of gestational diabetic mother rats. *Neuroreport* 1998;9: 4069–73.

Poston L, Briley AL, Seed PT, Kelly FJ, Shennan AH. Vitamin C and vitamin E in pregnant women at risk for pre-eclampsia (VIP trial): randomised placebo-controlled trial. *Lancet* 2006;367: 1145–54.

Poston L, Harthoorn L, Van Der Beek EM. Obesity in pregnancy; implications for the mother and lifelong health of the child. A consensus statement. *Pediatr Res* 2011;69:175–180.

Rahmouni K, Morgan DA, Morgan GM, Mark AL, Haynes WG. Role of selective leptin resistance in diet-induced obesity hypertension. *Diabetes* 2005;54 2012–8.

Rasmussen K, Yaktine A. Weight gain during pregnancy: reexamining the guidelines. Washington: National Academies Press, 2009.

Reilly JJ, Armstrong J, Dorosty AR, Emmett PM, Ness A, Rogers I, Steer C, Sherriff A. Early life risk factors for obesity in childhood: cohort study. *BMJ* 2005;330: 1357.

Reilly JJ, Methven E, Mcdowell ZC, Hacking B, Alexander D, Stewart L, Kelnar CJ. Health consequences of obesity. *Arch Dis Child* 2003;88: 748–52.

Ronnberg A, Nilsson K. Interventions during pregnancy to reduce excessive gestational weight gain: a systematic review assessing current clinical evidence using the Grading of Recommendations Assessment Development and Evaluation (GRADE) system. *BJOG* 2010;117: 1327–34.

Salsberry PJ, Reagan PB. Dynamics of early childhood overweight. *Pediatrics* 2005;116: 1329–38.

Samuelsson AM, Matthews PA, Argenton M, Christie MR, Mcconnell JM, Jansen EH, Piersma AH, Ozanne SE, Twinn DF, Remacle C, Rowlerson A, Poston L, Taylor PD. Diet-induced obesity in female mice leads to offspring hyperphagia adiposity hypertension and insulin resistance: a novel murine model of developmental programming. *Hypertension* 2008;51: 383–92.

Samuelsson AM, Morris A, Igosheva N, Kirk SL, Pombo JM, Coen CW, Poston L, Taylor PD. Evidence for sympathetic origins of hypertension in juvenile offspring of obese rats. *Hypertension* 2010;55: 76–82.

Sen S, Simmons RA. Maternal antioxidant supplementation prevents adiposity in the offspring of Western diet-fed rats. *Diabetes* 2010;59: 3058–65.

Sewell MF, Huston-Presley L, Super DM, Catalano P. Increased neonatal fat mass not lean body mass is associated with maternal obesity. *Am J Obstet Gynecol* 2006;195: 1100–3.

Shankar K, Harrell A, Liu X, Gilchrist JM, Ronis MJ, Badger TM. Maternal obesity at conception programs obesity in the offspring. *Am J Physiol Regul Integr Comp Physiol* 2008;294: R528–38.

Shelley P, Martin-Gronert MS, Rowlerson A, Poston L, Heales SJ, Hargreaves IP, Mcconnell JM, Ozanne SE, Fernandez-Twinn DS. Altered skeletal muscle insulin signaling and mitochondrial complex II-III linked activity in adult offspring of obese mice. *Am J Physiol Regul Integr Comp Physiol* 2009;297: R675–81.

Sivan E, Chen X, Homko CJ, Reece EA, Boden G. Longitudinal study of carbohydrate metabolism in healthy obese pregnant women. *Diabetes Care* 1997;20: 1470–5.

Smith J, Cianflone K, Biron S, Hould FS, Lebel S, Marceau S, Lescelleur O, Biertho L, Simard S, Kral JG, Marceau P. Effects of maternal surgical weight loss in mothers on intergenerational transmission of obesity. *J Clin Endocrinol Metab* 2009;94: 4275–83.

Srinivasan M, Aalinkeel R, Song F, Mitrani P, Pandya JD, Strutt B, Hill DJ, Patel MS. Maternal hyperinsulinemia predisposes rat fetuses for hyperinsulinemia and adult-onset obesity and maternal mild food restriction reverses this phenotype. *Am J Physiol Endocrinol Metab* 2006;290: E129-E134.

Sullivan EL, Grayson B, Takahashi D, Robertson N, Maier A, Bethea CL, Smith MS, Coleman K, Grove KL. Chronic consumption of a high-fat diet during pregnancy causes perturbations in the serotonergic system and increased anxiety-like behavior in nonhuman primate offspring. *J Neurosci* 2010;30: 3826–30.

Symonds ME, Sebert SP, Hyatt MA, Budge H. Nutritional programming of the metabolic syndrome. *Nat Rev Endocrinol* 2009;5: 604–10.

Tallam LS, Da Silva AA, Hall JE. Melanocortin-4 receptor mediates chronic cardiovascular and metabolic actions of leptin. *Hypertension* 2006;48: 58–64.

Walker CD, Naef L, D'asti E, Long H, Xu Z, Moreau A, Azeddine B. Perinatal maternal fat intake affects metabolism and hippocampal function in the offspring: a potential role for leptin. *Ann NY Acad Sci* 2008;1144: 189–202.

Wardle J, Brodersen NH, Cole TJ, Jarvis MJ, Boniface DR. Development of adiposity in adolescence: five year longitudinal study of an ethnically and socioeconomically diverse sample of young people in Britain. *BMJ* 2006;332: 1130–5.

Wardle J, Sanderson S, Guthrie CA, Rapoport L, Plomin R. Parental feeding style and the intergenerational transmission of obesity risk. *Obes Res* 2002;10: 453–62.

West NA, Crume TL, Maligie MA, Dabelea D. Cardiovascular risk factors in children exposed to maternal diabetes in utero. Diabetologia 2010, published ahead of print, accessed January 12, doi: 10.1007/s00125–010–2008–1.

Whitaker KL, Jarvis MJ, Beeken RJ, Boniface D, Wardle J. Comparing maternal and paternal intergenerational transmission of obesity risk in a large population-based sample. *Am J Clin Nutr* 2010;91: 1560–7.

Whitaker RC. Predicting preschooler obesity at birth: the role of maternal obesity in early pregnancy. *Pediatrics* 2004;114: e29–36.

White CL, Purpera MN, Morrison CD. Maternal obesity is necessary for programming effect of high-fat diet on offspring. *Am J Physiol Regul Integr Comp Physiol* 2009;296: R1464–72.

World Health Organization. Fact Sheet No 311: www.who.int/mediacentre/factsheets/fs311/en/index.html. 2006.

10 Short and long term effects of gestational obesity: Clinical observations

Patrick M. Catalano

There has been a significant increase of obesity in women of reproductive age in the past decades. Hence, compared to normal weight women there exists alterations in maternal metabolism prior to conception. Since obese women are more insulin resistant, when coupled with the increased insulin resistance of pregnancy, there is the additive effect making increased nutrients availability to the developing fetus.

The infant of the obese women weighs more at delivery because of increased fat and not lean body mass. In addition to adiposity, these neonates have increased insulin resistance. Increased insulin resistance in the neonate correlates with maternal insulin resistance and body fat. There has been a significant increase in children and adolescent obesity in the past decade. Multiple perinatal factors have been related to childhood obesity including maternal pre-pregnancy obesity, gestational weight gain and glucose intolerance, such as gestational diabetes. In our 8 year follow up of women with both normal glucose tolerance and gestational diabetes, maternal pregravid BMI was the strongest predictor of childhood obesity, independent of maternal glucose status or weight gain during pregnancy.

In summary our research group has been focusing on maternal factors facilitating fetal fat accretion. We hypothesize maternal obesity because of the increased insulin resistance, possibly mediated through inflammation, create a significant risk for the next generation because the process of obesity for the offspring is initiated in utero. Therefore if the treatment of obesity begins with prevention, then the perinatal period of development is an important focus for additional research.

10.1 Maternal metabolism in normal pregnancy

The metabolic alterations in normal human pregnancy can be considered as having two distinct phases. Early gestation can be considered as the time through about 28 weeks of gestation. Metabolically, early pregnancy is characterized as an anabolic state, manifested by a decrease in insulin sensitivity, increase in energy expenditure, accretion of maternal adipose tissue and placental growth and hormone production. Late gestation can be considered catabolic because of the further decreases in insulin sensitivity resulting in increased lipid mobilization for maternal energy needs and increased nutrient availability for fetal-placental energy needs and growth. However, because of the recent increases in overweight and obesity in women of reproductive age over the past few decades, these shifts in the population weight distribution have resulted in alterations in maternal metabolism during pregnancy and increased fetal growth.

10.2 Fetal growth and body composition

There has been a significant increase in obesity in the last 40 years not only in developed areas of the world but also in developing countries (World Health Organization, 2000). In the United States approximately 55% of the population is either overweight or obese and 30% are obese based on WHO BMI criteria (Ogden et al., 2006). Furthermore, 7% of women of reproductive age population have a BMI >40, or Class III obesity (Ogden et al., 2006). In Asian populations, because of differences in body composition, the criteria for risk of metabolic dysfunction such as diabetes and cardiovascular disease are different than in a Caucasian population. A BMI of 23–27.5 is designated as increased risk and a BMI greater than 27.5 as high risk for metabolic dysfunction (World Health Organization, 1999). Approximately 11% of US children are obese based on the Center for Disease Control and Prevention (CDC), i.e. weight for height greater than 2 standard deviations for age and gender (Ogden et al., 2008). Last, there has been reported a significant increase in the mean term birth weight in various European populations (Orskou et al., 2001; Surkan et al., 2004).

Anath has reported that between 1985 and 1998 in the United States there has been an 11 to 12% decrease in small for gestational age (birth weight less than the 10th percentile for gestational age) neonates, whereas there has been a 5–9% increase in large for gestational age neonates (birth weight greater than the 90th percentile for gestational age), in the white and black populations, respectively (Anath and Wen, 2002). In our own population in Cleveland Ohio, there has been a significant mean 116g increase in term birth weights from 1975 through 2005. The increases in birth weight reflect increases through the entire range of birth weights, i.e. there has been an increase from the 5th to 95th percentiles. These increases in birth weight remain after adjustment for gender, ethnicity and gestational age (Catalano, 2007).

In our research, we have elected to assess fetal growth using estimates of body composition. The rational for this is that at birth, we as humans have the greatest percent of body fat as compared with most other mammalian species. At birth the term human has approximately 12–16 percent body fat, depending on the methodology used. In contrast most murine models have 1–2% body fat (Widdowson, 1950). The increases in murine body fat occur during weaning. Non human primates at birth have in the order of 3–5 percent body fat (Ausman et al., 1982; Russo et al., 1980). Last guinea pigs have 8–10 percent body fat at birth. Of interest, humans share with guinea pigs a hemochorial type of placenta.

Based on animal husbandry studies and human autopsy data, lean body mass or fat free mass has a strong relationship with genetic factors for e.g. males weigh more at birth compared to females because of the increase in lean and not fat mass (Moulton, 1923; Sparks, 1984). In contrast fat mass at birth is strongly related to maternal environmental factors such as pre pregnancy obesity, weight gain and diabetes.

At birth infants of women with gestational diabetes (GDM) weigh more than women with normal glucose tolerance because of increased fat mass but not lean body mass (▶Tab. 10.1). This relationship holds when the data are adjusted for confounding variables such as gestational age and ethnicity.

Furthermore even when only considering those newborns whose weight for gestational age are appropriate for gestational age (AGA), the neonates of women with GDM have increased percent body fat as compared with the AGA neonates of women with

Tab. 10.1: Body composition in neonates of women with gestational diabetes (GDM) and normal glucose tolerance (NGT).

	GDM (n = 195)	NGT (n = 220)	p-value
Birth weight (g)	3398 ± 550	3337 ± 549	ns
Lean body mass (g)	2962 ± 405	2975 ± 408	ns
Fat mass (g)	436 ± 206	362 ± 198	0.0002
Body fat (%)	12.4 ± 4.6	10.4 ± 4.6	0.0001

Adapted from Catalano et al. (2003).

Tab. 10.2: Body composition in neonates of women with a pregravid BMI < 25 and BMI > 25.

	BMI < 25 (n = 144)	BMI > 25 (n = 76)	p-value
Birth weight (g)	3284 ± 534	3436 ± 567	ns
Lean body mass (g)	2951 ± 406	3023 ± 410	ns
Fat mass (g)	334 ± 179	416 ± 221	0.008
Body fat (%)	9.7 ± 4.3	11.6 ± 4.7	0.006

Adapted from Sewell et al. (2006).

normal glucose tolerance. Similarly, it has long been recognized that maternal pregravid obesity is a risk factor for fetal overgrowth or macrosomia. In a study by Sewell et al. they reported that in contrast to infants of women with a pregravid body mass index (BMI, kg/m²) BMI less than 25, overweight and obese women with a pregravid BMI greater than 25 had infants at birth whose weight were greater because of a significant increase in fat mass and not lean body mass (Sewell et al., 2006) (▶Tab. 10.2).

Furthermore, women with a BMI greater than 25 gained significantly less weight as compared to the lean or average weight women (BMI less than 25). Using a stepwise regression analysis maternal pregravid BMI was the strongest correlate and accounted for approximately 7% of the variance in neonatal body fat and percent body fat. Maternal well controlled GDM accounted less than 2% of the variance in fat mass and percent body fat (▶Tab. 10.3).

Maternal weight gain is a potentially modifiable variable in relationship to fetal growth. While increased weight gain in average weight women is associated with an increase in both lean and adipose tissue, in obese women excessive weight gain is associated primarily with an increase in adipose and not lean tissue. Therefore achievement of both normal pregravid weight and appropriate weight gain in pregnancy, (based on Institute of Medicine 2009 recommendations (Rasmussen and Yaktine, 2009)) are the optimal means to achieve appropriate fetal growth and prevent adiposity.

At birth the infants of obese women have an altered metabolic profile as compared with the infants of lean mothers (▶Tab. 10.4). At birth not only do these infants have significantly increased adiposity, but also higher umbilical cord leptin concentrations reflecting this increased adipokine production by the adipose tissue. Although there was no increase in cord blood TNF-alpha or C reactive protein, the neonates of the obese

Tab. 10.3: Stepwise regression analysis for factors relating to fetal adiposity at birth.

Fat Mass	r^2	delta r^2	
Pre-gravid BMI	0.066	–	
Gestational age	0.136	0.070	
Weight gain	0.171	0.035	
Group (GDM)	0.187	0.016	$p = 0.0001$
% Neonatal Body Fat			
Pre-gravid BMI	0.072	–	
Gestational age	0.116	0.044	
Weight gain	0.147	0.031	
Group (GDM)	0.166	0.019	$p = 0.0001$

Adapted from Catalano and Ehrenberg (2006).

Tab. 10.4: Metabolic profile of neonates from cord blood at time of elective cesarean delivery.

	Neonates of Lean mothers $n = 53$	Neonates of Obese mothers $n = 68$	p-value
Gestational age	38.8 ± 0.5	38.8 ± 0.6	ns
Birth weight (g)	3217 ± 452	3320 ± 460	ns
Neonatal body fat (%)	11.6 ± 2.9	13.1 ± 3.4	0.001
Placental weight (g)	614 ± 152	693 ± 184	0.01
Adiponectin (µg/mL)	30.8 ± 10.0	30.6 ± 9.7	ns
Leptin (ng/mL)	8.2 ± 4.7	14.7 ± 13.6	0.0001
IL-6 (ng/mL)	2.4 ± 1.4	3.5 ± 2.3	0.01
TNF-alpha (pg/mL)	1.7 ± 0.6	1.7 ± 0.3	ns
CRP (ng/mL)	121 ± 97	202 ± 286	ns
Cord plasma insulin (µU/mL)	7.0 ± 3.8	9.2 ± 4.7	0.02
Cord plasma glucose (mg/dL)	60 ± 13	66 ± 14	0.07

Adapted from Catalano et al. (2009a).

mothers had increased IL-6 concentrations, indicating the possibility of an early inflammatory milieu. Last the cord blood insulin concentrations were significantly greater and there was a trend towards an increase in cord blood glucose.

In neonates estimates of insulin resistance as estimated by clamp studies are very low and reflect primarily increased peripheral rather than hepatic insulin sensitivity (Farrag et al., 1997). Our group recently reported that at birth, neonates of obese women were significantly more insulin resistant (using HOMA estimates of insulin resistance) as compared with infants of lean women (▶Fig. 10.1).

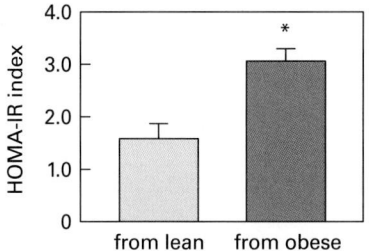

Fig. 10.1: HOMA-IR indexes in fetuses of lean and obese mothers. The fetuses of obese mothers have higher HOMA-IR indexes, i.e., they are more insulin resistant than those of lean mothers. *$p < 0.003$. Adapted from Catalano et al. (2009a).

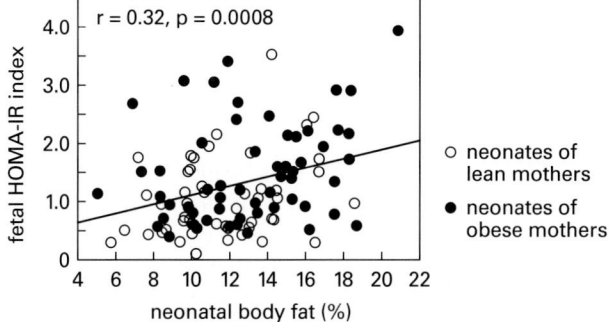

Fig. 10.2: Relationship of fetal insulin resistance with fetal adiposity. Regression analyses show a positive correlation between fetal insulin resistance estimated by HOMA-IR at birth and percent neonatal body fat of the fetus. Adapted from Catalano et al. (2009a).

These data are consistent with a recent report by Dyer et al, who using a minimal model technique, described increased insulin resistance in LGA term neonates compared with poorly grown neonates between 24 and 48 hours after birth (Dyer et al., 2007). There is a significant correlation between neonatal insulin resistance and neonatal percent body fat (▶Fig. 10.2). Last, maternal insulin resistance also had a strong correlation with fetal insulin resistance even when adjusted for various confounders such as fetal adiposity (Catalano et al., 2009a). These data suggest the possibility of genetic or epigenetic factors relating to neonatal insulin resistance.

10.3 The child of the obese woman

One of the goals of our research has to assess the perinatal factors related to the development of obesity and metabolic dysfunction in later life. Maternal glucose intolerance during pregnancy, gestational weight gain, maternal pregravid weight and fetal overgrowth have all have been implicated in childhood obesity (Boney et al. 2005; Dabelea et al., 2000; Oken et al., 2007). Our group has recently published the results

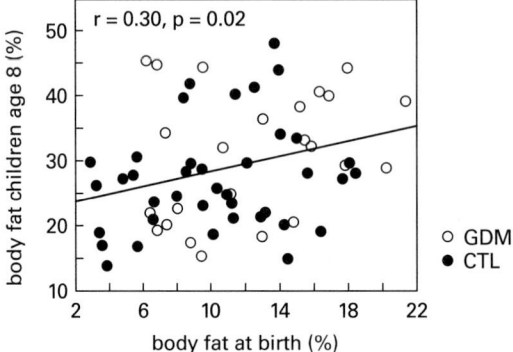

Fig. 10.3: Correlation between percentage body fat in neonates at birth and percentage body fat in children at follow-up, $r = 0.30$, $p = 0.02$ ($n = 63$). CTL – control; GDM – gestational diabetes. Adapted from Catalano et al. (2009b).

of a prospective longitudinal cohort evaluating the perinatal risk factors of childhood obesity. In this study we evaluated children of women with GDM and normal glucose tolerance (NGT) at birth and at approximately 8 years of age (Catalano et al. 2009b). At the time of follow up, the children were rank ordered into tertiles based on CDC criteria for overweight and obesity (Kuczmarski et al., 2002). A subset of the children had body composition estimated using dual-energy x-ray absorptiometry (DXA) and basal laboratory studies. Children in the upper tertile for height and weight had significantly greater energy intake, skinfold thickness and leptin concentrations than those in the first two tertiles. Children in the upper tertile for percent body fat had significantly greater waist circumference, insulin resistance, triglyceride concentrations and leptin concentrations as compared with children in tertiles 1 and 2. There was a significant correlation between percent body fat at birth and body fat at follow up (▶Fig. 10.3) but not between birth weight and weight of the child at follow-up. The strongest predictor for a child being in the upper tertile for CDC weight percentile was maternal pregravid BMI greater than 30. The odds ratio was 3.75 (95% CI of 1.39, 10.10). The risk for a child being in the upper tertile for percent body fat was maternal pregravid BMI greater than 30, with an odds ratio of 5.45 (95% CI of 1.62, 18.41). We concluded that although well controlled GDM during pregnancy is an important factor related to childhood obesity, that maternal pregravid obesity, independent of maternal glucose status or birth weight was the strongest predictor of childhood obesity in our study population.

10.4 Maternal factors facilitating fetal fat accretion

There are multiple factors related to the metabolism in obese women associated with fetal fat accretion. The longitudinal changes in insulin sensitivity during pregnancy in normal weight (BMI less than 25), overweight (BMI 25–29.9) and obese women (BMI greater than 30) are shown in ▶Fig. 10.4. There are significant ($p = 0.0004$) decreases in insulin sensitivity with advancing gestation in all women, regardless of pregravid BMI.

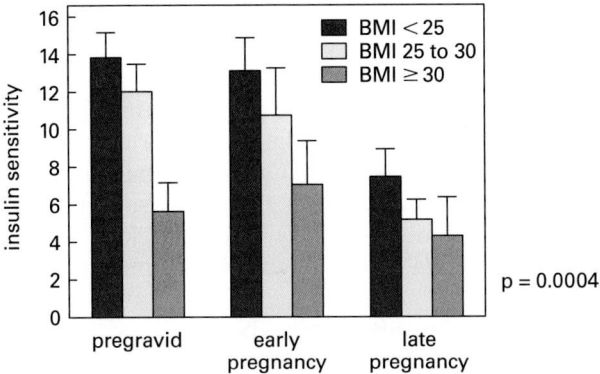

Fig. 10.4: The longitudinal changes in insulin sensitivity in lean, overweight and obese women, before conception and in early (12–14 weeks) and late (34–36 weeks) gestation. Adapted from Catalano and Ehrenberg (2006).

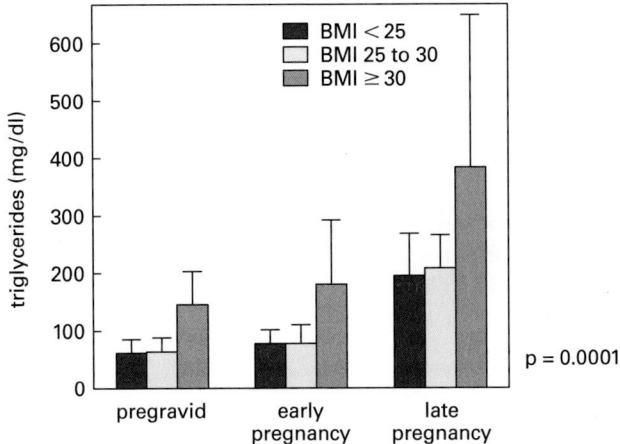

Fig. 10.5: The longitudinal changes in basal triglyceride concentration in lean, overweight and obese women, before conception and in early (12–14 weeks) and late (34–36 weeks) gestation.

However, obese women have significant decreased insulin sensitivity prior to conception as compared to normal and overweight women. Therefore, although there is a similar percent decrease in insulin sensitivity with advancing gestation, obese women have less of an actual net decrease in insulin sensitivity. Based on Pima Indian studies over a number of years, the decrease in net insulin sensitivity is inversely correlated with weight gain (Swinburn et al., 1991). This relationship between change in insulin sensitivity and weight gain are consistent with the epidemiological studies reporting decreased gestational weight gain in obese as compared with non-obese women during pregnancy (Chu et al., 2009).

The alterations in insulin sensitivity are not only relating to glucose metabolism but also other nutrients such as protein and lipids. ▶Fig. 10.5 shows the longitudinal changes in maternal fasting triglyceride concentrations in the same population. Again, although there is a significant increase basal triglyceride concentrations with advancing gestation, obese women have increased triglycerides before pregnancy, which are greatly increased by late gestation. This is because of a decreased ability of insulin to suppress lipolysis in late gestation. These metabolic alterations in obese women, both in early and late gestation result in an abnormal metabolic milieu for the developing placenta and fetus. These metabolic changes not only result in increased nutrient availability for the fetal growth/overgrowth but may alter fetal gene expression, which may become manifest as metabolic dysregulation in the future, i.e. perinatal programming.

The decrease in insulin sensitivity in pregnancy has been ascribed to various placental hormones. Because once the placenta has delivered there is a significant improvement in insulin sensitivity. Previously, the decrease in insulin sensitivity during pregnancy has been ascribed to placental hormones such as human placental lactogen and progesterone. However, more recent data points to cytokines and inflammation as putative factors. For example, tumor necrosis factor alpha (TNF-alpha) has a strong correlation with the changes in insulin sensitivity, as estimated by the euglycemic clamp, during pregnancy (Kirwan et al., 2002). Additionally, the post receptor defects in the insulin signaling cascade are consistent with the mechanism of cytokines relating to insulin resistance (Friedman et al., 2008).

Because of the macrophage infiltration of white adipose tissue (WAT), obesity is considered as an inflammatory condition. The increase in cytokines is one of the links between obesity and insulin resistance and constitutes a component of the metabolic syndrome. Furthermore pregnancy in and of itself is also considered an inflammatory state (▶Tab. 10.5). Therefore, maternal obesity in addition to the significant decreases in insulin sensitivity in late pregnancy results in a marked inflammatory state. Since to the best of our knowledge maternal cytokines do not cross the placenta (Aaltonen, 2005), any inflammation in the fetus is not a function of maternal inflammation but possibly endogenous to the fetus.

Tab. 10.5: Maternal systemic inflammation at time of elective cesarean delivery

	Lean $n = 53$	Obese $n = 68$	p-value
Pre-gravid BMI	22.0 ± 1.9	38.4 ± 6.3	
Gestational age	38.8 ± 0.5	38.8 ± 0.6	ns
Plasma plasma insulin (µU/mL)	11.8 ± 5.6	26.0 ± 14.6	0.0001
Plasma glucose (mg/dL)	74 ± 7	79 ± 11	0.006
Adiponectin (µg/mL)	10.7 ± 4.6	9.7 ± 4.0	ns
Leptin (ng/mL)	31.9 ± 20	72.1 ± 34.7	0.0001
IL-6 (ng/mL)	2.4 ± 1.4	4.6 ± 3.4	0.0001
TNF-alpha (pg/mL)	1.4 ± 0.9	1.3 ± 0.5	ns
CRP (ng/mL)	8074 ± 6467	12433 ± 7918	0.004

Adapted from Catalano et al. (2009a)

10.5 Summary

On the basis of the available evidence, our working hypothesis is that maternal obesity because of the increased insulin resistance, possibly mediated through inflammation, creates a significant risk for the next generation. At birth the fetus of the obese women has metabolic compromise already apparent because of increased adiposity. In childhood the strongest correlate with obesity and metabolic dysregulation is maternal pregravid obesity and not maternal weight gain, birth weight or well controlled GDM. If prevention is the goal to prevent further increases in obesity in the population, then the perinatal period of development is an important focus for additional research (Catalano, 2003).

Acknowledgment

Supported by NIH HD 22965 and Clinical Research Unit NCRR CTSA UL 1 RR 024989.

References

Aaltonen R, Heikkin T, Hakala K, Laine K, Alanen A. Transfer of proinflammatory cytokines across the placenta. *Obstet Gynecol* 2005;106: 802–7.

Ananth CV, Wen SW. Trends in fetal growth among singleton gestations in the United States and Canada. *Semin Perinatol* 2002;26: 260–7.

Ausman LM, Powell EM, Mercado DL, Samonds KW, Lozy M, Gallina DL. Growth and developmental body composition of the cebus monkey. *Am J Perinatol* 1982;3: 211–27.

Boney CM, Verner A, Tucker R, Vohr BR. Metabolic syndrome in childhood: Association with birth weight, maternal obesity and gestational diabetes mellitus. *Pediatrics* 2005;115: E290–6.

Catalano PM. Obesity and pregnancy – the propagation of a viscous cycle? *J Clin Endocrinol Metab* 2003;88: 3505–6.

Catalano PM, Thomas A, Huston-Presley L, Amini SB. Increased fetal adiposity: A very sensitive marker of abnormal in-utero development. *Am J Obstet Gynecol* 2003;189: 1698–704.

Catalano PM, Ehrenberg HM. The short and long term implications of maternal obesity on the mother and her offspring. *Br J Obstet Gynecol* 2006;113: 1126–33.

Catalano PM. Management of obesity in pregnancy. *Obstet Gynecol* 2007;109: 419–33.

Catalano P, Presley L, Minium J, De Mouzon SH. Fetuses of obese mothers develop insulin resistance in utero. *Diabetes Care* 2009a;32: 1076–80.

Catalano PM, Farrell K, Thomas A, Huston-Presley L, Mencin P, De Mouzon SH, Amini SB. Perinatal risk factors for childhood obesity and metabolic dysregulation. *Am J Clin Nutr* 2009b;90: 1303–13.

Chu SY, Callaghan WM, Bisch CC, D'Angelo D. Gestational weight gain by body mass index among US women delivering live births, 2004–2005. *Am J Obstet Gynecol* 2009;200: 271–7.

Dabelea D, Hanson RL, Lindsay RS, Pettitt DJ, Imperatore G, Gabir MM, Roumain J, Bennett PH, Knowler WC. Intrauterine exposure to obesity conveys risks for type 2 diabetes and obesity: A study of discordant sibships. *Diabetes* 2000;49: 2208–11.

Dyer JS, Rosenfeld CR, Rice J, Rice M, Hardin DS. Insulin resistance in Hispanic large-for-gestational-age neonates at birth. *J Clin Endocrinol Metab* 2007;92: 3836–43.

Farrag HM, Nawrath LM, Healey JE, Dorcus EJ, Rapoza RE, Oh W, Cowett RM. Persistent glucose production and greater peripheral sensitivity to insulin in the neonate vs. the adult. *Am J Physiol* 1997;272: E86–93.

Friedman JE, Kirwan JP, Jing M, Presley L, Catalano PM. Increased skeletal muscle tumor necrosis factor-alpha and impaired insulin signaling persist in obese women with gestational diabetes mellitus 1 year postpartum. *Diabetes* 2008;57: 606–13.

Kirwan JP, Hauguel-de Mouzon S, Lepercq J, Challier JC, Huston-Presley L, Friedman JE, Kalhan SC, Catalano PM. TNFalpha is a predictor of insulin resistance in human pregnancy. *Diabetes* 2002;51: 2207–13.

Kuczmarski RJ, Ogden CL, Guo SS, Grummer-Strawn LM, Flegal KM, Mei Z, Mei R, Curtin LR, Roche AF, Johnson CL. 2000 CDC growth charts for the United States: Methods and development. *Vital Health Stat* 2002;11: 1–190.

Moulton CR. Age and chemical development in mammals. *J Biol Chem* 1923;57: 79–97.

Ogden CC, Carroll MD, Curtin LR, McDowell MA, Tabak CJ, Flegal KM. Prevalence of overweight and obesity in the United States, 1999–2004. *JAMA* 2006;295: 1549–55.

Ogden CL, Caroll MD, Flegal KM. High body mass index for age among US children and adolescents 2003–2006. *JAMA* 2008;299: 2401–5.

Oken E, Taveras EM, Kleinman KP, Rich-Edwards JW, Gillman MW. Gestational weight gain and child adiposity at age 3 years. *Am J Obstet Gynecol* 2007;196: 322e1-e8.

Orskou J, Kesmodel U, Henrikson TB, Secker NJ. An increasing proportion of infants weight more than 4000 grams at birth. *Acta Obstet Gynecol Scand* 2001;80: 931–6.

Rasmussen KM, Yaktine AL, editors. Weight gain during pregnancy: Reexamining the guideline. Institute of Medicine and National Research Council of the National Academies. Washington, DC: National Academic Press, 2009.

Russo AR, Ausman LM, Gallina DL, Hegsted DM. Developmental body of composition of the squirrel monkey (Saimiri sciureus). *Growth* 1980;44: 271–86.

Sewell MF, Huston-Presley L, Super DM, Catalano P. Increased neonatal fat mass, not lean body mass, is associated with maternal obesity. *Am J Obstet Gynecol* 2006;195: 1100–3.

Sparks J. Human intrauterine growth and nutrient accretion. *Semin Perinatol* 1984;18: 74–93.

Surkan PJ, Hsieh CC, Johansson AL, Dickman PW, Cnattingius S. Reasons for increasing trends in large for gestational age births. *Obstet Gynecol* 2004;104: 720–6.

Swinburn BA, Nyomba BL, Saad MF, Zurlo F, Raz I, Knowler WC, Lillioja S, Bogardus C, Ravussin E. Insulin resistance associated with lower rates of weight gain in Pima Indians. *J Clin Invest* 1991;88: 168–73.

Widdowson EM. Chemical composition of newly born mammals. *Nature* 1950;166: 626–8.

World Health Organization. Definition, diagnosis and classification of diabetes mellitus and its complications: Report of a WHO Consultation. Part 1: Diagnosis and classification of diabetes mellitus. Geneva, Switzerland: World Health Organization, 1999.

World Health Organization. Obesity: Preventing and managing a global epidemic. *World Health Organization Tech Rep Ser* 2000;899: 1–4.

11 Emerging role of neuroendocrine programming in obesity

Sophie M. Steculorum and Sebastien G. Bouret

The incidence of obesity and diabetes in children and adults continues to rise at an alarming rate worldwide. Epidemiological and animal studies suggest that maternal, fetal, and postnatal health and nutrition, including obesity, diabetes, and malnutrition, may contribute to the development of these diseases. The precise biological mechanisms underlying this metabolic programming are still poorly understood. Nevertheless, there is compelling evidence that obesity and other related diseases may be a consequence of alterations in the developmental processes of neuroendocrine systems involved in energy balance regulation. Experimental data indicate that changes in nutrition during critical periods of development may affect the architecture and molecular signature of hypothalamic pathways involved in body weight and energy balance regulation. In addition, metabolic hormones, including leptin and insulin, are important mediators of the nutritional status and appear to exert profound organizational effects on hypothalamic appetite-related pathways.

11.1 Introduction

During the past three decades, the prevalences of obesity and type 2 diabetes have increased at alarming rates in the vast majority of developed countries (Ebbeling, Pawlak, and Ludwig, 2002; Wang et al., 2008). A number of obesity cases often manifest during childhood and early adulthood. Of particular concern is the finding that obese children and adolescents are more likely to become obese adults (Serdula et al., 1993; Whitaker et al., 1997). For example, epidemiological data indicate that approximately 80% of children who were overweight at ages of 10–15 years remained obese at age 25 (Whitaker et al., 1997). Despite an obvious relationship between obesity and a Western lifestyle, including a sedentary lifestyle and the overconsumption of energy-rich but nutrient-poor food, it is also clear that different individuals exposed to the same obesogenic environments display different responses in terms of obesity predispositions. There appears to be a genetic basis for a subpopulation of obese patients, but genetics alone cannot explain why obesity has increased so rapidly in recent decades. Recent epidemiological and animal studies have revealed that changes in the hormonal and nutritional environments during critical periods of development may increase the susceptibility for the development of obesity and diabetes in later life (Godfrey, Gluckman, and Hanson, 2010; Levin, 2006; McMillen and Robinson, 2005; Plagemann, 2006). Perinatal factors that contribute to lifelong obesity include both maternal and neonatal diabetes, obesity, and malnutrition (for review see Levin, 2006; McMillen and Robinson, 2005; Plagemann, 2006; Sullivan and Grove, 2010). The observation that both a surfeit and a paucity of energy supply during perinatal development are associated with similar metabolic outcomes suggests that the processes underlying programmed obesity may share common biological mechanisms.

The regulation of energy balance and glucose homeostasis is governed by a variety of organs and tissues. Among these tissues, a primary importance has been given to the hypothalamus, which contains sets of neurons that are devoted to metabolic regulation. Empirical experiments using physical lesions of specific hypothalamic structures and, more recently, studies using transgenic approaches have revealed the importance of neurons within the arcuate hypothalamic nucleus (ARC), the ventromedial hypothalamic nucleus (VMN), the dorsomedial nucleus (DMH), the paraventricular nucleus (PVH), and the lateral hypothalamic area (LHA) in the regulation of body weight and glucose levels (for review see Berthoud, 2006; Elmquist et al., 2005; Saper, Chou, and Elmquist, 2002; Sawchenko, 1998). The ARC appears to be a predominant site of integration of peripheral blood-born signals, including endocrine and metabolic factors. Neurons located in the ARC, such as the neurons coproducing neuropeptide Y (NPY) and agouti-related peptide (AgRP), or neurons containing proopiomelanocortin (POMC)-derived

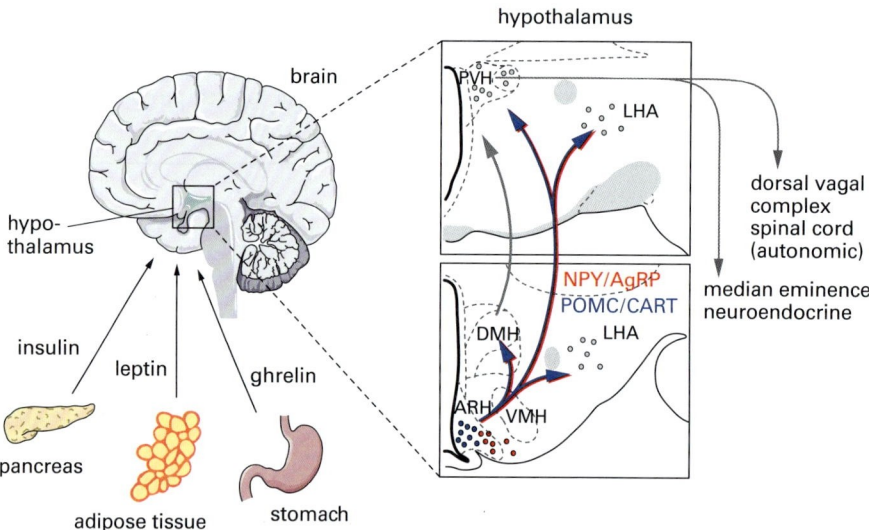

Fig. 11.1: Anatomy of neuroendocrine systems involved in feeding and body weight regulation. Highly simplified schematics illustrating the possible routes and neuronal populations relaying hormonal and nutrient signals from the periphery to the brain. Circulating hormones that reflect peripheral energy status, such as insulin, leptin, and ghrelin, act directly within a complex neuronal network in the hypothalamus to regulate energy balance and glucose homeostasis. The arcuate nucleus of the hypothalamus (ARC) contains a collection of heterogeneous neuronal populations, in particular neurons coexpressing neuropeptide Y (NPY) and agouti-related protein (AgRP) and another distinct neuronal population containing proopiomelanocortin (POMC). These neurons send extensive projections to other parts of the hypothalamus, including the paraventricular (PVH) and dorsomedial (DMH) nuclei of the hypothalamus, and the lateral hypothalamic area (LHA). These neuronal projections represent important routes for the actions of leptin, insulin, and ghrelin at the hypothalamic level. This figure was created in part using illustrations from "Servier Medical Art" with permission.

peptides, directly respond to peripheral hormonal signals, such as the adipocyte-derived hormone leptin, the pancreas-derived hormone insulin, and the gut-derived hormone ghrelin (►Fig. 11.1) (Elmquist et al., 2005; Myers Jr et al., 2009; Sawchenko, 1998).

In particular, leptin and insulin, which are anorexigenic hormones, activate POMC neurons and inhibit NPY neurons to reduce food intake and increase energy expenditure. In contrast, orexigenic hormones such as ghrelin stimulate NPY neurons and inhibit POMC neurons. Both NPY/AgRP- and POMC-containing neurons project extensively to other key hypothalamic nuclei, including the PVH, DMH, and LHA (►Fig. 11.1). These target nuclei contain subpopulations of neurons that also play a crucial role in energy balance regulation and include neurons that produce anorexigenic peptides, such as thyrotropin-releasing hormone (TRH), corticotropin-releasing hormone (CRH) and oxytocin in the PVH, and neurons that express orexigenic neuropeptides, such as orexins and melanin-concentrating hormone (MCH) in the LHA. Based on the critical role of the hypothalamus in the regulation of metabolism, it is clear that impairments of hypothalamic development during perinatal life may result in severe metabolic regulation. This chapter summarizes the developmental changes that have been observed in the hypothalamus in response to changes in the early nutritional and hormonal environment. It also discusses how the resetting of a diverse array of neuroendocrine systems may have long-term effects on the regulation of metabolism and energy balance.

11.2 Development of hypothalamic neuroendocrine pathways controlling appetite

The formation of the neuroendocrine hypothalamus is characterized by various developmental processes that fall into three major categories: (1) the birth of new neurons (i.e., neurogenesis), (2) the migration of these cells to their final destination, and (3) the formation of functional circuits that include axon growth and synaptogenesis (for review see Bouret, 2010a; Markakis, 2002). ►Fig. 11.2 provides a broad overview of the major developmental stages of hypothalamic nuclei and areas involved in appetite regulation.

Neurons that form hypothalamic nuclei originate from the proliferative zone of the third ventricle (Markakis, 2002). Classic experimental tools for the study of neurogenesis have included the administration of the thymidine analog, BrdU, during critical windows of development and have revealed that the majority of neurons that compose the hypothalamus are born between embryonic day (E) 12 and E14 in mice and between E12 and E17 in rats (►Fig. 11.2) (Altman and Bayer, 1986; Ishii, Gibbons, and Bouret, 2009; Padilla, Carmody, and Zeltser, 2010). Part of the complex process of hypothalamic development also includes the proper migration of neurons from their sites of origin (i.e., the proliferative zone of the third ventricle) to their final positions in the mature hypothalamus. This developmental process occurs primarily during late gestation in rodents (McClellana, Parker, and Tobet, 2006). In both rats and mice, the hypothalamus is still relatively immature at birth and continues to develop during the first 2 weeks of postnatal life when neurons send axonal projections to their target sites and form functional synapses. Axonal labeling experiments indicate that ARC axons reach each of their nuclei during the first 2 weeks of postnatal life (►Fig. 11.2) (Bouret et al., 2004a; Grove et al., 2003; Nilsson et al., 2005). The formation of synapses, which are the neurobiological substrates of almost all cell-to-cell communication, follows. In the

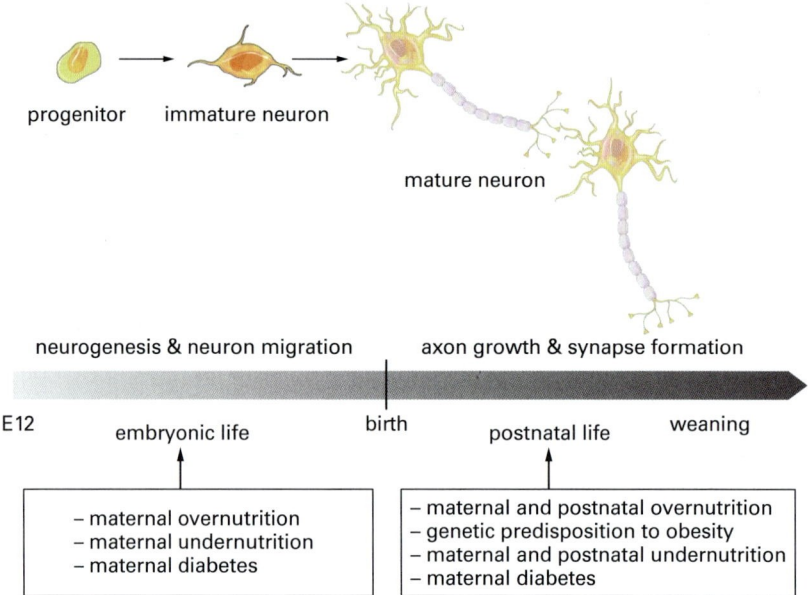

Fig. 11.2: Critical periods of development of neuroendocrine systems in rodents. Schematic illustrations summarizing major developmental stages governing the ultimate architecture of hypothalamic pathways involved in appetite regulation. The formation of a functional hypothalamus occurs in three major phases: (1) the birth of new neurons (neurogenesis), (2) the migration of these neurons to their final location, and (3) the formation of functional circuits that include neurite extension and the formation of functional synapses. Each of these developmental events appears sensitive to a variety of environmental insults that include maternal and neonatal obesity, diabetes, malnutrition, and genetic predispositions to obesity. This figure was created in part using illustrations from "Servier Medical Art" with permission.

rodent hypothalamus, synapses mature gradually from birth to adulthood (Matsumoto and Arai, 1976; Melnick et al., 2007). The considerable importance of postnatal hypothalamic development in rodents differs from humans and nonhuman primates (NHPs) in which the hypothalamus develops almost entirely during fetal life. Immunohistochemical studies performed in Japanese macaques have shown that arcuate projections containing NPY and POMC peptides are fully mature at birth and that the development of these projections is initiated as early as the late second trimester of gestation (Grayson et al., 2006). These results suggest that different species may display different periods of vulnerability to environmental insults based on the temporal and regional maturation patterns of the hypothalamus.

11.3 Animal models of metabolic programming

Animal models of metabolic programming, which include maternal and/or postnatal obesity, undernutrition, and diabetes, represent valuable tools for the study of the mechanisms by which changes in the perinatal nutritional and hormonal environments predispose individuals to obesity (▶Tab. 11.1).

11.3.1 Perinatal obesity

Maternal high-fat diet (HFD) feeding during pregnancy is probably the most widely used approach for studying the consequences of maternal obesity in both rodents and in NHPs. Offspring born to obese females fed an HFD (45% to 60% of calories from fat) during gestation only or during both gestation and lactation become progressively overweight, hyperphagic, and glucose intolerant and display an increase in adiposity (Chen, Simar, and Morris, 2009; Kirk et al., 2009). Remarkably, a short exposure to an HFD during pregnancy without development of metabolic syndrome also predisposes the offspring to obesity, which includes an increase in body weight, fat mass, and food intake (Chang et al., 2008). These data suggest that maternal obesity per se is not required for metabolic programming, but transient and short exposures to nutritional and hormonal challenges during gestation are sufficient to induce long-term metabolic alterations in the offspring. Because of the importance of postnatal organ development, including the brain, in rodents, animal models of postnatal metabolic programming have been developed to specifically target this developmental period. An approach that has proven extremely fruitful for the study of postnatal overfeeding is a reduction of litter size. Pups raised in small litters (SL) display accelerated growth during the preweaning period. Accordingly, pups raised in small litters exhibit heavier body weight as early as the second week of postnatal life, and these animals remain heavier throughout life (Bouret et al., 2007; Davidowa and Plagemann, 2000; Glavas et al., 2010). In addition, postnatally overfed animals show accelerated and exacerbated weight gain when fed an HFD (Glavas et al., 2010). The model of diet-induced obesity (DIO) developed by Barry Levin (Levin et al., 1997) is particularly well-suited for the study of the underlying biological processes that contribute to the development of obesity in humans because Levin's DIO rats share several features with human obesity, including polygenic inheritance. This animal model is also useful for the study of the relative contribution of genetic versus environmental factors in metabolic programming. In this model, the offspring of mothers genetically predisposed to DIO are obese, hyperphagic, and glucose intolerant when fed a high-energy diet compared to offspring born to diet resistant mothers (Levin et al., 2003; Ricci and Levin, 2003).

11.3.2 Maternal diabetes

Almost all animal models of maternal obesity are associated with hyperglycemia and insulin resistance. Accordingly, it is often difficult to determine whether the metabolic abnormalities of pups born to obese dams are caused by changes in the dams' diet or whether they are a consequence of maternal diabetes. The manipulation of glucose levels without an alteration of the diet can be performed experimentally by injecting streptozotocin (STZ), a pancreatic beta-cell toxin. Using this approach, rodent studies indicate that dams (either rats or mice) treated with STZ during early gestation are hypoinsulinemic and hyperglycemic and give birth to pups that are overweight, hyperphagic, and hyperglycemic (Plagemann et al., 1998; Steculorum and Bouret, 2009).

Tab. 11.1: Animal models of nutritional and hormonal programming and long-term consequences on metabolism.

Animal Model				Metabolic Effects			
Model	Preconception	Gestation	Lactation	Growth Curves	Food Intake	Glucose Homeostasis	References
Overnutrition							
Maternal high-fat diet (HFD)	HFD or chow diet	HFD	HFD or chow diet	↑	↑	Glucose intolerant	Chen et al., 2008, 2009; Chang et al., 2008; Kirk et al., 2009; McCurdy et al., 2009
Polygenic model of obesity (diet-induce obesity prone rat, DIO)	High-energy diet (HE) or chow diet	HE or chow diet	HE or chow diet	↑	↑	Glucose intolerant	Gorski, Dunn-Meynell, and Levin, 2007; Levin and Govek, 1998; Levin et al., 2003
Pups raised in small litters	Chow diet	Chow diet	Litter size n = 3	↑	↑	Glucose intolerant	Glavas et al., 2010; Plagemann et al., 1999
High carbohydrate milk formula (HC)	Chow diet	Chow diet	Artificial HC milk formula	↑	↑	Glucose intolerant	Hiremagalur et al., 1993; Srinivassan et al., 2008
Maternal Diabetes							
Maternal streptozotocin injections (STZ)	Control	Insulin-deficient diabetes induced during early gestation	Diabetes persisted during lactation	↑	↑	Hyperglycemic	Plagemann et al., 1999; Steculorum & Bouret, 2009

Malnutrition

Maternal food restriction (FR)	Chow diet *ad libitum*	Food restriction	FR or Chow diet *ad libitum*	↓ birth weight followed by catch up growth	↑	Glucose intolerant	Manuel-Apolinar et al., 2010; Vickers et al., 2000, 2005; Yura et al., 2005
Maternal protein restriction (PR)	Chow diet *ad libitum*	Protein restriction	PR or Chow diet *ad libitum*	↓ birth weight followed by catch up growth	↑	Glucose intolerant	Coupe et al., 2009; Cripps et al., 2009; Plagemann et al., 2000
Pups raised in large litters	Chow diet *ad libitum*	Chow diet *ad libitum*	Litter size n = 12/20	↓ pre- and post-weaning body weights	→	No data	Lopez et al., 2005; Remmers et al., 2008

11.3.3 Perinatal malnutrition

Well-validated rodent models of intrauterine growth retardation include animals born to dams that were either caloric-restricted (food-restricted, FR) or fed a low protein diet (protein-restricted, PR) during pregnancy and lactation. The offspring born of and raised by FR or PR mothers have a low birth weight and slow growth during the preweaning period. In contrast, pups born to FR or PR dams but raised by lactating mothers fed *ad libitum* display a rapid catch-up growth during the first postnatal week (Coupe et al., 2009; Cripps et al., 2009; Yura et al., 2005). Although adult animals born to malnourished mothers display normal body weight, they are hyperphagic and glucose intolerant and display an increased sensitivity to diet-induced obesity (Coupe et al., 2009; Vickers et al., 2000; Yura et al., 2005). The rodent models of divergent litter size can also be used to specifically study the role of postnatal undernutrition on metabolic and developmental outcomes. For example, raising pups in large litters (LL) decreases milk availability and attenuates preweaning growth. Interestingly, pups raised in LLs display rapid weaning-to-adult weight gain that is associated with an increase in adiposity and glucose intolerance (Bouret et al., 2007).

11.4 Assessment of neuroendocrine regulation in metabolically malprogrammed animals

Resistance to the regulatory action of metabolic hormones is a hallmark of obesity in adult individuals. For example, most forms of obesity are associated with a diminished response of the hypothalamus to the appetite-suppressing effects of leptin (Enriori et al., 2006; Myers, Cowley, and Munzberg, 2008) (▶Tab. 11.2).

Interestingly, animals perinatally predisposed to obesity also exhibit leptin resistance. Therefore, adult offspring born to obese (HFD and DIO) and undernourished dams display a blunted response to the anorectic effects of leptin (Kirk et al., 2009; Levin and Dunn-Meynell, 2002; Yura et al., 2005) (▶Tab. 11.3). Moreover, this diminished response to leptin is associated with a reduced ability of leptin to induce pSTAT3, a marker of LepRb activation, in arcuate neurons, which demonstrates that this is a centrally mediated phenomenon (Bouret et al., 2008; Kirk et al., 2009, Yura et al., 2005). Insulin sensitivity also appears to be affected in rats selectively bred to develop DIO (Clegg et al., 2005). Remarkably, DIO rats are leptin- and insulin-resistant before they become obese (Bouret et al., 2008; Clegg et al., 2005), which suggests that this hormonal resistance may initiate the development and maintenance of obesity. Leptin and insulin resistance have also been described in arcuate neurons of adult rats subjected to chronic postnatal overnutrition (Davidowa and Plagemann, 2000, 2007). Electrophysiological studies indicate that the arcuate neurons of rats raised in small litters are less inhibited by leptin and insulin, and some of these neurons are actually partially activated by these hormones (Davidowa and Plagemann, 2000, 2007). A likely mechanism underlying the hormonal resistance is an alteration in receptor expression and/or signaling. For example, a downregulation of hypothalamic leptin receptor mRNA has been described in several animal models of nutritional programming, including SL, DIO, and maternal malnutrition, and an altered leptin binding has been reported in the hypothalamus of DIO rats (Chen et al., 2009; Cripps et al., 2009; Irani, Dunn-Meynell, and Levin, 2007; Levin et al., 2003, 2004).

Tab. 11.2: Hormonal alterations reported in animal models of nutritional and hormonal programming.

Model	Leptin sensitivity	Postnatal leptin surge/Preweaning leptin levels	Preweaning insulin levels	References
Overnutrition				
Maternal high-fat diet (HFD)	↓ anorectic effect ↓ leptin-induced pSTAT3 in the ARH (pups and adults)	↑ and prolonged	↑	Kirk et al., 2009; Chen et al., 2008, Gupta et al., 2009
Polygenic model of obesity	↓ anorectic ↓ leptin-induced pSTAT3 in the ARH (pups and adults)	↑ (at P16)	↑	Bouret et al., 2008; Gorski et al., 2007; Levin et al., 2002, 2004
Pups raised in small litters	↓ leptin sensitivity (adults, electrophysiology); ↓ leptin-induced pSTAT3 in the ARH (pups)	↑	↑	Bouret et al., 2007; Davidowa and Plagemann, 2000; Glavas et al., 2010; Plagemann et al., 1999
High carbohydrate milk formula (HC)	No data	↓ (PND12)	↑	Srinivassan et al., 2008
Diabetes				
Maternal streptozotocin injections	↓ anorectic effects of leptin (adults) ↓ leptin-induced pSTAT3 in the ARH (pups)	= (at P21)	↑	Franke et al., 2005; Plagemann et al., 1998; Steculorum & Bouret, 2009

(Continued)

Tab. 11.2 (*Continued*)

Model	Leptin sensitivity	Postnatal leptin surge/Preweaning leptin levels	Preweaning insulin levels	References
Malnutrition				
Maternal food restriction (FR)/ protein restriction (PR)	↓ anorectic effect of leptin (adults) ↓ leptin-induced pSTAT3 in the ARH (adults); ↓ leptin-induced pSTAT3/cfos in ARH (pups)	Premature and ↑ (mouse) ↓ (rat)	↑ (mouse) ↓ (rat)	Coupe et al., 2010; Delahaye et al., 2007; Desai et al., 2007; Plagemann et al., 2000; Yura et al., 2005
Pups raised in large litter (LL)	No data	→	→	Bouret et al., 2007

Tab. 11.3: Molecular, neurodevelopmental, and structural alterations reported in animal models of nutritional and hormonal programming.

Model	Orexigenic/Anorexigenic mRNA Pre-weaning	Neurogenesis/Number of Neurons	Hypothalamic Projections	References
Overnutrition				
Maternal high-fat diet (HFD)	↑ (adults and preweaning)	↑ neurogenesis ↑ # orexigenic neurons	↓ AgRP fiber density	Chang et al., 2008; Beck et al., 2006; Grayson et al., 2010; Gupta et al., 2009; Kirk et al., 2009; Morris and Chen, 2009
Polygenic model of obesity	↑ NPY mRNA (adults)	No data	↓ AgRP fiber density	Bouret et al., 2008; Levin et al., 1997, 2002
Pups raised in small litters	↑ (adults)	↓ # CCK neurons and ↑ # GAL in neurons PVH	↓ AgRP fiber density ↓ α-MSH fiber density	Bouret et al., 2007; Plagemann et al., 1998, 1999; Lopez et al., 2005
High carbohydrate milk formula	↑ (preweaning and adult)	No data	No data	Srinivassan et al., 2008
Diabetes				
Maternal streptozotocin injections	No data	↑ # NPY neurons	↓ AgRP fiber density ↓ α-MSH fiber density	Plagemann et al., 1998; Steculorum & Bouret, 2009
Malnutrition				
Maternal food restriction (FR)	↑ (young adult)	↓ # NPY neurons in ARH	↑ NPY, CART fiber density ↓ POMC fibers fiber density	Delahaye et al., 2008; Garcia et al., 2010; Yura et al., 2005

(Continued)

Tab. 11.3 (Continued)

Model	Orexigenic/ Anorexigenic mRNA Pre-weaning	Neurogenesis/ Number of Neurons	Hypothalamic Projections	References
Maternal protein restriction (PR)	↑ (preweaning and adult)	↓ # NPY neurons ARC, ↓ # of GAL neurons in PVH	↓ ↓α-MSH fiber density ↓ AgRP fiber density	Coupe et al., 2009, 2010; Cripps et al., 2009; Plagemann et al., 2000
Pups raised in large litters	↑ (preweaning and adult)	No data	↓ AgRP fiber density ↓ α-MSH fiber density	Bouret et al., 2007; Remmers et al., 2008; Lopez et al., 2005

Other regulatory processes are also perturbed in animals born in an obesogenic environment, such as an imbalance in the hypothalamic expression of appetite regulators (▶Tab. 11.3). In most cases, programmed overweight is associated with an elevated ratio of orexigenic to anorexigenic neuropeptide expression in the hypothalamus. For example, both maternal obesity and undernutrition as well as postnatal overnutrition and undernutrition cause an overall increase in the expression of orexigenic neuropeptides, such as NPY and AgRP, and a decrease in the expression of anorexigenic neuropeptides, such as POMC and cocaine and amphetamine-regulated transcript peptide (CART) (Chen et al., 2009; Coupe et al., 2009; Cripps et al., 2009; López et al., 2005; Remmers et al., 2008; Srinivasan et al., 2008). It has been postulated that the elevated ratio of orexigenic to anorexigenic neuropeptides may explain the increased drive to eat in perinatally malprogrammed animals. However, the application and generalization of the results of mRNA studies warrant a good degree of caution until the relationships between mRNA and protein levels are well characterized. In other words, gene expression approaches may be useful for mechanistic studies, but unless they are used in conjunction with an examination of protein levels and localization, these studies may not always prove useful for the prediction of an adverse effect. Nevertheless, it appears that the observed changes in neuropeptide gene expression reflect an acquired mechanism that originates from a malprogramming of hypothalamic neuropeptidergic systems during early life rather than being a consequence of metabolic dysfunctions, such as overweight and hyperphagia. Consistent with this idea, changes in neuropeptide gene expression are often observed as early as embryonic life and/or during the first postnatal weeks, that is, prior to the development of overweight and hyperphagia (Chen et al., 2009; Cripps et al., 2009; Gupta et al., 2009; Morris and Chen, 2009; Remmers et al., 2010; Srinivasan et al., 2008; Terroni et al., 2005). In addition to its adverse effects on the expression of appetite-regulating genes, postnatal overfeeding affects neuronal response to neuropeptides. For example, PVH neurons of chronically overfed pups display reduced electrophysiological responses to arcuate neuropeptides, such as NPY, AgRP, alpha-melanocyte stimulating hormone (alpha-MSH), and CART (Davidowa, Li, and Plagemann, 2003).

11.5 Structural influences of perinatal nutrition on hypothalamic appetite-related networks

As described previously, the developing hypothalamus is exposed to two distinct environments: one *in utero* and the other *extra utero*. These developmental periods represent important windows of sensitivity during which alterations of the nutritional and metabolic environments may lead to structural abnormalities in the hypothalamus, such as changes in cell numbers and/or neuronal connectivity.

11.5.1 Determination of neuronal cell numbers

The capacity of diet to alter proliferation in the neuroepithelium has been demonstrated recently in rodents. In the case of maternal high-fat feeding, hypothalamic cell proliferation is increased in rats and results in higher numbers of neurons containing orexigenic neuropeptides (i.e., galanin, enkephalin, dynorphin, MCH, and orexin) in the PVH and

LHA (Chang et al., 2008). In general, rodent studies indicate that the adverse effects of a maternal obesogenic environment are similar on hypothalamic cell numbers when they occur either during gestation or during gestation and lactation. For example, offspring of HFD mothers cross-fostered with control mothers during lactation exhibit similar changes in orexigenic cell numbers and metabolic outcomes compared with pups raised by HFD mothers during pregnancy and lactation (Chang et al., 2008). Increased nutrition and growth, specifically during early postnatal life, also influences neural cell numbers in the hypothalamus and results in higher number of neurons that produce orexigenic neuropeptides (Plagemann et al., 1999c). In sharp contrast to perinatal overfeeding, maternal undernutrition is associated with a reduction in the number of orexigenic neurons (García et al., 2010). However, whether this change in neuronal cell numbers is the result of a reduction of neurogenesis and cell migration or an enhancement of programmed cell death remains to be investigated. The observation that the thickness of the neuroepithelium of the cortical plate is reduced in the fetuses of undernourished mothers supports the idea that maternal malnutrition may reduce cell proliferation during embryonic life (Gressens et al., 1997). Moreover, expression screening indicates that a maternal low protein diet downregulates various genes involved in brain development, including cell proliferation and differentiation genes (Coupe et al., 2010). Furthermore, astrocytogenesis, which directly follows the neurogenic period, is also affected by maternal diet. At weaning, the offspring of protein-restricted mothers have a reduced number of astrocytes and a reduction in the glia-to-neuron ratio (Plagemann et al., 2000). These findings are particularly interesting because of the reported role of glial cells in the development of the nervous system and in processes such as synaptic plasticity and synaptogenesis (see Lemke, 2001).

11.5.2 Determination of neuronal connectivity

Impaired organization of hypothalamic circuits is a common feature of nutritional malprogramming. In particular, perturbations in the establishment of ARC neural projections have been reported in virtually all animals subjected to nutritional insults during perinatal life (▶Tab. 11.3). However, the degree of alterations may differ depending on the nature of the nutritional insult. In both rodents and NHPs, the chronic consumption of an HFD during pregnancy induces a reduction in the density of ARC AgRP fibers that innervate the PVH (Grayson et al., 2010; Kirk et al., 2009). Similarly, maternal diabetes alone (i.e., without maternal obesity) causes a reduction in the density of arcuate orexigenic (AgRP)- and anorexigenic (aMSH)-containing fibers that innervate the PVH (Steculorum and Bouret, 2009). Moreover, maternal undernutrition affects the overall organization of hypothalamic neural projections (Coupe et al., 2010; Delahaye et al., 2008; Yura et al., 2005). Therefore, both a surfeit and a paucity of nutrition during gestation impair hypothalamic neural projections. This paradoxical observation is exemplified in animal models of chronic postnatal overnutrition and undernutrition. Animals raised in either small or large litters display a disruption of arcuate projections containing aMSH and AgRP peptides (Bouret et al., 2007). Moreover, in intrauterine growth-retarded animals, the timing of catch-up growth is an important determinant for postnatal hypothalamic development. Whereas early catch-up growth ameliorates the abnormal organization of hypothalamic pathways and is highly beneficial for markers of brain development, including markers of cell adhesion and axon elongation, late catch-up growth causes more detrimental neurodevelopmental effects in the hypothalamus (Coupe et al., 2010).

It is important to recognize that the nervous system, including the hypothalamus, continues to remodel and change not just early in development but throughout the entire period of development and even during adulthood in response to environmental influences and genetically programmed events. Consistent with this idea, recent data from Horvath and collaborators (2010) have shown a significant remodeling of synapses in obese-prone (DIO) rats, particularly in response to nutritional challenges. First, obese-prone DIO rats fed a chow diet display increased inhibitory inputs to POMC neurons compared to obesity-resistant (diet-resistant, DR) rats. Second, POMC neurons of obese-prone DIO rats exposed to an HFD lose synapses, whereas control (obesity-resistant) rats show an increase in POMC synaptic coverage (Horvath et al., 2010).

11.6 Developmental signals influencing the ultimate architecture of neuroendocrine feeding pathways

An important number of developmental signals control the ultimate architecture of hypothalamic feeding pathways. These signals can influence one or multiple components of hypothalamic development, including neurogenesis, axonal growth, and synaptogenesis. Among this array of signals, particular attention has been paid to the importance of hormones in hypothalamic development. A particular salient example is the role of leptin in hypothalamic development (for review see Bouret, 2010b; Udagawa et al., 2007). Recent data from our laboratory indicate that embryos that lack leptin (Lep^{ob}/Lep^{ob}) have a decrease in cell proliferation in the neuroepithelium of the third ventricle (Ishii et al., 2009), which is the embryonic brain structure that ultimately generates hypothalamic neurons. Consistent with these data, the number of neurons involved in feeding regulation, in particular POMC, orexin A, and MCH neurons, is reduced in the hypothalamus of Lep^{ob}/Lep^{ob} mice (Ishii et al., 2009). These observations are consistent with the finding that fetuses of HFD dams, which are hyperleptinemic, display an enhanced neurogenesis in the developing hypothalamus (Chang et al., 2008; Gupta et al., 2009). The organizational effects of leptin are not restricted to a cell number determination. Leptin also influences the strength of axonal projections of neuroendocrine systems that are involved in appetite regulation. One hypothalamic nucleus that has received a significant amount of attention with respect to the leptin influence on hypothalamic circuit development is the ARC. As noted previously, ARC neural projections develop primarily postnatally in rodents, and leptin is a required hormonal signal for the normal development of these pathways. Mice lacking leptin or leptin receptors show excessive reductions in the density of arcuate axons that innervate the PVH (Bouret et al., 2004b). Similarly, obese leptin receptor-deficient Zucker rats have a reduced density of AgRP-immunoreactive nerve fibers in the PVH (Bouret and Simerly, 2007). The magnitude of leptin levels during the first postnatal weeks is particularly important for the proper development of ARC axonal projections. Therefore, animals raised in SLs or animals born to obese dams show elevated postnatal leptin levels that are associated with the disrupted development of ARC projections (Bouret et al., 2007; Kirk et al., 2009). Similarly, animals raised in LLs or pups born to undernourished mothers exhibit blunted postnatal leptin levels that are also associated with perturbations in the development of ARC axonal projections (Bouret et al., 2007; Delahaye et al., 2008; Yura et al., 2005). Remarkably, daily leptin treatment during early postnatal life in pups born to undernourished dams normalizes their metabolic abnormalities (Vickers et al., 2005), which indicates that metabolic malprogramming is potentially reversible with leptin administration during specific phases of developmental plasticity. Leptin continues to remodel hypothalamic circuits not just early in development but throughout the entire life span. For example, the seminal work of Pinto and colleagues (2004) demonstrated a significant and rapid synaptic remodeling in the ARC of Lep^{ob}/Lep^{ob} mice in response to leptin injections during adult life.

In fact, a variety of hormones play orchestrated roles in the development of the neuroendocrine systems. For example, insulin has long been associated with brain development. Interestingly, a reduced number of arcuate neurons has been reported in the offspring of diabetic mothers, and this reduction of neuronal cell number is preventable by the normalization of glycemia using pancreatic islet transplantation (Franke et al., 2005). These key observations suggest that maternal insulin and/or glucose levels are critical for the proper determination of neuronal cell number in the hypothalamus. Correct insulin levels during early postnatal life also appear to be an important determinant for proper hypothalamic development. Cross-fostering experiments have shown that normal neonates raised by diabetic mothers during the lactating period have an alteration in the number of arcuate neurons (Fahrenkrog et al., 2004). Also, intra-hypothalamic hyperinsulinism induced experimentally during early postnatal life causes structural alterations in the hypothalamus and life-long metabolic dysregulation (Plagemann et al., 1992, 1999b). Neonatal insulin levels can not only determine hypothalamic neuronal cell numbers but also influence the number of astrocytes in the hypothalamus. Whereas hypoinsulinemic pups born to protein-restricted dams display a reduction in the number of astrocytes (Plagemann et al., 2000), the offspring of diabetic mothers have increased insulin levels that are associated with an increase in the numbers of astrocytes (Plagemann et al., 1992, 1999a). The observation that insulin simulates glial fibrillary acidic protein (GFAP) expression further supports a role for this hormone in astrocyte development and function (Toran-Allerand et al., 1991). In addition, insulin is an important axonotrophic factor. The incubation of hypothalamic explants in vitro with insulin causes neurite extension (Toran-Allerand et al., 1988). Furthermore, in vivo experiments indicate that insulin acts in synapse development (Kessler et al., 1984), which suggests a role for insulin in synaptogenesis. Other hormones, such as ghrelin and corticosterone, also have organizational effects on hypothalamic neural circuits by modulating the synaptic inputs of arcuate POMC and NPY neurons in adult mice (Gyengesi et al., 2010; Pinto et al., 2004).

11.7 Perspectives and conclusions

It is now clear from several different fields of research that the disruption of neurodevelopmental processes can lead to diseases later in life. The current stage of knowledge of neuroendocrine programming is probably just the tip of the iceberg considering the important potential for this emerging field and the complexity of hypothalamic development. A comprehensive understanding of perinatally acquired obesity will require a map of the neuroendocrine system's intricate wiring diagram, the breakdown of which will ultimately be responsible for the emergence of a particular metabolic phenotype. A better understanding of how neuroendocrine pathways develop under a particular intrauterine and/or extrauterine environment is also critical for the development of interventional studies to ameliorate and hopefully reverse the metabolic malprogramming of the fetus and/or neonate.

References

Altman J, Bayer SA. The development of the rat hypothalamus. *Adv Anat Embryol Cell Biol* 1986;100: 1–178.

Beck B, Kozak R, Moar KM, Mercer JG. Hypothalamic orexigenic peptides are overexpressed in young Long-Evans rats after early life exposure to fat-rich diets. *Biochem Biophys Res Commun* 2006;342: 452–8.

Berthoud HR. Homeostatic and non-homeostatic pathways involved in the control of food intake and energy balance. *Obesity* 2006;14: 197S–200S.

Bouret SG, Draper SJ, Simerly RB. Formation of projection pathways from the arcuate nucleus of the hypothalamus to hypothalamic regions implicated in the neural control of feeding behavior in mice. *J Neurosci* 2004a;24: 2797–805.

Bouret SG, Draper SJ, Simerly RB. Trophic action of leptin on hypothalamic neurons that regulate feeding. *Science* 2004b;304: 108–10.

Bouret SG, Burt-Solorzano C, Wang CH, Simerly RB. Impact of neonatal nutrition on development of brain metabolic circuits in mice. Proc of the 37th Annual Meeting The Society For Neuroscience, San Diego, CA. 2007.

Bouret S, Simerly RB. Development of leptin-sensitive circuits. *J Neuroendocrinology* 2007;19: 575–82.

Bouret SG, Gorski JN, Patterson, CM, Chen, S, Levin, BE, Simerly RB. Hypothalamic neural projections are permanently disrupted in diet-induced obese rats. *Cell Metabolism* 2008;7: 179–85.

Bouret SG. Development of hypothalamic neural networks controlling appetite. *Forum Nutr* 2010a;63: 84–93.

Bouret SG. Neurodevelopmental actions of leptin. *Brain Research* 2010b;350: 2–9.

Chang GQ, Gaysinskaya V, Karatayev O, Leibowitz SF. Maternal high-fat diet and fetal programming: increased proliferation of hypothalamic peptide-producing neurons that increase risk for overeating and obesity. *J Neurosci* 2008;28: 12107–19.

Chen H, Simar D, Lambert K, Mercier J, Morris, MJ. Maternal and postnatal overnutrition differentially impact appetite regulators and fuel metabolism. *Endocrinology* 2008;149: 5348–56.

Chen H, Simar D, Morris MJ. Hypothalamic neuroendocrine circuitry is programmed by maternal obesity: interaction with postnatal nutritional environment. *PLoS ONE* 2009;4: e6259.

Clegg DJ, Benoit SC, Reed JA, Woods SC, Dunn-Meynell A, Levin BE. Reduced anorexic effects of insulin in obesity-prone rats fed a moderate-fat diet. *Am J Physiol Regul Integr Comp Physiol* 2005;288: R981–6.

Coupe B, Grit I, Darmann D, Parnet P. The timing of "catch-up growth" affects metabolism and appetite regulation in male rats born with intrauterine growth restriction. *Am J Physiol Regul Integr Comp Physiol* 2009;297: R813–24.

Coupe B, Amarger V, Grit I, Benani A, Parnet P. Nutritional programming affects hypothalamic organization and early response to leptin. *Endocrinology* 2010;151: 702–13.

Cripps RL, Martin Äëgronert MS, Archer ZA, Hales CN, Mercer JG, Ozanne SE. Programming of hypothalamic neuropeptide gene expression in rats by maternal dietary protein content during pregnancy and lactation. *Clin Sci* 2009;117: 85–93.

Davidowa H, Plagemann A. Decreased inhibition by leptin of hypothalamic arcuate neurons in neonatally overfed young rats. *Neuroreport* 2000;11: 2795–8.

Davidowa H, Li Y, Plagemann A. Altered responses to orexigenic (AGRP, MCH) and anorexigenic (a-MSH, CART) neuropeptides of paraventricular hypothalamic neurons in early postnatally overfed rats. *Eur J Neurosci* 2003;18: 613–21.

Davidowa H, Plagemann A. Insulin resistance of hypothalamic arcuate neurons in neonatally overfed rats. *Neuroreport* 2007;18: 521–4.

Delahaye F, Breton C, Risold PY, et al. Maternal perinatal undernutrition drastically reduces post-natal leptin surge and affects the development of arcuate nucleus proopiomelanocortin neurons in neonatal male rat pups. *Endocrinology* 2008;149: 470–5.

Desai M, Gayle D, Han G, Ross MG. Programmed hyperphagia due to reduced anorexigenic mechanisms in intrauterine growth-restricted offspring. *Reprod Sci* 2007;14: 329–37.

Ebbeling CB, Pawlak DB, Ludwig DS. Childhood obesity: public-health crisis, common sense cure. *Lancet* 2002;360: 473–82.

Elmquist JK, Coppari R, Balthasar N, Ichinose M, Lowell BB. Identifying hypothalamic pathways controlling food intake, body weight, and glucose homeostasis. *J Comp Neurol* 2005;493: 63–71.

Enriori PJ, Evans AE, Sinnayah P, Cowley MA. Leptin resistance and obesity. *Obesity* 2006;14: 254S–8.

Fahrenkrog S, Harder T, Stolaczyk E, et al. Cross-fostering to diabetic rat dams affects early develop-ment of mediobasal hypothalamic nuclei regulating food intake, body weight, and metabolism. *J Nutr* 2004;134: 648–54.

Franke K, Harder T, Aerts L, et al. "Programming" of orexigenic and anorexigenic hypothalamic neurons in offspring of treated and untreated diabetic mother rats. *Brain Res* 2005;1031: 276–83.

García AP, Palou M, Priego T, Sánchez J, Palou A, Picó C. Moderate caloric restriction during gesta-tion results in lower arcuate nucleus NPY- and alpha MSH-neurons and impairs hypothalamic response to fed/fasting conditions in weaned rats. *Diabetes Obes Metab* 2010;12: 403–13.

Glavas MM, Kirigiti MA, Xiao XQ, et al. Early overnutrition results in early-onset arcuate leptin resistance and increased sensitivity to high-fat diet. *Endocrinology* 2010;151: 1598–610.

Godfrey KM, Gluckman PD, Hanson MA. Developmental origins of metabolic disease: life course and intergenerational perspectives. *Trends Endocr Metab* 2010;21: 199–205.

Gorski JN, Dunn-Meynell AA, Levin BE. Maternal obesity increases hypothalamic leptin receptor expression and sensitivity in juvenile obesity-prone rats. *Am J Physiol Regul Integr Comp Physiol* 2007;292: R1782–91.

Grayson BE, Allen SE, Billes SK, Williams SM, Smith MS, Grove KL. Prenatal development of hypothalamic neuropeptide systems in the nonhuman primate. *Neuroscience* 2006;143: 975–86.

Grayson BE, Levasseur PR, Williams SM, Smith MS, Marks DL, Grove KL. Changes in melanocortin expression and inflammatory pathways in fetal offspring of nonhuman primates fed a high-fat diet. *Endocrinology* 2010;151: 1622–32.

Gressens P, Muaku SM, Besse L, et al. Maternal protein restriction early in rat pregnancy alters brain development in the progeny. *Dev Brain Res* 1997;103: 21–35.

Grove KL, Allen S, Grayson BE, Smith MS. Postnatal development of the hypothalamic neuropep-tide Y system. *Neuroscience* 2003;116: 393–406.

Gupta A, Srinivasan M, Thamadilok S, Patel MS. Hypothalamic alterations in fetuses of high fat diet-fed obese female rats. *J Endocrinol* 2009;200: 293–300.

Gyengesi E, Liu ZW, D'agostino G, et al. Corticosterone regulates synaptic input organization of POMC and NPY/AgRP neurons in adult mice. *Endocrinology* 2010;151: 5395–402.

Hiremagalur BK, Vadlamudi S, Johanning GL, Patel MS. Long-term effects of feeding high carbo-hydrate diet in pre-weaning period by gastrostomy: a new rat model for obesity. *Int J Obes Relat Metab Disord* 1993;17: 495–502.

Horvath TL, Sarman B, García-Cáceres C, et al. Synaptic input organization of the melanocortin system predicts diet-induced hypothalamic reactive gliosis and obesity. *Proc Natl Acad Sci USA* 2010;107: 14875–80.

Irani BG, Dunn-Meynell AA, Levin BE. Altered hypothalamic leptin, insulin, and melanocortin binding associated with moderate-fat diet and predisposition to obesity. *Endocrinology* 2007;148: 310–6.

Ishii Y, Gibbons MB, Bouret SG. Neurogenic actions of leptin on hypothalamic structures involved in feeding regulation. Proc of the 39th Annual Meeting of The Society For Neuroscience, Chicago, IL. 2009.

Kessler JA, Spray DC, Saez JC, Bennett MV. Determination of synaptic phenotype: insulin and cAMP independently initiate development of electrotonic coupling between cultured sympathetic neurons. *Proc Natl Acad Sci USA* 1984;81: 6235–9.

Kirk SL, Samuelsson AM, Argenton M, et al. Maternal obesity induced by diet in rats permanently influences central processes regulating food intake in offspring. *PLoS ONE* 2009;4: e5870.

Lemke G. Glial control of neuronal development. *Annu Rev Neurosci* 2001;24: 87–105.

Levin B. Metabolic imprinting: critical impact of the perinatal environment on the regulation of energy homeostasis. *Phil Trans R Soc Lond B* 2006;361: 1107–21.

Levin BE, Dunn-Meynell AA, Balkan B, Keesey RE. Selective breeding for diet-induced obesity and resistance in Sprague-Dawley rats. *Am J Physiol Regul Integr Comp Physiol* 1997;273: R725–30.

Levin BE, Dunn-Meynell AA. Reduced central leptin sensitivity in rats with diet-induced obesity. *Am J Physiol Regul Integr Comp Physiol* 2002;283: R941–8.

Levin BE, Dunn-Meynell AA, Ricci MR, Cummings DE. Abnormalities of leptin and ghrelin regulation in obesity-prone juvenile rats. *Am J Physiol Endocrinol Metab* 2003;285: E949–57.

Levin BE, Dunn-Meynell AA, Banks WA. Obesity-prone rats have normal blood-brain barrier transport but defective central leptin signaling before obesity onset. *Am J Physiol Regul Integr Comp Physiol* 2004;286: R143–50.

Levin BE, Govek E. Gestational obesity accentuates obesity in obesity-prone progeny. *Am J Physiol* 1998;275: R1374–9.

López M, Seoane LM, Tovar S, et al. A possible role of neuropeptide Y, agouti-related protein and leptin receptor isoforms in hypothalamic programming by perinatal feeding in the rat. *Diabetologia* 2005;48: 140–8.

Manuel-Apolinar L, Zarate A, Rocha L, Hernández M. Fetal malnutrition affects hypothalamic leptin receptor expression after birth in male mice. *Arch Med Res* 2010;41: 240–5.

Markakis EA. Development of the neuroendocrine hypothalamus. *Front Neuroendocrinol* 2002;23: 257–91.

Matsumoto A, Arai Y. Developmental changes in synaptic formation in the hypothalamic arcuate nucleus of female rats. *Cell Tissue Res* 1976;14: 143–56.

McClellana KM, Parker KL, Tobet SA. Development of the ventromedial nucleus of the hypothalamus. *Frontiers in Neuroendocrinology* 2006;27: 193–209.

McCurdy CE, Bishop JM, Williams SM, et al. Maternal high-fat diet triggers lipotoxicity in the fetal livers of nonhuman primates. *J Clin Invest* 2009;119: 323–35.

McMillen IC, Robinson JS. Developmental origins of the metabolic syndrome: prediction, plasticity, and programming. *Physiol Rev* 2005;85: 571–633.

Melnick I, Pronchuck N, Cowley MA, Grove KL, Colmers WF. Developmental switch in neuropeptide Y and melanocortin effects in the paraventricular nucleus of the hypothalamus. *Neuron* 2007;56: 1103–15.

Morris MJ, Chen H. Established maternal obesity in the rat reprograms hypothalamic appetite regulators and leptin signaling at birth. *Int J Obes* 2009;33: 115–22.

Myers MG, Cowley MA, Munzberg H. Mechanisms of leptin action and leptin resistance. *Ann Rev Physiol* 2008;70: 537–56.

Myers MG, Jr, Münzberg H, Leinninger GM, Leshan RL. The geometry of leptin action in the brain: more complicated than a simple ARC. *Cell Metab* 2009;9: 117–23.

Nilsson I, Johansen JE, Schalling M, Hokfelt T, Fetissov SO. Maturation of the hypothalamic arcuate agouti-related protein system during postnatal development in the mouse. *Dev Brain Res* 2005;155: 147–54.

Padilla SL, Carmody JS, Zeltser LM. Pomc-expressing progenitors give rise to antagonistic neuronal populations in hypothalamic feeding circuits. *Nature Med* 2010;16: 403–5.

Pinto S, Roseberry AG, Liu H, et al. Rapid rewiring of arcuate nucleus feeding circuits by leptin. *Science* 2004;304: 110–5.

Plagemann A, Heidrich I, Götz F, Rohde W, Dörner G. Lifelong enhanced diabetes susceptibility and obesity after temporary intrahypothalamic hyperinsulinism during brain organization. *Exp Clin Endocrinol* 1992;99: 91–5.

Plagemann A, Harder T, Rake A, et al. Hypothalamic insulin and neuropeptide Y in the offspring of gestational diabetic mother rats. *Neuroreport* 1998;9: 4069–73.

Plagemann A, Harder T, Janert U, et al. Malformations of hypothalamic nuclei in hyperinsulinemic offspring of rats with gestational diabetes. *Dev Neurosci* 1999a;21: 58–67.

Plagemann A, Harder T, Rake A, et al. Morphological alterations of hypothalamic nuclei due to intrahypothalamic hyperinsulinism in newborn rats. *Int J Dev Neurosci* 1999b;17: 37–44.

Plagemann A, Harder T, Rake A, et al. Observations on the orexigenic hypothalamic neuropeptide Y-system in neonatally overfed weanling rats. *J Neuroendocrinol* 1999c;11: 541–6.

Plagemann A, Harder T, Rake A, Melchior K, Rohde W, Dörner, GN. Hypothalamic nuclei are malformed in weanling offspring of low protein malnourished rat dams. *J Nutr* 2000;130: 2582–9.

Plagemann A. Perinatal nutrition and hormone-dependent programming of food intake. *Horm Res* 2006;65: 83–9.

Remmers F, Verhagen LA, Adan RA, Delemarre-van de Waal HA. Hypothalamic neuropeptide expression of juvenile and middle-aged rats after early postnatal food restriction. *Endocrinology* 2008;149: 3617–25.

Ricci MR, Levin BE. Ontogeny of diet-induced obesity in selectively bred Sprague-Dawley rats. *Am J Physiol Regul Integr Comp Physiol* 2003;285: R610–8.

Saper C, Chou T, Elmquist JK. The need to feed: homeostatic and hedonic control of eating. *Neuron* 2002;36: 199–211.

Sawchenko PE. Toward a new neurobiology of energy balance, appetite, and obesity: the anatomists weigh in. *J Comp Neurol* 1998;402: 435–41.

Serdula MK, Ivery D, Coates RJ, Freedman DS, Williamson DF, Byers T. Do obese children become obese adults? A review of the literature. *Prev Med* 1993;22: 167–77.

Srinivasan M, Mitrani P, Sadhanandan G, et al. A high-carbohydrate diet in the immediate postnatal life of rats induces adaptations predisposing to adult-onset obesity. *J Endocrinol* 2008;197: 565–74.

Steculorum SM, Bouret SG. Maternal diabetes compromises organization of hypothalamic neural projections and induces leptin resistance in the offspring. Proc of the 39th Annual Meeting of The Society For Neuroscience, Washington, DC. 2009.

Sullivan EL, Grove KL. Metabolic imprinting in obesity. *Forum Nutr* 2010;63: 186–94.

Terroni PL, Anthony FW, Hanson MA, Cagampang FR. Expression of agouti-related peptide, neuropeptide Y, pro-opiomelanocortin and the leptin receptor isoforms in fetal mouse brain from pregnant dams on a protein-restricted diet. *Brain Res* 2005;140: 111–5.

Toran-Allerand CD, Ellis L, Pfenninger KH. Estrogen and insulin synergism in neurite growth enhancement in vitro: mediation of steroid effects by interactions with growth factors? *Dev Brain Res* 1988;41: 87–100.

Toran-Allerand CD, Bentham W, Miranda RC, Anderson JP. Insulin influences astroglial morphology and glial fibrillary acidic protein (GFAP) expression in organotypic cultures. *Brain Res* 1991;558: 296–304.

Udagawa J, Hatta T, Hashimoto R, Otani H. Roles of leptin in prenatal and perinatal brain development. *Congenit Anom* (Kyoto) 2007;47: 77–83.

Vickers MH, Breier BH, Cutfield WS, Hofman PL, Gluckman PD. Fetal origins of hyperphagia, obesity, and hypertension and postnatal amplification by hypercaloric nutrition. *Am J Physiol Endocrinol Metab* 2000;279: E83–7.

Vickers MH, Gluckman PD, Coveny AH, et al. Neonatal leptin treatment reverses developmental programming. *Endocrinology* 2005;146: 4211–6.

Wang Y, Beydoun MA, Liang L, Caballero B, Kumanyika SK. Will all Americans become overweight or obese? Estimating the progression and cost of the US obesity epidemic. *Obesity* 2008;16: 2323–30.

Whitaker RC, Wright JA, Pepe MS, Seidel KD, Dietz WH. Predicting obesity in young adulthood from childhood and parental obesity. *N Engl J Med* 1997;337: 869–73.

Yura S, Itoh H, Sagawa N, et al. Role of premature leptin surge in obesity resulting from intrauterine undernutrition. *Cell Metabolism* 2005;1: 371–8.

12 Genetic influences on the long-term effects of the perinatal environment on energy homeostasis and offspring obesity

Barry E. Levin

Much of human obesity is inherited as a polygenic disorder which can then be influenced by perinatal factors. In rodents, perinatal manipulations can have a major impact on the development of neural systems that regulate energy homeostasis, i.e. the balance among energy intake, expenditure and storage. To assess gene-environment interactions, we selectively bred rats to develop diet-induced obesity (DIO) or to be diet-resistant (DR) when fed a high fat diet. Maternal obesity throughout gestation and lactation in DIO, but not DR dams augments the development of obesity in their offspring. However, if DR neonates are fostered to obese DIO dams, they do become obese on high fat diet possibly due to high insulin levels in the milk of obese DIO dams. Importantly, alterations of the early postnatal and pre-pubertal environments can also have major, long-term effects on the development neural pathways and the sensitivity to hormones involved in the regulation of energy homeostasis. Although the development of these pathways differs temporally between humans and rodents, animal models offer the potential for identifying factors in the perinatal environment that might become therapeutic targets to prevent the development of obesity in genetically predisposed individuals. More importantly, such models might provide clues for the prevention of obesity as primary goal for stemming the obesity epidemic.

12.1 Introduction

The idea that the perinatal nutritional environment can affect the metabolic status of offspring arose from epidemiological studies in offspring of mothers who were exposed to gestational undernutrition during the famine that followed World War II in Holland (Ravelli and Belmont, 1979; Ravelli et al., 1976; Ravelli et al., 1998; Stein et al., 1995) and Germany (Dorner, 1973). Although the results varied with regard to outcome, these and other studies (Barker, 1995; Barker, 1998) suggested that undernutrition during various stages of gestation is associated with an increased risk of adverse metabolic outcomes in offspring. These include obesity, diabetes, hypertension, stroke and other metabolic outcomes (Gillman et al., 2001; O'Tierney et al., 2009; Plagemann et al., 2002; Ravelli et al., 2000). However, as might be expected from a heterogeneous population, such outcomes vary considerably. This is not surprising with regard to obesity since almost 70% of human obesity is inherited as a polygenic trait (Bouchard and Tremblay, 1990; Stunkard et al., 1986) and the most common forms of human obesity arise from the interactions of multiple genes, environmental factors, and behavior (Comuzzie and

Allison, 1998). Thus, different long-term outcomes would be expected in offspring depending upon the interaction of their perinatal environment and genetic backgrounds.

In addition to gestational undernutrition, maternal obesity can also predispose to offspring obesity. Although it is known that parental obesity has a high correlation with offspring obesity (Maffeis et al., 1994; Schaefer-Graf et al., 2005), the inability to identify individual obesity-prone humans accurately before they become obese makes interpretation of such data difficult with regard to the role of environment x gene interactions. Finally, although strides have been made with sophisticated imaging techniques to link obesity with altered brain function (Baicy et al., 2007; Batterham et al., 2007; Del Parigi et al., 2002; Farooqi et al., 2007; Matsuda et al., 1999; Wang et al., 2001), these techniques still lack sufficient resolution to assess the function of complex brain regions that regulate energy homeostasis such as the hypothalamus and brainstem. Thus, many of the advances in our understanding of how genotype interacts with the brain – body-external environment interface to alter the regulation of energy homeostasis in offspring have utilized animal models. These interactions are the subject of this review with a specific focus on the perinatal and pre-pubescent periods since this is the time during which the development of these systems are highly susceptible to environmental perturbations.

12.2 Neural control of energy homeostasis

Energy homeostasis is the balance between intake and expenditure, where adipose depots act as the buffer for any imbalance between the two. The regulation of energy homeostasis reflects an ongoing dialogue among the internal and external environments and the brain. The brain senses and integrates a multitude of hormonal, metabolic and hard wired neural signals from peripheral sensors and organs to regulate both the control of individual meals and the long-term balance between intake and expenditure. Leptin, which is produced by adipose depots in proportion to their size, acts as the prototypic signal for informing the brain as to the status of peripheral adipose stores (Zhang et al., 1994). As depot size increases due to energy excess, leptin levels increase to provide a tonic, negative feedback on anabolic, and a positive feedback on catabolic neural circuits. Insulin, although produced by the pancreas, indirectly reflects adipose levels (Bagdade et al., 1967; Polonsky et al., 1988) and acts as an additional long-term negative feedback signal. A variety of gut neuropeptides are produced in response to both pre- and postingestive factors to modulate short-term regulation of individual meals (Shin et al., 2009). Many of these peptides are sensed by vagal and sympathetic afferents which terminate in critical brainstem areas (Shin et al., 2009). In addition, peripheral metabolic substrates such as glucose, fatty acids, ketone bodies and lactate, as well as cytokines, signal the brain via these same autonomic afferents, as well as by direct transport across the blood-brain barrier (Levin, 2006; Levin et al., 2004b; Patterson and Levin, 2008). These signals are sensed and integrated by a distributed network of "metabolic sensing" neurons located in discrete areas throughout the brain. These include critical hypothalamic nuclei such as the arcuate (ARC) and ventromedial (VMN) nuclei (Levin, 2006; Levin et al., 2004b; Patterson and Levin, 2008). The integrated signals from this network are relayed to neuroendocrine and autonomic output areas of the hypothalamus (paraventricular nucleus (PVN) and lateral hypothalamic area (LHA)) and hindbrain. In addition, neurons in areas of the brain involved in motivation, reward and memory are engaged by many of the same afferent signals from the periphery (Levin, 2006; Levin et al., 2004b; Patterson and Levin, 2008).

12.3 Development of neural systems controlling energy homeostasis

Progenitor cells arise in a number of sites throughout the nervous system and differentiate during development into glial and neural elements. In the hypothalamus, new neuron formation (neurogenesis) takes place in the neuroepithelial lining of the third cerebral ventricle from which they migrate to their final destination (Altman and Bayer, 1978; Cottrell et al., 2009; Kokoeva et al., 2005; Kokoeva et al., 2007; Xu et al., 2005). At this point, neurons send out axons to their target areas. Neurons whose axons that form functional target connections survive and those that do not undergo apoptotic cell death (Botchkina and Morin, 1995; Fujioka et al., 1999). While there are many similarities, there are critical differences in the temporal patterns of central nervous system development between humans and rodents. For example, whereas the human hypothalamus is completely developed at birth (Ackland et al., 1983; Bugnon et al., 1982; Burford and Robinson, 1982; Koutcherov et al., 2002; Mai et al., 1997), most rodent hypothalamic neurons are born during late gestation (Markakis, 2002) but ARC projections to the PVN are not completed until postnatal day (P)12–14 in rodents (Bouret et al., 2004a; Grove et al., 2003; Grove and Smith, 2003). Also, while some hypothalamic neurogenesis continues into early postnatal, and, in some cases, adult life in rodents (Cottrell et al., 2009; Kokoeva et al., 2005; Kokoeva et al., 2007), it is unknown whether similar continued neurogenesis occurs in humans. Finally, other brain areas also undergo different temporal patterns of this developmental sequence and these patterns are different in human vs. rodent brains.

Regardless of the temporal sequences, there are numerous factors that can influence neural development. Importantly, both leptin and insulin can affect the migration (Udagawa et al., 2006), survival (neurotropic) and process outgrowth (neurotrophic) of developing neurons (Bouret et al., 2004b; Bouret et al., 2008; Puro and Agardh, 1984; Recio-Pinto et al., 1984; Tanaka et al., 1995; Udagawa et al., 2006). Rodents with deficient leptin signaling have abnormal development of ARC-PVN axonal projections of anabolic neuropeptide Y (NPY/ agouti-related peptide (AgRP) and catabolic proopiomelanocortin (POMC) neurons involved in the regulation of energy homeostasis (Bouret et al., 2004b; Bouret et al., 2008). On the other hand, injection of insulin into the dam during the last week of gestation (Jones and Dayries, 1990; Jones et al., 1995; Jones et al., 1996) or directly into the hypothalamus on or before P8, produces obesity and associated alterations in hypothalamic development (Plagemann et al., 1992; Plagemann et al., 1999b). Thus, during early development, leptin and insulin play a primary role in neural development. Later, their primary roles involve the regulation of metabolic function and energy homeostasis.

12.4 Gene x environment interactions in the development of obesity

Both maternal undernutrition (caloric or protein) or obesity, as well as offspring overnutrition can lead to obesity and/or diabetes in adult offspring of both humans and rodents (Buckley et al., 2005; Faust et al., 1980; Fernandez-Twinn et al., 2004; Guo and Jen, 1995; Jones and Friedman, 1982; Jones et al., 1984; Jones et al., 1986; Kennedy, 1957; Levin et al., 2005; Ozanne et al., 2004; Ravelli et al., 1998; Ravelli et al., 1999; Samuelsson et al., 2008). In rodents, such perinatal environmental manipulations have lasting effects on the development and function of hypothalamic pathways and systems involved in the regulation of energy homeostasis (Cripps et al., 2009; Gorski et al., 2006; Heidel et al., 1999; Irani et al., 2009; Jones et al., 1995; Le Foll et al., 2009; Levin and Dunn-Meynell, 2002; Plagemann et al., 1998a; Plagemann et al., 1998b; Plagemann et al., 1999a). With the exception of one rodent study (Reifsnyder et al., 2000), most others were carried out either retrospectively in humans or in animal models where genetic predispositions towards obesity were not considered. This lack of such gene x environment interaction studies first led us to develop substrains of rats which we selectively bred for their propensity to develop diet-induced obesity (DIO) or to be diet-resistant (DR) when fed a 31%, 25% sucrose high energy (HE) diet (Levin et al., 1997). The resulting phenotypic traits have been remarkably stable due to their polygenic mode of inheritance (Levin et al., 2003a). The obesity of DIO rats occurs only after exposure to diets similar to the HE diet. This obesity is associated with hyperphagia, insulin resistance, hypertension and hyperlipidemia (Ricci and Levin, 2003). Thus, this rat strain has many of the characteristics of a polygenically inherited metabolic syndrome seen in a majority of obese humans (Bouchard and Perusse, 1993; Stunkard et al., 1986).

Importantly, selectively bred DIO rats have an early postnatal resistance to the behavioral and physiological effects of leptin on neural development and energy homeostasis. By P10 they have reduced signaling downstream of the long, signaling form of the leptin receptor (Lepr-b) in the ARC (Bouret et al., 2008). Before they become obese they have reduced Lepr-b gene expression (Levin et al., 2003b; Levin et al., 2004a), binding of leptin to its receptor (Irani et al., 2007) and the excitatory effects of leptin on their ARC and/or VMN neurons (Irani et al., 2009). These early postnatal molecular and cellular aspects of leptin resistance are associated with a reduced trophic effect on the outgrowth of ARC-PVN AgRP and alpha-MSH axonal projections (Bouret et al., 2008). In the VMN, they also have reduced dendritic arborizations (Labelle et al., 2009) and numbers of neurons (Levin, 1996) and sensitivity to the effects of glucose and fatty acids (Le Foll et al., 2009). After weaning, leptin resistance in non-obese DIO rats is associated with reduced anorectic and thermogenic effects of leptin as compared to DR rats (Gorski et al., 2007). In addition to this inherent leptin resistance, DIO rats have both reduced ARC binding of insulin to its receptors (Irani et al., 2009) and a reduced anorectic response to centrally administered insulin (Clegg et al., 2005). DIO rats also have altered hypothalamic norepinephrine, dopamine and serotonin function before they become obese (Hassanain and Levin, 2002; Levin, 1995; Levin, 1996; Wilmot et al., 1988).

Using this model, we showed that making DIO dams obese during gestation and lactation caused their adult offspring to become obese and insulin resistant when fed only a low fat diet and further accentuated their obesity when placed on HE diet (Levin and Govek, 1998). In addition, these offspring had fewer PVN norepinephrine reuptake transporters (Levin and Dunn-Meynell, 2002). Since these transporters remove norepinephrine from the synapse and since PVN norepinephrine infusions cause hyperphagia and obesity (Leibowitz et al., 1984), the reduced complement of PVN transporters in offspring of obese DIO dams would be predicted to increase PVN NE levels and to increase their adiposity. On the other hand, neither maternal intake of HE diet nor obesity during gestation and lactation caused DR offspring to become obese (Levin and Govek, 1998). These studies show the critical importance of gene x environment interactions in determining the obesity phenotype of offspring.

These interactions also affect the sensitivity to leptin and metabolic substrates on metabolic sensing neurons in the hypothalamus. Offspring of lean DIO dams have fewer VMN neurons that are excited and more that are inhibited by leptin than do offspring of lean DR dams. Maternal intake of HE diet during gestation and lactation reduces the number of leptin-excited neurons in both DIO and DR offspring but has a much greater inhibitory effect on neurons from offspring of obese DIO dams (Irani et al., 2009). The VMN is also enriched in metabolic sensing neurons which respond to both glucose and long chain fatty acids. Whereas offspring of lean DIO dams have two fold more VMN neurons that are inhibited by glucose (GI neurons) than do those of lean DR dams, this difference is eliminated in offspring of obese DIO dams (Le Foll et al., 2009). Similarly, while offspring of lean DIO dams have more GI neurons that are either excited or inhibited by oleic acid than do lean DR offspring, maternal obesity exaggerates this difference in offspring of obese DIO dams (Le Foll et al., 2009). Thus, VMN neurons in DIO rats are generally less responsive to both hormonal and metabolic signals from the periphery than are those from DR rats and this difference is exaggerated by maternal intake of HE diet and the development of obesity in DIO dams.

Since a great deal of hypothalamic development occurs postnatally in rodents (Bouret and Simerly, 2007), manipulation of the postnatal environment can have major effects on this development in genetically predisposed animals. Cross-fostering obesity-resistant DR pups to obese (but not lean) DIO dams causes them to become obese and insulin resistant when fed HE diet as adults (Gorski et al., 2006). Their obesity is associated with an anabolic profile in their hypothalamus (increased ARC AgRP and decreased VMN Lepr-b and insulin receptor mRNA expression) (Gorski et al., 2006). This adverse effect of fostering DR pups to obese DIO dams may be due to the high insulin levels present in their milk (Gorski et al., 2006) since rat pups absorb insulin from milk during the early postnatal period (Koldovsky et al., 1995; Sanchez et al., 2005) and increasing hypothalamic insulin levels during this period causes obesity in adult offspring (Plagemann et al., 1992). Unfortunately, while DR rats can be made more obese by raising them in an obesogenic environment, the opposite is not true. Fostering offspring of either lean or obese DIO dams to DR dams does not prevent their development of obesity when they are later exposed to HE diet (Gorski et al., 2006). Thus, these studies demonstrate a potent, genotype-specific effect of the postnatal environment on altering the phenotype of offspring.

Even though most postnatal hypothalamic development is thought to be completed during the first 2 weeks of life (Bouret and Simerly, 2007), it is likely that both hypothalamic and other brain area development continues over longer postnatal periods (Burnett et al., 2009; Ellgren et al., 2008; Kim et al., 2009; Kokoeva et al., 2005; Kokoeva et al., 2007; Lehmann et al., 2009). Although exercise causes weight loss in obese adult male rodents, (Levin and Dunn-Meynell, 2004; Levin and Dunn-Meynell, 2006; Mayer et al., 1954), they regain their lost weight as soon as exercise ceases (Applegate et al., 1984). In light of the continued brain development during early life, we hypothesized that beginning exercise prior to puberty might have a persistent effect on lowering body weight in DIO rats. Thus, when male DIO rats were fed HE diet and given access to a running wheel for only three weeks, beginning at four weeks of age, they gained less weight than sedentary DIO rats. Moreover, when the wheels were removed, they maintained their lower body weight and adiposity for up to two and a half months (Patterson et al., 2008). Their obesity resistance was associated with an increased sensitivity to the anorectic effects of leptin and increased binding of leptin and signaling downstream of the leptin receptor in the ARC (Patterson et al., 2009). Unexpectedly, although this early onset exercise did not correct the defective development of the ARC-PVN pathways of exercising DIO rats, caloric restriction during this same period further decreased the density of ARC axons in the PVN in association with increased weight gain above that seen in sedentary rats when ad libitum food intake was restored (Patterson et al., 2008). Thus, interventions begun as late as weaning, but prior to puberty onset, can have long lasting positive or negative effects on brain function and structure and body weight gain phenotype in genetically obese DIO rats.

12.5 Summary and conclusions

Once it develops, only surgical intervention has proven effective as a treatment for obesity in humans. For that reason, prevention is the best strategy to fight the world-wide epidemic of obesity. Because energy homeostasis is regulated by the brain and because the development of neural systems that regulate energy homeostasis are affected by a number of perinatal and early pre-pubertal interventions, this developmental period provides a potential time window for identification of factors that might prevent the development of obesity. Since human obesity has a strong underlying genetic predisposition, a focus on gene x environment interactions in surrogate rodent models is a reasonable approach to identifying potential preventive strategies. Of course, to apply lessons learned from such animal models would require that we prospectively be able to identify humans who are at high risk for becoming obese. Thus, research in this field should also focus on early identification of common traits shared by obesity-prone animal models and humans and on factors that alter the likelihood that such individuals will become obese. Our studies suggest that a profitable area for exploration is the identification of specific factors produced by alterations of the perinatal nutritional and metabolic environments and physiological interventions such as exercise that increase the inhibitory feedback of signals such as leptin as a strategy for producing pharmacological interventions to prevent and/or treat early onset obesity.

References

Ackland J, Ratter S, Bourne GL, Rees LH. Characterisation of immunoreactive somatostatin in human fetal hypothalamic tissue. *Regul Pept* 1983;5: 95–101.

Altman J, Bayer SA. Development of the diencephalon in the rat. III. Ontogeny of the specialized ventricular linings of the hypothalamic third ventricle. *J Comp Neurol* 1978;182: 995–1015.

Applegate EA, Upton DE, Stern JS. Exercise and detraining: effect on food intake, adiposity and lipogenesis in Osborne-Mendel rats made obese by a high fat diet. *J Nutr* 1984;114: 447–59.

Bagdade JD, Bierman EL, Porte D Jr. The significance of basal insulin levels in the evaluation of the insulin response to glucose in diabetic and nondiabetic subjects. *J Clin Invest* 1967;46: 1549–57.

Baicy K, London ED, Monterosso J, Wong ML, Delibasi T, Sharma A, Licinio J. Leptin replacement alters brain response to food cues in genetically leptin-deficient adults. *Proc Natl Acad Sci U S A* 2007;104: 18276–9.

Barker DJ. The Wellcome Foundation Lecture, 1994. The fetal origins of adult disease. *Proc Royal Soc Lond* 1995;262: 37–43.

Barker DJ. In utero programming of chronic disease. *Clin Sci* 1998;95: 115–28.

Batterham RL, Ffytche DH, Rosenthal JM, Zelaya FO, Barker GJ, Withers DJ, Williams SC. PYY modulation of cortical and hypothalamic brain areas predicts feeding behaviour in humans. *Nature* 2007;450: 106–9.

Botchkina GI, Morin LP. Organization of permanent and transient neuropeptide Y-immunoreactive neuron groups and fiber systems in the developing hamster diencephalon. *J Comp Neurol* 1995;357: 573–602.

Bouchard C, Tremblay A. Genetic effects in human energy expenditure components. *Int J Obes* 1990; 14 Suppl: 1–55.

Bouchard C, Perusse L. Genetics of obesity. *Ann Rev Nutr* 1993;13: 337–54.

Bouret SG, Draper SJ, Simerly RB. Formation of projection pathways from the arcuate nucleus of the hypothalamus to hypothalamic regions implicated in the neural control of feeding behavior in mice. *J Neurosci* 2004a;24: 2797–805.

Bouret SG, Draper SJ, Simerly RB. Trophic action of leptin on hypothalamic neurons that regulate feeding. *Science* 2004b;304: 108–10.

Bouret SG, Simerly RB. Development of leptin-sensitive circuits. *J Neuroendocrinol* 2007;19: 575–82.

Bouret SG, Gorski JN, Patterson CM, Chen S, Levin BE, Simerly RB. Hypothalamic neural projections are permanently disrupted in diet-induced obese rats. *Cell Metab* 2008;7: 179–85.

Buckley AJ, Keseru B, Briody J, Thompson M, Ozanne SE, Thompson CH. Altered body composition and metabolism in the male offspring of high fat-fed rats. *Metabolism* 2005;54: 500–7.

Bugnon C, Fellmann D, Bresson JL, Clavequin MC. [Immunocytochemical study of the ontogenesis of the CRF-containing neuroglandular system in the human hypothalamus (author's transl)]. *C R Seances Acad Sci III* 1982;294: 491–6.

Burford GD, Robinson IC. Oxytocin, vasopressin and neurophysins in the hypothalamo-neurohypophysial system of the human fetus. *J Endocrinol* 1982;95: 403–8.

Burnett S, Bird G, Moll J, Frith C, Blakemore SJ. 2009. Development during adolescence of the neural processing of social emotion. *J Cogn Neurosci* 2009;21: 1736–50.

Clegg DJ, Benoit SC, Reed JA, Woods SC, Dunn-Meynell A, Levin BE. Reduced anorexic effects of insulin in obesity-prone rats fed a moderate-fat diet. *Am J Physiol Regul Integr Comp Physiol* 2005;288: R981–6.

Comuzzie AG, Allison DB. The search for human obesity genes. *Science* 1998;280: 1374–7.

Cottrell EC, Cripps RL, Duncan JS, Barrett P, Mercer JG, Herwig A, Ozanne SE. Developmental changes in hypothalamic leptin receptor: relationship with the postnatal leptin surge and energy balance neuropeptides in the postnatal rat. *Am J Physiol Regul Integr Comp Physiol* 2009;296: R631–9.

Cripps RL, Martin-Gronert MS, Archer ZA, Hales CN, Mercer JG, Ozanne SE. Programming of hypothalamic neuropeptide gene expression in rats by maternal dietary protein content during pregnancy and lactation. *Clin Sci* (Lond) 2009;117: 85–93.

Del Parigi A, Gautier JF, Chen K, Salbe AD, Ravussin E, Reiman E, Tataranni PA. Neuroimaging and obesity: mapping the brain responses to hunger and satiation in humans using positron emission tomography. *Ann NY Acad Sci.* 2002;967: 389–97.

Dorner G. [Possible significance of prenatal and-or perinatal nutrition for the pathogenesis of obesity]. *Acta Biol Med Ger* 1973;30: K19–22.

Ellgren M, Artmann A, Tkalych O, Gupta A, Hansen HS, Hansen SH, Devi LA, Hurd YL. Dynamic changes of the endogenous cannabinoid and opioid mesocorticolimbic systems during adolescence: THC effects. *Eur Neuropsychopharmacol* 2008;18: 826–34.

Farooqi IS, Bullmore E, Keogh J, Gillard J, O'Rahilly S, Fletcher PC. Leptin regulates striatal regions and human eating behavior. *Science* 2007;317: 1355.

Faust IM, Johnson PR, Hirsch J. Long-term effects of early nutritional experience on the development of obesity in the rat. *J Nutr* 1980;110: 2027–34.

Fernandez-Twinn DS, Wayman A, Ekizoglou S, Martin MS, Hales CN, Ozanne SE. Maternal protein restriction leads to hyperinsulinemia and reduced insulin signalling protein expression in 21 month-old female rat offspring. *Am J Physiol Regul Integr Comp Physiol* 2004;288: R368–73.

Fujioka T, Sakata Y, Yamaguchi K, Shibasaki T, Kato H, Nakamura S. The effects of prenatal stress on the development of hypothalamic paraventricular neurons in fetal rats. *Neuroscience* 1999;92: 1079–88.

Gillman MW, Rifas-Shiman SL, Camargo CA Jr, Berkey CS, Frazier AL, Rockett HR, Field AE, Colditz GA. Risk of overweight among adolescents who were breastfed as infants. *JAMA* 2001;285: 2461–7.

Gorski J, Dunn-Meynell AA, Hartman TG, Levin BE. Postnatal environment overrides genetic and prenatal factors influencing offspring obesity and insulin resistance. *Am J Physiol* 2006;291: R768–78.

Gorski JN, Dunn-Meynell AA, Levin BE. Maternal obesity increases hypothalamic leptin receptor expression and sensitivity in juvenile obesity-prone rats. *Am J Physiol Regul Integr Comp Physiol* 2007;292: R1782–91.

Grove KL, Allen S, Grayson BE, Smith MS. Postnatal development of the hypothalamic neuropeptide Y system. *Neuroscience* 2003;116: 393–406.

Grove KL, Smith MS. Ontogeny of the hypothalamic neuropeptide Y system. *Physiol Behav* 2003;79: 47–63.

Guo F, Jen KL. High-fat feeding during pregnancy and lactation affects offspring metabolism in rats. *Physiol Behav* 1995;57: 681–6.

Hassanain M, Levin BE. Dysregulation of hypothalamic serotonin turnover in diet-induced obese rats. *Brain Res* 2002;929: 175–80.

Heidel E, Plagemann A, Davidowa H. Increased response to NPY of hypothalamic VMN neurons in postnatally overfed juvenile rats. *Neuroreport* 1999;10: 1827–31.

Irani BG, Dunn-Meynell AA, Levin BE. Altered hypothalamic leptin, insulin and melanocortin binding associated with moderate fat diet and predisposition to obesity. *Endocrinology* 2007;148: 310–6.

Irani BG, Le Foll C, Dunn-Meynell AA, Levin BE. Ventromedial nucleus neurons are less sensitive to leptin excitation in rats bred to develop diet-induced obesity. *Am J Physiol Regul Integr Comp Physiol* 2009;296: R521–7.

Jones AP, Friedman MI. Obesity and adipocyte abnormalities in offspring of rats undernourished during pregnancy. *Science* 1982;215: 1518–9.

Jones AP, Simson EL, Friedman MI. Gestational undernutrition and the development of obesity in rats. *J Nutr* 1984;114: 1484–92.

Jones AP, Assimon SA, Friedman MI. The effect of diet on food intake and adiposity in rats made obese by gestational undernutrition. *Physiol Behav* 1986;37: 381–6.

Jones AP, Dayries M. Maternal hormone manipulations and the development of obesity in rats. *Physiol Behav* 1990;47: 1107–10.

Jones AP, Pothos EN, Rada P, Olster DH, Hoebel BG. Maternal hormonal manipulations in rats cause obesity and increase medial hypothalamic norepinephrine release in male offspring. *Dev Brain Res* 1995;88: 127–31.

Jones AP, Olster DH, States B. Maternal insulin manipulations in rats organize body weight and noradrenergic innervation of the hypothalamus in gonadally intact male offspring. *Dev Brain Res* 1996;97: 16–21.

Kennedy GC. The development with age of hypothalamic restraint upon the appetite of the rat. *J Endocrinol* 1957;16: 9–17.

Kim JH, Hamlin AS, Richardson R. Fear extinction across development: the involvement of the medial prefrontal cortex as assessed by temporary inactivation and immunohistochemistry. *J Neurosci* 2009;29: 10802–8.

Kokoeva MV, Yin H, Flier JS. Neurogenesis in the hypothalamus of adult mice: potential role in energy balance. *Science* 2005;310: 679–83.

Kokoeva MV, Yin H, Flier JS. Evidence for constitutive neural cell proliferation in the adult murine hypothalamus. *J Comp Neurol* 2007;505: 209–20.

Koldovsky O, Illnerova H, Macho L, Strbak V, Stepankova R. Milk-borne hormones: possible tools of communication between mother and suckling. *Physiol Res* 1995;44: 349–51.

Koutcherov Y, Mai JK, Ashwell KW, Paxinos G. Organization of human hypothalamus in fetal development. *J Comp Neurol* 2002;446: 301–24.

Labelle DR, Cox JM, Dunn-Meynell AA, Levin BE, Flanagan-Cato LM. Genetic and dietary effects on dendrites in the rat hypothalamic ventromedial nucleus. *Physiol Behav* 2009;98: 511–6.

Le Foll C, Irani BG, Magnan C, Dunn-Meynell AA, Levin BE. Effects of maternal genotype and diet on offspring glucose and fatty acid sensing ventromedial hypothalamic nucleus neurons. *Am J Physiol Regul Integr Comp Physiol* 2009;297: R1351–7.

Lehmann K, Grund T, Bagorda A, Bagorda F, Grafen K, Winter Y, Teuchert-Noodt G. Developmental effects on dopamine projections and hippocampal cell proliferation in the rodent model of postweaning social and physical deprivation can be triggered by brief changes of environmental context. *Behav Brain Res* 2009;205: 26–31.

Leibowitz SF, Roissin P, Rosenn M. Chronic norepinephrine injection into the hypothalamic paraventricular nucleus produces hyperphagia and increased body weight in the rat. *Pharmacol Biochem Behav* 1984;21: 801–8.

Levin BE. Reduced norepinephrine turnover in organs and brains of obesity-prone rats. *Am J Physiol* 1995;268: R389–94.

Levin BE. Reduced paraventricular nucleus norepinephrine responsiveness in obesity-prone rats. *Am J Physiol* 1996;270: R456–61.

Levin BE, Dunn-Meynell AA, Balkan B, Keesey RE. Selective breeding for diet-induced obesity and resistance in Sprague-Dawley rats. *Am J Physiol* 1997;273: R725–30.

Levin BE, Govek E. Gestational obesity accentuates obesity in obesity-prone progeny. *Am J Physiol* 1998;275: R1374–9.

Levin BE, Dunn-Meynell AA. Maternal obesity alters adiposity and monoamine function in genetically predisposed offspring. *Am J Physiol* 2002;283: R1087–93.

Levin BE, Dunn-Meynell AA, McMinn E, Alperovich M, Cunningham-Bussel A, Chua S Jr. A new obesity-prone, glucose-intolerant rat strain (F.DIO). *Am J Physiol Regul Integr Comp Physiol* 2003a;285: R1184–91.

Levin BE, Dunn-Meynell AA, Ricci MR, Cummings DE. Abnormalities of leptin and ghrelin regulation in obesity-prone juvenile rats. *Am J Physiol* 2003b;285: E949–57.

Levin BE, Dunn-Meynell AA. Chronic exercise lowers the defended body weight gain and adiposity in diet-induced obese rats. *Am J Physiol* 2004;286: R771–8.

Levin BE, Dunn-Meynell AA, Banks WA. Obesity-prone rats have normal blood-brain barrier transport but defective central leptin signaling prior to obesity onset. *Am J Physiol* 2004a;286: R143–50.

Levin BE, Routh VH, Kang L, Sanders NM, Dunn-Meynell A. Neuronal glucosensing: what do we know after 50 years? *Diabetes* 2004b;53: 2521–8.

Levin BE, Magnan C, Migrenne S, Chua Jr SC, Dunn-Meynell AA. The F-DIO obesity-prone rat is insulin resistant prior to obesity onset. *Am J Physiol* 2005;289: R704–11.

Levin BE. Metabolic sensing neurons and the control of energy homeostasis. *Physiol Behav* 2006;89: 486–9.

Levin BE, Dunn-Meynell AA. Differential effects of exercise on body weight gain and adiposity in obesity-prone and -resistant rats. *Int J Obes* 2006;30: 722–7.

Maffeis C, Micciolo R, Must A, Zaffanello M, Pinelli L. Parental and perinatal factors associated with childhood obesity in north-east Italy. *Int J Obes* 1994;18: 301–5.

Mai JK, Lensing-Hohn S, Ende AA, Sofroniew MV. Developmental organization of neurophysin neurons in the human brain. *J Comp Neurol* 1997;385: 477–89.

Markakis EA. Development of the neuroendocrine hypothalamus. *Front Neuroendocrinol* 2002; 23:257–91.

Matsuda M, Liu Y, Mahankali S, Pu Y, Mahankali A, Wang J, DeFronzo RA, Fox PT, Gao JH. Altered hypothalamic function in response to glucose ingestion in obese humans. *Diabetes* 1999;48: 1801–6.

Mayer J, Marshall NB, Vitale JJ, Christensen JH, Mashayekhi MB, Stare FJ. Exercise, food intake and body weight in normal rats and genetically obese adult mice. *Am J Physiol* 1954;177: 544–8.

O'Tierney PF, Barker DJ, Osmond C, Kajantie E, Eriksson JG. Duration of breast-feeding and adiposity in adult life. *J Nutr* 2009;139: 422S-5S.

Ozanne SE, Lewis R, Jennings BJ, Hales CN. Early programming of weight gain in mice prevents the induction of obesity by a highly palatable diet. *Clin Sci* (Lond) 2004;106: 141–5.

Patterson CM, Dunn-Meynell AA, Levin BE. Three weeks of early-onset exercise prolongs obesity resistance in DIO rats after exercise cessation. *Am J Physiol Regul Integr Comp Physiol* 2008;294: R290–301.

Patterson CM, Levin BE. Role of exercise in the central regulation of energy homeostasis and in the prevention of obesity. *Neuroendocrinology* 2008;87: 65–70.

Patterson CM, Bouret SG, Dunn-Meynell AA, Levin BE. Three-weeks of post-weaning exercise in DIO rats produces prolonged increases in central leptin sensitivity and signaling. *Am J Physiol Regul Integr Comp Physiol* 2009;296: R537–49.

Plagemann A, Heidrich I, Gotz F, Rohde W, Dorner G. Lifelong enhanced diabetes susceptibility and obesity after temporary intrahypothalamic hyperinsulinism during brain organization. *Exp Clin Endocrinol* 1992;99: 91–5.

Plagemann A, Harder T, Rake A, Melchior K, Rittel F, Rohde W, Dorner G. Hypothalamic insulin and neuropeptide Y in the offspring of gestational diabetic mother rats. *NeuroReport* 1998a;9: 4069–73.

Plagemann A, Rake A, Harder T, Melchior K, Rohde W, Dorner G. Reduction of cholecystokinin-8S-neurons in the paraventricular hypothalamic nucleus of neonatally overfed weanling rats. *Neurosci Lett* 1998b;258: 13–6.

Plagemann A, Harder T, Janert U, Rake A, Rittel F, Rohde W, Dorner G. Malformations of hypothalamic nuclei in hyperinsulinemic offspring of rats with gestational diabetes. *Dev Neurosci* 1999a;21: 58–67.

Plagemann A, Harder T, Rake A, Janert U, Melchior K, Rohde W, Dorner G. Morphological alterations of hypothalamic nuclei due to intrahypothalamic hyperinsulinism in newborn rats. *Int J Dev Neurosci* 1999b;17: 37–44.

Plagemann A, Harder T, Franke K, Kohlhoff R. Long-term impact of neonatal breast-feeding on body weight and glucose tolerance in children of diabetic mothers. *Diabetes Care* 2002;25: 16–22.

Polonsky KS, Given BD, Van Cauter E. Twenty-four-hour profiles and pulsatile patterns of insulin secretion in normal and obese subjects. *J Clin Invest* 1988;81: 442–8.

Puro DG, Agardh E. Insulin-mediated regulation of neuronal maturation. *Science* 1984;225: 1170–2.

Ravelli AC, van der Meulen JH, Michels RP, Osmond C, Barker DJ, Hales CN, Bleker OP. Glucose tolerance in adults after prenatal exposure to famine. *Lancet* 1998;351: 173–7.

Ravelli AC, van der Meulen JH, Osmond C, Barker DJ, Bleker OP. Obesity at the age of 50 years in men and women exposed to famine prenatally. *Am J Clin Nutr* 1999;70: 811–6.

Ravelli AC, van der Meulen JH, Osmond C, Barker DJ, Bleker OP. Infant feeding and adult glucose tolerance, lipid profile, blood pressure, and obesity. *Arch Dis Child* 2000;82: 248–52.

Ravelli GP, Stein ZA, Susser MW. Obesity in young men after famine exposure in utero and early infancy. *N Engl J Med* 1976;295: 349–53.

Ravelli GP, Belmont L. Obesity in nineteen-year-old men: family size and birth order associations. *Am J Epidemiol* 1979;109: 66–70.

Recio-Pinto E, Lang FF, Ishii DN. Insulin and insulin-like growth factor II permit nerve growth factor binding and the neurite formation response in cultured human neuroblastoma cells. *Proc Natl Acad Sci USA* 1984;81: 2562–6.

Reifsnyder PC, Churchill G, Leiter EH. Maternal environment and genotype interact to establish diabesity in mice. *Genome Res* 2000;10: 1568–78.

Ricci MR, Levin BE. Ontogeny of diet-induced obesity in selectively bred Sprague-Dawley rats. *Am J Physiol Regul Integr Comp Physiol* 2003;285: R610–8.

Samuelsson AM, Matthews PA, Argenton M, Christie MR, McConnell JM, Jansen EH, Piersma AH, Ozanne SE, Twinn DF, Remacle C, Rowlerson A, Poston L, Taylor PD. Diet-induced obesity in female mice leads to offspring hyperphagia, adiposity, hypertension, and insulin resistance: a novel murine model of developmental programming. *Hypertension* 2008;51: 383–92.

Sanchez J, Oliver P, Miralles O, Ceresi E, Pico C, Palou A. Leptin orally supplied to neonate rats is directly uptaken by the immature stomach and may regulate short-term feeding. *Endocrinology* 2005;146: 2575–82.

Schaefer-Graf UM, Pawliczak J, Passow D, Hartmann R, Rossi R, Buhrer C, Harder T, Plagemann A, Vetter K, Kordonouri O. Birth weight and parental BMI predict overweight in children from mothers with gestational diabetes. *Diabetes Care* 2005;28: 1745–50.

Shin AC, Zheng H, Berthoud HR. An expanded view of energy homeostasis: neural integration of metabolic, cognitive, and emotional drives to eat. *Physiol Behav* 2009;97: 572–80.

Stein AD, Ravelli AC, Lumey LH. Famine, third-trimester pregnancy weight gain, and intrauterine growth: the Dutch Famine Birth Cohort Study. *Hum Biol* 1995;67: 135–50.

Stunkard AJ, Foch TT, Hrubec Z. A twin study of human obesity. *JAMA* 1986;256: 51–4.

Tanaka M, Sawada M, Yoshida S, Hanaoka F, Marunouchi T. Insulin prevents apoptosis of external granular layer neurons in rat cerebellar slice cultures. *Neurosci Lett* 1995;199: 37–40.

Udagawa J, Hashimoto R, Hioki K, Otani H. The role of leptin in the development of the cortical neuron in mouse embryos. *Brain Res* 2006;1120: 74–82.

Wang GJ, Volkow ND, Logan J, Pappas NR, Wong CT, Zhu W, Netusil N, Fowler JS. Brain dopamine and obesity. *Lancet* 2001;357: 354–7.

Wilmot CA, Sullivan AC, Levin BE. Effects of diet and obesity on brain a_1- and a_2-noradrenergic receptors in the rat. *Brain Res* 1988;453: 157–66.

Xu Y, Tamamaki N, Noda T, Kimura K, Itokazu Y, Matsumoto N, Dezawa M, Ide C. Neurogenesis in the ependymal layer of the adult rat 3rd ventricle. *Exp Neurol* 2005;192: 251–64.

Zhang Y, Proenca R, Maffei M, Barone M, Leopold L, Friedman JM. Positional cloning of the mouse obese gene and its human homologue. *Nature* 1994;372: 425–32.

13 Perinatal programming in offspring of diabetic mothers: Clinical data

Peter Damm, Louise Kelstrup, Elisabeth R. Mathiesen, and Tine Dalsgaard Clausen

The epidemic of obesity and type 2 diabetes has a major impact on public health and underlines the urgency for identification of risk groups to target preventive strategies. Studies of developmental origins of health and disease have highlighted the possible role of intrauterine exposure to maternal diabetes in the pathogenesis of overweight, type 2 diabetes, and cardiovascular disease. Furthermore, diabetes in pregnancy may also affect cognitive function in the offspring. This review primarily includes human studies of long-term implications for the offspring of maternal diabetes during pregnancy – with special focus on recent studies performed in Copenhagen. We find that fetuses exposed to intrauterine hyperglycemia have a significantly increased risk of development of type 2 diabetes/prediabetes, overweight, and the metabolic syndrome in childhood and adult life.

Thus, based on literature and own studies, we conclude that women with gestational diabetes or type 1 diabetes during pregnancy should be informed about the excess risk of overweight, type 2 diabetes, and the metabolic syndrome in their offspring and that preventive strategies toward diabetes and cardiovascular disease are urgently needed in the next generation.

13.1 Introduction

Studies of developmental origins of health and disease have put focus on the possible role of intrauterine exposure to maternal diabetes in the pathogenesis of overweight, type 2 diabetes, and cardiovascular disease (Dabelea, 2007; Gillman, 2005), and diabetes in pregnancy may also affect cognitive function in the offspring (Rizzo et al., 1991).

The majority of previous studies have been performed in ethnically mixed populations, and data from Caucasians are limited.

The aim of this chapter is to summarize the possible long-term implications of maternal diabetes for the human offspring followed into adulthood with special focus on recent studies performed in Copenhagen. As described previously in this book, low birth weight is strongly associated with later development of diabetes and cardiovascular disease, but, in fact, the relationship between birth weight and subsequent development of diabetes is U-shaped. This has been found in animal studies as well as in humans (Aerts, Holemans, and Van Assche, 1990; Egeland, Skjaerven, and Irgens, 2000; Pettitt and Knowler, 1998), and over the years, parallel studies of developmental origins of health and disease have focused also on the possible role of *fetal overnutrition* as seen in relation to maternal diabetes in pregnancy (Gillman, 2005).

13.2 Short-term implications for the offspring

Both pregestational diabetes (type 1 as well as type 2 diabetes) and gestational diabetes (GDM) imply increased risk of several perinatal complications. The most severe and frequent include perinatal mortality, congenital malformations, prematurity, macrosomia, shoulder dystocia, neonatal hypoglycemia, respiratory difficulties, and jaundice.

Several studies have shown associations between increasing maternal glucose values during pregnancy and increasing risk of perinatal complications (Clausen et al., 2005; Jensen et al., 2001, 2003, 2004; Lauenborg et al., 2003; Metzger et al., 2008). It is now well established that intensified maternal glucose control improves the short-term/perinatal outcome of both pregestational diabetic pregnancy (DCCT Research Group, 1996) and GDM (Crowther et al., 2005; Landon et al., 2009).

13.3 Long-term implications for the offspring

In animal studies, intrauterine hyperglycemia increases the risk of abnormal glucose tolerance, diabetes, overweight, and insulin-resistance in the offspring (Plagemann, 2005). Transplantation of islet cells, before the last third of pregnancy, normalizes maternal glycemia and prevents harmful effects (Aerts and Van Assche, 1992; Harder et al., 2001).

At present there are no animal studies of cognitive function in offspring exposed to intrauterine hyperglycemia, but in rodent models of type 1 diabetes cognitive function in adult animals is adversely affected by hyperglycemia in fetal life (Biessels and Gispen, 2005). Deleterious effects of hyperglycemia are related to the severity of glycemic derangement (Biessels et al., 1996) and are furthermore preventable through immediate insulin treatment (Biessels et al., 1998).

In animal models it is possible to separate genetic and environmental factors when long-term effects of intrauterine exposure to intrauterine hyperglycemia are studied. In contrast, this is more complicated in human studies, for example, because ideal control groups are very difficult to identify, and in fact, many published studies do not have optimal control groups. In our recent studies we aimed to separate the effect of genes and environment.

13.3.1 Studies in adults

Overall, there is only sparse literature addressing the risk of type 2 diabetes, overweight, and other cardiovascular risk factors in adult offspring of women with diabetes during pregnancy (Dabelea, Knowler, and Pettitt, 2000; Franks et al., 2006; Gautier et al., 2001; Nilsson, 1999; Pettitt et al., 1988, 1991; Pribylova and Dvorakova, 1996; Sobngwi et al., 2003), and only one study evaluates cognitive function in the offspring (Nielsen et al., 2007).

Findings are not uniform; the studies did not report data on lipid metabolism in the offspring, and only papers on the Pima Indians (Franks et al., 2006; Pettitt et al., 1991) as well as the study on cognitive function (Nielsen et al., 2007) included data on estimates of maternal glycemic control during pregnancy.

The population of Pima Indians in Arizona has been followed prospectively with oral glucose tolerance tests (OGTT) since 1965 (Pettitt et al., 1993). Papers have been published demonstrating that diabetes in pregnancy and the level of 2-hour blood glucose during OGTT in pregnancy are strong predictors of overweight and type 2 diabetes in the offspring (Dabelea et al., 2000; Franks et al., 2006; Pettitt et al., 1988, 1991), and signs of impaired insulin sensitivity have been reported in the form of elevated levels of fasting insulin (Pettitt et al., 1991). However, Pima Indians have very specific genetics, with a prevalence of overweight and type 2 diabetes each reaching 70% by the age of 25, making it difficult to apply these findings to other populations.

In a study from Prague, 148 offspring of women with type 1 diabetes were compared with 31 matched controls of healthy mothers without a family history of diabetes (Pribylova and Dvorakova, 1996). Offspring of women with type 1 diabetes had significantly higher blood glucose and insulin levels during OGTT as well as higher BMI and blood pressure. Of the offspring studied, 9% had impaired glucose tolerance (IGT) or type 2 diabetes, and 5% had type 1 diabetes. A French study compared 15 offspring of mothers with type 1 diabetes (exposed) with 16 offspring of fathers with type 1 diabetes (unexposed) and found no difference concerning BMI, fat mass, waist – hip ratio, or blood pressure (Sobngwi et al., 2003). However, 33% of the exposed offspring compared with none of the nonexposed offspring had IGT. Exposed offspring with IGT had the overall lowest early insulin secretion index compared with exposed without IGT as well as unexposed. Exposed offspring had lower C-peptide levels than unexposed, and those with IGT had the lowest level of all, but none of the offspring had autoantibodies known to be associated with type 1 diabetes. The three groups had comparable insulin sensitivity.

Finally, a Danish study linked data from hospital records with data from the Danish Medical Birth Registry and the Conscript Registry (Nielsen et al., 2007). The study included 227 men 18 to 20 years old, born to women with gestational and pregestational diabetes. Controls were 736 unexposed men matched on birth year and maternal residence at time of birth. Offspring of women with diabetes during pregnancy had a significantly higher army rejection rate and insignificantly lower test-scores at conscription (3.0 points on the commonly used IQ-scale, $P = 0.12$) than controls. In a subgroup with available measures of maternal HbA1c during pregnancy, HbA1c was inversely associated with cognitive performance.

13.3.2 Studies in children

There are markedly more follow-up studies in children up to adolescence (Aberg and Westbom, 2001; Boney et al., 2005; Bunt, Tataranni, and Salbe, 2005; Cho et al., 2000; Churchill, Berendes, and Nemore, 1969; Cummins and Norrish, 1980; Dahlquist and Kallen, 2007; Gillman et al., 2003; Hadden et al., 1984; Haworth, McRae, and Dilling, 1976; Hillier et al., 2007; Hod et al., 1999; Hunter et al., 2004; Kowalczyk et al., 2002; Malcolm et al., 2006; Manderson et al., 2002; Metzger et al., 1990; Ornoy et al., 1998, 1999, 2001; Persson and Gentz, 1984; Persson, Gentz, and Moller, 1984; Petersen et al., 1988; Pettitt et al., 1983, 1985, 1987; Plagemann et al., 1997a, 1997b, 2005; Rizzo et al., 1990, 1991, 1994, 1995; Rodekamp et al., 2006; Schaefer-Graf et al., 2005; Sells et al., 1994; Silverman et al., 1995, 1998; Stehbens, Baker, and Kitchell, 1977; Vohr and McGarvey, 1997; Vohr, McGarvey, and Tucker, 1999; Weiss et al., 2000; Whitaker et al., 1998). Several papers are from studies of the Pima Indians or from the Chicago group, but literature covers populations from most parts of the Western World.

Many studies are relatively small and include less than 100 exposed offspring or no internal control groups. Furthermore, some of the studies have limitations due to analysis, including maternal type 1 and type 2 diabetes together or high numbers lost to follow-up. Only one follow-up study of children from a small randomized trial in women with GDM has been performed, without definitive conclusions (Malcolm et al., 2006). The future will bring results from follow-up of offspring of mothers involved in the two trials on GDM treatment (Crowther et al., 2005; Landon et al., 2009).

There are several studies concerning glucose metabolism; the majority found increased risk of prediabetes or type 2 diabetes in offspring exposed to intrauterine hyperglycemia, but others found no such indications.

There are also several studies evaluating overweight and cardiovascular risk factors in children born to women with diabetes in pregnancy, but only one study included all components of the metabolic syndrome and found increased risk of the metabolic syndrome in 6–11-year-old offspring of women with GDM (Boney et al., 2005). The majority of studies report an increased offspring risk of overweight (Cho et al., 2000; Hillier et al., 2007; Hunter et al., 2004; Malcolm et al., 2006; Metzger et al., 1990; Pettitt et al., 1987; Plagemann et al., 1997b; Schaefer-Graf et al., 2005; Silverman et al., 1998; Vohr and McGarvey, 1997; Vohr et al., 1999; Weiss et al., 2000), though others are not consistent with this (Bunt et al., 2005; Gillman et al., 2003; Whitaker et al., 1998). According to individual cardiovascular risk factors, studies have reported increased systolic blood pressure, increased total cholesterol and LDL, decreased HDL-cholesterol, and increased waist-circumference in children of women with diabetes during pregnancy. However, findings are ambiguous as cholesterol, HDL, and waist circumference have also been found to be comparable between exposed and unexposed children, and levels of cholesterol and LDL-cholesterol have even been found to be significantly lower in exposed offspring. Levels of triglycerides as well as diastolic blood pressure have uniformly been found unaffected.

Most studies have found indications of impaired insulin sensitivity in diabetes-exposed offspring, however, one found signs of insulin secretion deficiency (Plagemann et al., 1997a), and two studies found no indication of either (Bunt et al., 2005; Manderson et al., 2002).

When it comes to studies of cognitive function in the offspring several different tests have been applied to children in different age groups, making it difficult to draw general conclusions because some subtests might be affected and others not. The following section, therefore, summarizes findings of the different studies in very general terms. Around half of the studies have found indications of impaired cognitive function in offspring of women with diabetes in pregnancy (Aberg and Westbom, 2001; Churchill et al., 1969; Dahlquist and Kallen, 2007; Haworth et al., 1976; Hod et al., 1999; Kowalczyk et al., 2002; Ornoy et al., 1998, 1999, 2001; Petersen et al., 1988; Sells et al., 1994; Stehbens et al., 1977), whereas the other half have not found this (Cummins and Norrish, 1980; Hadden et al., 1984; Persson and Gentz, 1984; Plagemann et al., 2005; Rizzo et al., 1990, 1991, 1994, 1995; Rodekamp et al., 2006; Silverman et al., 1998).

The most impressive studies are from the Chicago group and a group from Berlin as well as two large Swedish register studies; however, findings are to some extent not concordant. The Chicago group prospectively followed 200 children of women with GDM or pregestational diabetes and 30 controls of nondiabetic women with several tests from birth until the age of 16 years (Silverman et al., 1991). Test scores did not at any age differ between diabetes-exposed children and controls, but there were inverse associations between estimates of maternal metabolism and offspring scores in cognitive tests. The group from Berlin found no difference according to speech development in 240 2-year-old diabetes-exposed offspring compared with the background population (Plagemann et al., 2005; Rodekamp et al., 2006). However, they found a dose – response relationship between ingestion of breast milk from diabetic mothers during the first neonatal week and speech delay. Dahlquist and Kallen (2007) found lower school marks and an increased risk of not completing compulsory school in 6,400 16-year-old offspring of women with unspecified diabetes during pregnancy compared with 1.3 million unexposed controls. Aberg and Westbom (2001) found an increased risk of hospitalizations for neurological/developmental disorders in 10-year-old offspring of women with pregestational diabetes ($N = 3,874$) as well as GDM ($N = 8,684$) compared with 1.2 million control-children of women without diabetes.

Finally, some studies in children demonstrate a direct association between estimates of maternal metabolism and overweight or other cardiovascular risk factors in the offspring; others fail to do so. As mentioned previously, the Chicago-group found several significant inverse associations between estimates of maternal glucose metabolism (i.e., fasting plasma glucose, HbA1c, b-hydroxybutyrate, and free fatty acids) and offspring scores in cognitive tests, and this has also been found in other studies.

13.4 Own studies

We aimed to study the risk of type 2 diabetes and prediabetes, as well as overweight and the metabolic syndrome and the cognitive function in adult offspring exposed to intrauterine hyperglycemia, focusing on associations between maternal glucose levels during pregnancy and offspring outcome.

A total of 597 subjects aged 18–27 years were studied. Four groups were chosen to represent various degrees of genetic disposition to type 2 diabetes and exposure to intrauterine hyperglycemia.

1. Offspring of women with GDM (O-GDM), representing intrauterine hyperglycemia and a relatively high genetic predisposition to type 2 diabetes.
2. Offspring of women who were screened for GDM because of risk indicators and elevated fasting blood glucose but had a normal OGTT (O-NoGDM), representing normal intrauterine glycemia and a relatively high genetic predisposition to type 2 diabetes.
3. Offspring of women with type 1 diabetes (O-Type 1), representing intrauterine hyperglycemia and a relatively low genetic predisposition to type 2 diabetes.
4. Offspring of women from the background population (O-BP), representing normal intrauterine glycemia and a relatively low genetic predisposition to type 2 diabetes.

Of the eligible offspring, 56% participated, and no major demographic differences were found between participants and nonparticipants.

The subjects were examined thoroughly by OGTT, anthropometric examinations, blood tests, and testing of cognitive function. Furthermore, information on health, medication, smoking habits, and physical activity as well as information concerning current parental education and occupation and paternal diabetes status was collected (Clausen et al., 2008, 2009). Diabetes and prediabetes were classified according to the World Health Organization (WHO) criteria (WHO, 1999), and the metabolic syndrome was diagnosed based on the International Diabetes Federation (IDF) criteria (Alberti, Zimmet, and Shaw, 2006).

We used five different estimates of intrauterine glycemia. In analyses based on all participants the *assignment into four groups* (O-GDM, O-NoGDM, O-Type1, and O-BP) was used as a surrogate measure of different levels of intrauterine glycemia. In analyses restricted to offspring of women who underwent an OGTT during pregnancy we used maternal *fasting* or *2-hour blood glucose*. In analyses restricted to O-Type1, we used the mean maternal blood glucose in the *first* or *third trimester* as exposure variables. We tried carefully to correct for confounding in extensive statistical analyses. The prevalence of type 2 diabetes/prediabetes was 21% in O-GDM, 12% in O-NoGDM, and 11% in O-Type1 compared to 4% in O-BP. The prevalence of type 1 diabetes was 1% in O-NoGDM and 4% in O-Type1, whereas no O-GDM or O-BP had type 1 diabetes (▶Fig. 13.1).

Only 1 of the 11 cases of type 2 diabetes was known before the study, and the remaining were diagnosed during the study. Two of the nine cases of type 1 diabetes were diagnosed during the study. O-GDM had significantly higher fasting and 2-hour plasma glucose than O-BP, and also O-NoGDM had significantly higher fasting plasma glucose than O-BP. Finally O-Type1 had significantly higher 2-hour plasma glucose than O-BP.

The adjusted odds ratios (OR) for type 2 diabetes/prediabetes were markedly increased in O-GDM (OR 7.76 (95% CI 2.58–23.39)), O-NoGDM (4.46 (1.38–14.46)) and O-Type1 (4.02 (1.31–12.33)) compared with O-BP.

A positive association between maternal glucose level and offspring risk of type 2 diabetes/prediabetes was found.

The prevalence of offspring overweight (BMI > 25kg/m²) was 40% in O-GDM, 30% in O-NoGDM, 41% in O-Type1, and 24% in O-BP, while the prevalence of the metabolic syndrome was 24%, 15%, 14%, and 6%, respectively (▶Fig. 13.2).

In adjusted analyses the risk of overweight was significantly higher in O-GDM (OR 1.79 (CI 95% 1.00–3.24)) and O-Type1 (OR 2.27 (1.30–3.98)) but not in O-NoGDM (OR 1.47 (0.78–2.78)) compared with O-BP. The risk of the metabolic syndrome was significantly higher in O-GDM, adjusted OR (4.12 (1.69–10.06)), O-NoGDM (2.74 (1.08–6.97)), as well as in O-Type1 (2.59 (1.04–6.45)) compared with O-BP. A positive

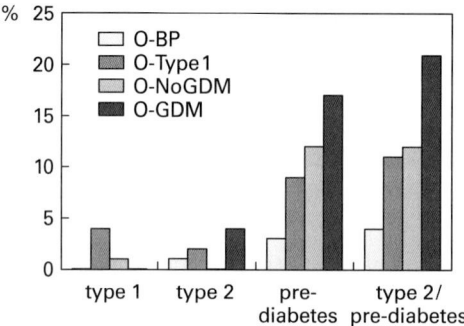

Fig. 13.1: Prevalence of diabetes and prediabetes in 18–27-year-old offspring of mothers with type 1 diabetes (O-Type 1), gestational diabetes (O-GDM), normoglycemic women with risk factors for GDM (O-NoGDM), or from the background population (O-BP).

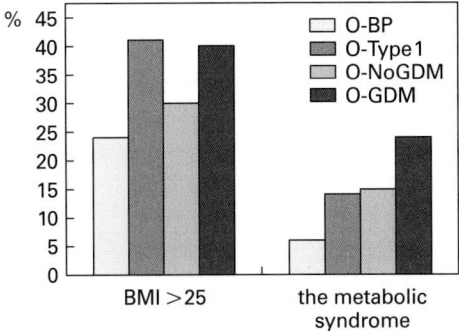

Fig. 13.2: Prevalence of overweight (BMI 25 kg/m²) and the metabolic syndrome (IDF criteria) in 18–27-year-old-offspring of mothers with type 1 diabetes (O-Type 1), gestational diabetes (O-GDM), normoglycemic women with risk factors for GDM (O-NoGDM), or from the background population (O-BP).

association was found between maternal glucose levels and risk of the metabolic syndrome.

We find that our four groups are enriched with different combinations of exposure to intrauterine hyperglycemia and other risk factors for overweight and the metabolic syndrome, which enables us to some extent to evaluate the possible impact of intrauterine hyperglycemia in a human model. In this context, we hypothesize that differences according to outcome between O-GDM and O-NoGDM as well as between O-Type1 and O-BP could be partly explained by a lasting effect of intrauterine hyperglycemia. On the other hand, the difference between O-GDM and O-Type1 as well as between O-NoGDM and O-BP could be interpreted as a reflection of genetics and other risk factors.

13.5 Concluding remarks

The Copenhagen study (Clausen et al., 2008, 2009) demonstrated a high risk of type 2 diabetes/prediabetes in adult offspring of mothers with GDM in a primarily Caucasian population, and data is in accordance with results from high-risk populations (Pettitt et al., 1988) as well as studies of children from Caucasian populations (Plagemann et al., 1997a; Silverman et al., 1998).

The findings of a higher risk of type 2 diabetes/prediabetes, overweight, and the metabolic syndrome in O-Type1 compared with O-BP as well as several associations between maternal glucose values during pregnancy and adverse outcome in the offspring support the hypothesis that a hyperglycemic intrauterine environment play a role in the pathogenesis of type 2 diabetes, overweight, and the metabolic syndrome, in addition to genetics and other risk factors. Aiming at glycemic levels as normal as possible in women with diabetes during pregnancy would prevent many of the perinatal complications and may reduce the risk of type 2 diabetes, overweight, the metabolic syndrome, and cognitive deficits in the offspring, but randomized trials are needed to prove this.

Mothers with gestational diabetes as well as type 1 diabetes in pregnancy should receive information about the increased risk in their offspring, and preventive strategies for diabetes and cardiovascular disease in these offspring are urgently needed.

References

Aberg A, Westbom L. Association between maternal pre-existing or gestational diabetes and health problems in children. *Acta Paediatr* 2001;90: 746–50.

Aerts L, Holemans K, Van Assche FA. Maternal diabetes during pregnancy: consequences for the offspring. *Diabetes Metab Rev* 1990;6: 147–67.

Aerts L, Van Assche FA. Islet transplantation in diabetic pregnant rats normalizes glucose homeostasis in their offspring. *J Dev Physiol* 1992;17: 283–87.

Alberti KG, Zimmet P, Shaw J. Metabolic syndrome – a new world-wide definition. A consensus statement from the International Diabetes Federation. *Diabet Med* 2006;23: 469–80.

Biessels GJ, Kamal A, Ramakers GM, et al. Place learning and hippocampal synaptic plasticity in streptozotocin-induced diabetic rats. *Diabetes* 1996; 45: 1259–66.

Biessels GJ, Kamal A, Urban IJ, Spruijt BM, Erkelens DW, Gispen WH. Water maze learning and hippocampal synaptic plasticity in streptozotocin-diabetic rats: effects of insulin treatment. *Brain Res* 1998;800: 125–35.

Biessels GJ, Gispen WH. The impact of diabetes on cognition: what can be learned from rodent models? *Neurobiol Aging* 2005;26: 36–41.

Boney CM, Verma A, Tucker R, Vohr BR. Metabolic syndrome in childhood: association with birth weight, maternal obesity, and gestational diabetes mellitus. *Pediatrics* 2005;115: 290–6.

Bunt JC, Tataranni PA, Salbe AD. Intrauterine exposure to diabetes is a determinant of hemoglobin A(1)c and systolic blood pressure in Pima Indian children. *J Clin Endocrinol Metab* 2005;90: 3225–9.

Cho NH, Silverman BL, Rizzo TA, Metzger BE. Correlations between the intrauterine metabolic environment and blood pressure in adolescent offspring of diabetic mothers. *J Pediatrics* 2000;136: 587–92.

Churchill JA, Berendes HW, Nemore J. Neuropsychological deficits in children of diabetic mothers: A report from the Collaborative Study of Cerebral Palsy. *Am J Obstet Gynecol* 1969;105: 257–68.

Clausen TD, Mathiesen E, Ekbom P, Hellmuth E, Mandrup-Poulsen T, Damm P. Poor pregnancy outcome in women with type 2 diabetes. *Diabetes Care* 2005;28: 323–8.

Clausen TD, Mathiesen ER, Hansen T, et al. High prevalence of type 2 diabetes and pre-diabetes in adult offspring of women with gestational diabetes mellitus or type 1 diabetes: the role of intrauterine hyperglycemia. *Diabetes Care* 2008;31: 340–6.

Clausen TD, Mathiesen ER, Hansen T, et al. Overweight and the metabolic syndrome in adult offspring of women with diet-treated gestational diabetes mellitus or type 1 diabetes. *J Clin Endocrinol Metab* 2009; 94: 2464–70.

Crowther CA, Hiller JE, Moss JR, McPhee AJ, Jeffries WS, Robinson JS. Effect of treatment of gestational diabetes mellitus on pregnancy outcomes. *N Engl J Med* 2005;352: 2477–86.

Cummins M, Norrish M. Follow-up of children of diabetic mothers. *Arch Dis Child* 1980;55: 259–64.

Dabelea D, Knowler WC, Pettitt DJ. Effect of diabetes in pregnancy on offspring: follow-up research in the Pima Indians. *J Matern Fetal Med* 2000;9: 83–8.

Dabelea D. The predisposition to obesity and diabetes in offspring of diabetic mothers. *Diabetes Care* 2007;30: 169–74.

Dahlquist G, Kallen B. School marks for Swedish children whose mothers had diabetes during pregnancy: a population-based study. *Diabetologia* 2007;50: 1826–31.

DCCT Research Group. Pregnancy outcomes in the diabetes control and complications trial. *Am J Obstet Gynecol* 1996;174: 1343–53.

Egeland GM, Skjaerven R, Irgens LM. Birth characteristics of women who develop gestational diabetes: population based study. *BMJ* 2000;321: 546–7.

Franks PW, Looker HC, Kobes S, et al. Gestational glucose tolerance and risk of type 2 diabetes in young Pima Indian offspring. *Diabetes* 2006;55: 460–5.

Gautier JF, Wilson C, Weyer C, et al. Low acute insulin secretory responses in adult offspring of people with early onset type 2 diabetes. *Diabetes* 2001;50: 1828–33.

Gillman MW, Rifas-Shiman S, Berkey CS, Field AE, Colditz GA. Maternal gestational diabetes, birth weight, and adolescent obesity. *Pediatrics* 2003;111: 221–6.

Gillman MW. Developmental origins of health and disease. *N Engl J Med* 2005;353: 1848–50.

Hadden DR, Byrne E, Trotter I, Harley JM, McClure G, McAuley RR. Physical and psychological health of children of Type 1 (insulin-dependent) diabetic mothers. *Diabetologia* 1984;26: 250–4.

Harder T, Aerts L, Franke K, Van BR, Van Assche FA, Plagemann A. Pancreatic islet transplantation in diabetic pregnant rats prevents acquired malformation of the ventromedial hypothalamic nucleus in their offspring. *Neurosci Lett* 2001;299: 85–8.

Haworth JC, McRae KN, Dilling LA. Prognosis of infants of diabetic mothers in relation to neonatal hypoglycaemia. *Dev Med Child Neurol* 1976;18: 471–9.

Hillier TA, Pedula KL, Schmidt MM, Mullen JA, Charles MA, Pettitt, DJ. Childhood obesity and metabolic imprinting: the ongoing effects of maternal hyperglycemia. *Diabetes Care* 2007;30: 2287–92.

Hod M, Levy-Shiff R, Lerman M, Schindel B, Ben Rafael Z, Bar J. Developmental outcome of offspring of pregestational diabetic mothers. *J Pediatr Endocrinol Metab* 1999;12: 867–72.

Hunter WA, Cundy T, Rabone D, et al. Insulin sensitivity in the offspring of women with type 1 and type 2 diabetes. *Diabetes Care* 2004;27:1148–52.

Jensen DM, Damm P, Sorensen B, et al. Clinical impact of mild carbohydrate intolerance in pregnancy: a study of 2904 nondiabetic Danish women with risk factors for gestational diabetes mellitus. *Am J Obstet Gynecol* 2001;185: 413–9.

Jensen DM, Damm P, Sorensen B, et al. Proposed diagnostic thresholds for gestational diabetes mellitus according to a 75-g oral glucose tolerance test maternal and perinatal outcomes in 3260 Danish women. *Diabet Med* 2003;20: 51–7.

Jensen DM, Damm P, Molsted-Pedersen L, et al. Outcomes in type 1 diabetic pregnancies: a nationwide, population-based study. *Diabetes Care* 2004;27: 2819–23.

Kowalczyk M, Ircha G, Zawodniak-Szalapska M, Cypryk K, Wilczynski J. Psychomotor development in the children of mothers with type 1 diabetes mellitus or gestational diabetes mellitus. *J Pediatr Endocrinol Metab* 2002;15: 277–81.

Landon MB, Spong CY, Thom E, et al. A multicenter, randomized trial of treatment for mild gestational diabetes. *N Engl J Med* 2009;361: 1339–48.

Lauenborg J, Mathiesen E, Ovesen P, et al. Audit on stillbirths in women with pregestational type 1 diabetes. *Diabetes Care* 2003;26: 1385–9.

Malcolm JC, Lawson ML, Gaboury I, Lough G, Keely E. Glucose tolerance of offspring of mother with gestational diabetes mellitus in a low-risk population. *Diabet Med* 2006;23: 565–70.

Manderson JG, Mullan B, Patterson CC, Hadden DR, Traub AI, McCance DR. Cardiovascular and metabolic abnormalities in the offspring of diabetic pregnancy. *Diabetologia* 2002; 45: 991–6.

Metzger BE, Silverman BL, Freinkel N, Dooley SL, Ogata ES, Green OC. Amniotic fluid insulin concentration as a predictor of obesity. *Arch Dis Child* 1990; 65: 1050–2.

Metzger BE, Lowe LP, Dyer AR, et al. Hyperglycemia and adverse pregnancy outcomes. *N Engl J Med* 2008;358: 1991–2002.

Nielsen GL, Dethlefsen C, Sorensen HT, Pedersen JF, Molsted-Pedersen L. Cognitive function and army rejection rate in young adult male offspring of women with diabetes: a Danish population-based cohort study. *Diabetes Care* 2007;30: 2827–31.

Nilsson PM. Increased weight and blood pressure in adolescent male offspring to mothers with pre-pregnancy diabetes-a genetic link? *J Hum Hypertens* 1999;13: 793–5.

Ornoy A, Ratzon N, Greenbaum C, Peretz E, Soria D, Dulitzky M. Neurobehaviour of school age children born to diabetic mothers. *Arch Dis Child Fetal Neonatal Ed* 1998; 79: 94–9.

Ornoy A, Wolf A, Ratzon N, Greenbaum C, Dulitzky M. Neurodevelopmental outcome at early school age of children born to mothers with gestational diabetes. *Arch Dis Child Fetal Neonatal Ed* 1999;81: 10–4.

Ornoy A, Ratzon N, Greenbaum C, Wolf A, Dulitzky M. School-age children born to diabetic mothers and to mothers with gestational diabetes exhibit a high rate of inattention and fine and gross motor impairment. *J Pediatr Endocrinol Metab* 2001;14: 681–9.

Persson B, Gentz J. Follow-up of children of insulin-dependent and gestational diabetic mothers neuropsychological outcome. *Acta Paediatr Scand* 1984;73: 349–58.

Persson B, Gentz J, Moller E. Follow-up of children of insulin dependent (type I) and gestational diabetic mothers growth pattern, glucose tolerance, insulin response, and HLA types. *Acta Paediatr Scand* 1984;73: 778–84.

Petersen MB, Pedersen SA, Greisen G, Pedersen JF, Molsted-Pedersen L. Early growth delay in diabetic pregnancy: relation to psychomotor development at age 4. *Br Med J* 1988;296: 598–600.

Pettitt DJ, Baird HR, Aleck KA, Bennett H, Knower WC. Excessive obesity in offspring of Pima Indian women with diabetes during pregnancy. *N Engl J Med* 1983;308: 242–5.

Pettitt DJ, Bennett PH, Knowler WC, Baird HR, Aleck KA. Gestational diabetes mellitus and impaired glucose tolerance during pregnancy – long-term effects on obesity and glucose tolerance in the offspring. *Diabetes* 1985;34: 119–22.

Pettitt DJ, Knowler WC, Bennett PH, Aleck KA, Baird HR. Obesity in offspring of diabetic Pima Indian women despite normal birth weight. *Diabetes Care* 1987;10: 76–80.

Pettitt DJ, Aleck KA, Baird HR, Carraher MJ, Bennett PH, Knowler WC. Congenital susceptibility to NIDDM role of intrauterine environment. *Diabetes* 1988;37: 622–8.

Pettitt DJ, Bennett PH, Saad MF, Charles MA, Nelson RG, Knowler WC. Abnormal glucose tolerance during pregnancy in Pima Indian women long-term effects on offspring. *Diabetes* 1991;40: 126–30.

Pettitt DJ, Nelson RG, Saad MF, Bennett PH, Knowler WC. Diabetes and obesity in the offspring of Pima Indian women with diabetes during pregnancy. *Diabetes Care* 1993;16: 310–4.

Pettitt DJ, Knowler WC. Long-term effects of the intrauterine environment, birth weight, and breast-feeding in Pima Indians. *Diabetes Care* 1998;21: 138–41.

Plagemann A, Harder T, Kohlhoff R, Rohde W, Dorner G. Glucose tolerance and insulin secretion in children of mothers with pregestational IDDM or gestational diabetes. *Diabetologia* 1997a; 40: 1094–100.

Plagemann A, Harder T, Kohlhoff R, Rohde W, Dorner G. Overweight and obesity in infants of mothers with long-term insulin-dependent diabetes or gestational diabetes. *Int J Obes Relat Metab Disord* 1997b;21: 451–6.

Plagemann A. Perinatal programming and functional teratogenesis: impact on body weight regulation and obesity. *Physiol Behav* 2005;86: 661–8.

Plagemann A, Harder T, Kohlhoff R, et al. Impact of early neonatal breast-feeding on psychomotor and neuropsychological development in children of diabetic mothers. *Diabetes Care* 2005;28: 573–8.

Pribylova H, Dvorakova L. Long-term prognosis of infants of diabetic mothers: Relationship between metabolic disorders in newborns and adult offspring. *Acta Diabetol* 1996;33: 30–4.

Rizzo T, Freinkel N, Metzger BE, Hatcher R, Burns WJ, Barglow P. Correlations between antepartum maternal metabolism and newborn behavior. *Am J Obstet Gynecol* 1990;163: 1458–64.

Rizzo T, Metzger BE, Burns WJ, Burns K. Correlations between antepartum maternal metabolism and child intelligence. *N Engl J Med* 1991;325: 911–6.

Rizzo TA, Ogata ES, Dooley SL, Metzger BE, Cho NH. Perinatal complications and cognitive development in 2- to 5-year-old children of diabetic mothers. *Am J Obstet Gynecol* 1994;171: 706–13.

Rizzo TA, Dooley SL, Metzger BE, Cho NH, Ogata ES, Silverman BL. Prenatal and perinatal influences on long-term psychomotor development in offspring of diabetic mothers. *Am J Obstet Gynecol* 1995;173: 1753–8.

Rodekamp E, Harder T, Kohlhoff R, Dudenhausen JW, Plagemann A. Impact of breast-feeding on psychomotor and neuropsychological development in children of diabetic mothers: role of the late neonatal period. *J Perinat Med* 2006;34: 490–6.

Schaefer-Graf UM, Pawliczak J, Passow D, et al. Birth weight and parental BMI predict overweight in children from mothers with gestational diabetes. *Diabetes Care* 2005;28: 1745–50.

Sells CJ, Robinson NM, Brown Z, Knopp RH. Long-term developmental follow-up of infants of diabetic mothers. *J Pediatr* 1994;125: 9–17.

Silverman BL, Rizzo T, Green OC, et al. Long-term prospective evaluation of offspring of diabetic mothers. *Diabetes* 1991;40: 121–5.

Silverman BL, Metzger BE, Cho NH, Loeb CA. Impaired glucose tolerance in adolescent offspring of diabetic mothers relationship to fetal hyperinsulinism. *Diabetes Care* 1995;18: 611–7.

Silverman BL, Rizzo TA, Cho NH, Metzger BE. Long-term effects of the intrauterine environment The northwestern University diabetes in pregnancy center. *Diabetes Care* 1998;21: 142–9.

Sobngwi E, Boudou P, Mauvais-Jarvis F, et al. Effect of a diabetic environment in utero on predisposition to type 2 diabetes. *Lancet* 2003;361: 1861–5.

Stehbens JA, Baker GL, Kitchell M. Outcome at ages 1, 3, and 5 years of children born to diabetic women. *Am J Obstet Gynecol* 1977;127: 408–13.

Vohr BR, McGarvey ST. Growth patterns of large-for-gestational-age and appropriate-for-gestational-age infants of gestational diabetic mothers and control mothers at age 1 year. *Diabetes Care* 1997;20: 1066–72.

Vohr BR, McGarvey ST, Tucker R. Effects of maternal gestational diabetes on offspring adiposity at 4–7 years of age. *Diabetes Care* 1999;22: 1284–91.

Weiss PA, Scholz HS, Haas J, Tamussi KF, Seissler J, Borkenstein MH. Long-term follow-up of infants of mothers with type 1 diabetes: evidence for hereditary and nonhereditary transmission of diabetes and precursors. *Diabetes Care* 2000;23: 905–11.

Whitaker RC, Pepe MS, Seidel KD, Wright JA, Knopp RH. Gestational diabetes and the risk of offspring obesity. *Pediatrics* 1998;101: 9.

World Health Organization [WHO]. Definition, diagnosis and classification of diabetes mellitus and its complications. Geneva: Author; 1999.

14 Experimental observations on perinatal programming in offspring of diabetic mothers

*Thomas Harder, Leona Aerts, Andreas Plagemann,
and F. André Van Assche*

Since the 1970s, epidemiological and experimental studies provided evidence that exposure to a diabetic intrauterine environment increases the risk of developing overweight and diabetes in the offspring. Animal models of diabetes during pregnancy may discover the specific effects of exposure to a diabetic intrauterine environment, independent of inherited trails. First evidence came from animal research in 1979, when it was demonstrated that mild diabetes in the pregnant rat induced gestational diabetes in the second generation and, as a consequence, macrosomia, increased insulin secretion, and B-cell hyperplasia in the fetuses of the third generation. It was postulated that overstimulation of the insulin producing B-cells in utero leads to a reduced capacity of insulin secretion in conditions of increased demand in later life, such as obesity and pregnancy. Beyond alterations in the periphery, overweight and metabolic disturbances in offspring of diabetic rat dams were found to be associated with perinatally acquired and persisting malformation of the ventromedial hypothalamic nucleus (VMN) and alterations of hypothalamic neurons expressing orexigenic neuropeptides like neuropeptide Y (NPY) in the arcuate hypothalamic nucleus (ARC). We hypothesized that these hypothalamic alterations could at least be coresponsible for increased risk of overweight and diabetes in offspring of diabetic rat dams. Consequently, normalization of maternal glycemia during pregnancy must be able to prevent this "neuro-endocrine phenotype" and its metabolic consequences. Therefore, in a collaborative study we investigated the consequences of treatment of maternal diabetes by pancreatic islet transplantation in rats for the development of the aforementioned hypothalamic circuits. Our data showed that both disorganization of the VMN as well as increased expression of NPY in the ARC can be prevented by treatment of maternal hyperglycemia, accompanied by normalization of the long-term metabolic risk.

   In summary, animal models support the hypothesis that maternal diabetes during pregnancy has an independent and long-lasting effect on risk of overweight and diabetes in the offspring. Beyond unraveling the biological mechanisms responsible, animal studies demonstrate that these alterations are accessible to measures of primary prevention.

14.1 Introduction

Two major pathophysiological paradigms have paved the way toward our current understanding of perinatal programming. Whereas one of these issues – the relationship between prenatal undernutrition, low birth weight, and later metabolic and cardiovascular diseases – was brought into the focus of the scientific community not more than about 20 years ago, the other paradigm is much older and dates back to the middle of the last century. The potential long-term consequences of exposure to a diabetic intrauterine environment came into focus relatively soon after the formulation of the hypothesis named after J. Pedersen. He proposed that in diabetic pregnancies increased glucose passes along its concentration gradient to the fetus, where it leads to macrosomia due to increased fetal pancreatic insulin secretion (Pedersen, Bojsen-Moller, and Poulsen, 1954), which was shown to go along with pancreatic B-cell hyperplasia (Van Assche and Gepts, 1971). Given these and other pathognomonic short-term consequences of maternal diabetes during pregnancy, such as hypoglycemia, hyperbilirubinemia, and shoulder dystocia, the question quickly arose whether the long-term perspective of these infants might also be impaired. In this chapter, we give an overview of the results, hypotheses, and pathophysiological concepts developed since these days in the field of experimental research on perinatal programming in offspring of diabetic mothers (ODM), with a particular emphasis on the development of body weight and glucose metabolism.

In the first part of this chapter, we briefly review major epidemiological and clinical findings regarding the long-term outcome of ODM. In the second part, we present data from experimental approaches on animal (mainly rodent) models of exposure to maternal diabetes and its long-term consequences for the offspring. This second part not only provides phenomenological data but also discusses etiological and pathophysiological models developed during recent years to explain the epidemiological and experimental findings. We conclude with a short summary and an outlook that highlights possible directions for future research.

14.2 Epidemiological and clinical studies

14.2.1 Historical notes

Probably the first epidemiological – clinical study that investigated a long-term impact of exposure to a diabetic intrauterine environment was published by Farquhar in 1969, reporting an increased risk of overweight in these offspring during childhood. These observations were confirmed a few years later by other investigators (Amendt, Michaelis, and Hildmann, 1976; Toeller et al., 1981) and were preceded by studies showing alterations of insulin secretion in ODM (Dörner et al., 1973). Historically, a second line of evidence indicating that maternal diabetes during pregnancy might be a risk factor for the later development of diabetes in the offspring came from epidemiological studies that investigated patterns of diabetes manifestation within families of patients with diabetes. In particular, the pioneering studies by Dörner et al. (1973) revealed that there is a significantly higher prevalence of diabetes in the maternal than in the paternal ascendance of patients with diabetes, which could later on also be shown to be present explicitly in patients having type 1 diabetes (Dörner, Plagemann, and Reinagel, 1987). Particularly regarding type 2 diabetes, more recent studies could clearly confirm an aggregation of diabetes cases in the maternal ascendance of patients with type 2 diabetes (Alcolado and Alcolado, 1991; Riley et al., 1997).

14.2.2 Contemporary studies

Two more recent epidemiological studies can be regarded as the break-through for the public attention on the field of epidemiological research on long-term consequences of exposure to maternal diabetes during pregnancy for the offspring. In the first one, Pettitt and coworkers (1983) analyzed the prevalences of obesity in 5–19-year-old Pima Indians depending on whether the mothers of these participants have had type 2 diabetes during pregnancy, had no diabetes, or developed diabetes after the index pregnancy. This study showed that those offspring who were exposed to diabetes in utero had a higher prevalence of obesity during childhood and adolescence than those whose mothers did not have diabetes or developed diabetes only *after* the index pregnancy. Subsequently, the group of Metzger from Chicago (Silverman et al., 1991) reported an increased risk of overweight in a Caucasian population of ODM and showed that the degree of fetal hyperinsulinism, measured by amniocentesis, was positively correlated to the extent of overweight in the offspring during childhood. Remarkably, the same group subsequently published data that provided evidence for a long-term effect of adequate treatment of maternal diabetes. This study revealed that ODM who had fetal hyperinsulinism, as an indicator of maternal gestational hyperglycemia, displayed higher prevalences of impaired glucose tolerance (IGT) during adolescence than ODM who had normal fetal insulin levels. Moreover, the latter had prevalences of IGT that were very similar to those of the control group of offspring of nondiabetic women (Silverman et al., 1995).

Subsequent epidemiological studies also indicated that the risk of overweight and IGT in ODM does not depend on the genetic background, that is, it develops independent of whether the mother has type 1 diabetes or gestational diabetes (Claussen et al., 2008; Plagemann et al., 1997a, 1997b; Weiss et al., 2000). Independency of genetic factors was further confirmed by an elegant study performed in the Pima Indian population. Dabelea and coworkers analyzed body weight and prevalence of type 2 diabetes in pairs of siblings born to women who had no diabetes during the pregnancy of the first sibling but were diabetic during the pregnancy of the second one. Those siblings who had been exposed to maternal diabetes in utero had a higher body mass index and increased risk of type 2 diabetes compared to siblings from the normoglycemic pregnancies (Dabelea et al., 2000).

Beyond overweight and impaired glucose metabolism, epidemiological studies also provided evidence for an increased cardiovascular risk in ODM, as indicated by increased systolic blood pressure (Tam et al., 2008) and altered blood lipid profiles (Weiss et al., 2000). Furthermore, there are also epidemiological studies indicating that the risk of developing type 1 diabetes is increased in offspring of women with gestational diabetes (Dörner et al., 1984, 1985, 1987, 2000; for review see Dörner and Plagemann, 1994). However, impairments in long-term prognosis in ODM are not restricted to overweight, diabetes, and cardiometabolic diseases. A number of studies have shown that ODM also have, for example, an impaired cognitive (Rizzo et al., 1991; Sells et al., 1994) and psychomotor development (Rizzo et al., 1995).

Taken together, a huge number of epidemiological and clinical studies performed on different geographical, ethnical, and genetic backgrounds strongly suggest that exposure to a diabetic intrauterine environment increases the risk of developing adipogenic, cardiometabolic, and psychological alterations during later life. However, due to the observational nature of these studies, confounding and bias cannot be completely excluded. Animal models may help to clarify the specific effects of exposure to maternal hyperglycemia and unravel underlying pathophysiological mechanisms.

14.3 Animal studies

14.3.1 Historical notes

The history of animal models of diabetes during pregnancy goes back, at least, to studies using pancreatectomy (Hultquist, 1948) or alloxan (Bartelheimer and Kloos, 1952; Dunn and McLetchie, 1943) to induce hyperglycemia in pregnant rats. However, these models were complicated by high maternal and fetal mortality, thereby limiting their value for studies on long-term effects in the offspring. Therefore, subsequently, the majority of investigators used streptozotocin (STZ) to induce diabetes in pregnant rats. STZ induces a selective destruction of pancreatic beta-cells (Rakieten, Rakieten, and Nadkarni, 1963), leading to a rapid reduction of pancreatic insulin content (Junod et al., 1969). Rishi, Golob, and Becker (1969) were the first to use this substance to experimentally induce diabetes in pregnant rats. The biological half-time of STZ lies within some minutes (Reynolds et al., 1974), therefore, when given on the day of conception, as it has been done by the majority of investigators, a direct effect on the fetus can be excluded.

Application of a single dose of STZ on the day of conception prevents the development of the physiological pancreatic beta-cell hypertrophy in pregnant rat dams (De Vlieger, Casteels, and Van Assche, 2008; Van Assche, Gepts, and Aerts, 1980). As in the human, increased maternal blood glucose concentrations pass the placenta, following the concentration gradient of glucose, and stimulate fetal insulin secretion (Asplund, 1973). This leads to a sharp increase in fetal pancreatic insulin concentrations during late gestation (De Gasparo and Milner, 1980). Furthermore, this early stimulation of the functionally immature beta-cells results in pancreatic islet hypertrophy (Aerts and Van Assche, 1977). However, these effects vary according to the dose of STZ used to induce hyperglycemia. Higher doses are known to induce more severe degrees of maternal hyperglycemia, which rather lead to decreased fetal pancreatic insulin concentrations (Kervran, Guillaume, and Jost, 1978) and increased beta-cell degranulation (Aerts and Van Assche, 1977). This also has consequences for the development of macrosomia in the offspring: depending on the severity of maternal gestational hyperglycemia, either macrosomia (Eriksson et al., 1980), normal birth weights (Björntorp et al., 1974), or even decreased birth weights (Aerts and Van Assche, 1981; Plagemann et al., 1998a) were observed in offspring of STZ-diabetic rat dams.

14.3.2 Epigenetic intergenerational transmission of increased diabetes and overweight risk due to exposure to maternal diabetes

Already in the very first experiments performed by Bartelheimer and Kloos (1952) it was noted that offspring of (alloxan-) diabetic rat dams had increased body weight in adulthood. In the same model, Goldner and Spergel (1972) described the development of impaired glucose tolerance and hyperinsulinemia in the adult offspring. In the

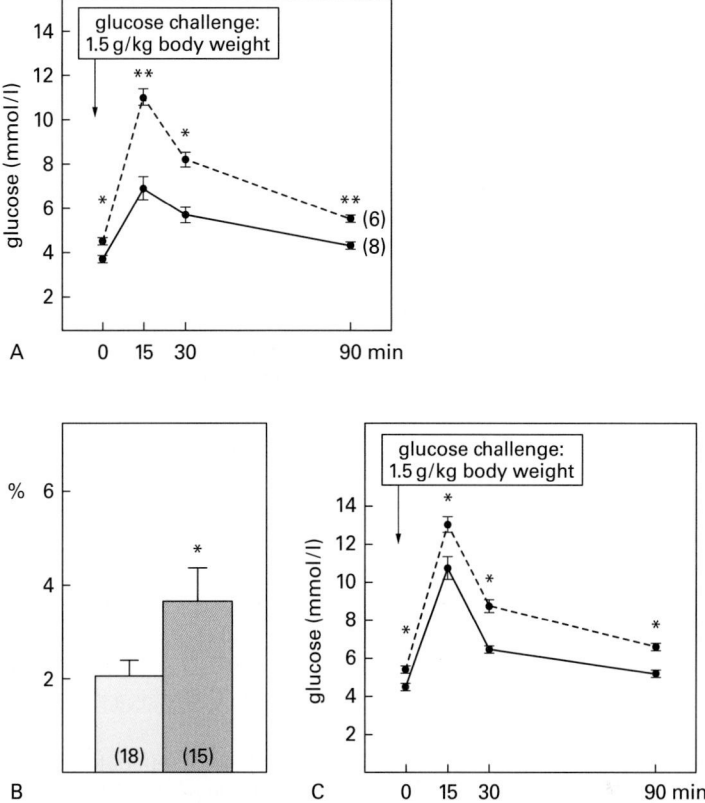

Fig. 14.1: Epigenetic intergenerational transmission of increased diabetes risk due to exposure to maternal diabetes during pregnancy. (A) Glucose tolerance during pregnancy in female F1 offspring of F0 diabetic pregnant rat dams (dashed line), as compared to F1 offspring of F0 control dams (solid line). (B) Percentage of pancreatic endocrine tissue at birth, as indicator of perinatal hyperinsulinism, in F2 offspring of F1 spontaneously diabetic dams (dark grey bar), as compared to F2 offspring of F1 control dams (light grey bar). (C) Glucose tolerance in adulthood in F2 offspring of F1 spontaneously diabetic dams (dashed line), as compared to F2 offspring of F1 control dams (solid line). *$p < 0.05$; **$p < 0.01$. Adapted from Aerts and Van Assche (1979) and Dörner et al. (1988).

STZ model, Aerts and Van Assche proved in 1979 that exposure to maternal diabetes has long-term consequences for glucose homeostasis in the offspring. Moreover, in this publication it has been described that the diabetic phenotype is transmitted over more than one generation on the maternal side. F1 offspring show impaired glucose tolerance, as compared to offspring of control dams. This impaired glucose tolerance is also present during pregnancy, that is, when F1 females are mated to control males (▶Fig. 14.1A; Aerts and Van Assche, 1979; Dörner et al., 1988). Thereby, the F2 offspring are again exposed to a hyperglycemic intrauterine environment that is generated by their (F1) mothers who spontaneously developed diabetes during pregnancy. As a direct consequence of this exposure, the F2 offspring develop perinatal hyperinsulinism (▶Fig. 14.1B). And again, this perinatal hyperinsulinism is followed by impaired glucose tolerance in adulthood (▶Fig. 14.1C; for review, see Dörner and Plagemann, 1994). Remarkably, such an intergenerational transmission of increased diabetes risk is restricted to the maternal line because F2 offspring that resulted from mating male F1 offspring of F0 diabetic rat dams with normoglycemic female F1 offspring of control dams have normal glucose tolerance (Dörner et al., 1988).

Although Bartelheimer and Kloos (1952) reported an increased body weight in offspring of rat dams with experimentally induced diabetes, only a limited number of studies investigated the development of body weight in these models. Nevertheless, it has been shown that offspring of STZ-diabetic rat dams develop overweight in adulthood, resulting at least in part from increased food intake (▶Fig. 14.2B, C; Plagemann et al., 1999a). Remarkably, the latter finding is supported by epidemiological data showing an increased daily caloric intake in infantile and adolescent ODM (Mughal et al., 2010).

Beyond the development of metabolic-syndrome – like symptoms, such as overweight and impaired glucose tolerance, offspring of diabetic rat dams also have an increased disposition to type 1 diabetes: after application of a single "subdiabetogenic" dose of STZ, that is, a dose that does not induce hyperglycemia in control rats, offspring of diabetic rat dams show permanently increased basal glucose concentrations, speaking for an increased vulnerability against beta-cell destroying agents (Plagemann et al., 1992a). This hypothesis of an increased susceptibility to type 1 diabetes after exposure to maternal gestational hyperglycemia is supported by epidemiological studies that, on the one hand, found an increased prevalence of gestational diabetes in mothers of children with type 1 diabetes (Dörner et al., 1987; see also 2.2) and, on the other hand, revealed that macrosomia at birth, being a key feature of ODM, is a risk factor for type 1 diabetes during childhood (Harder et al., 2009).

Taken together, these data strongly speak for an epigenetic effect transmitted through the maternal line and indicate that the observed effects are produced in each generation *de novo* by exposure to a hyperglycemic intrauterine environment, which, itself, is the result of a disposition to diabetes, which, in turn, was induced by previous exposure to diabetes in utero and so on.

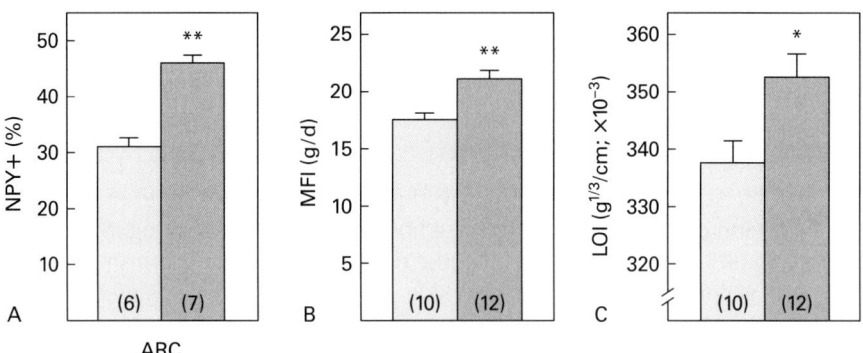

Fig. 14.2: Adult offspring of diabetic rat dams develop hyperphagia and overweight due to increased expression of neuropeptide Y (NPY) in the arcuate hypothalamic nucleus (ARC). (A) Immunopositivity of NPY in the ARC, (B) mean food intake (MFI), and (C) Lee obesity index (LOI) in adult offspring of diabetic rats dams (dark grey bars), as compared to offspring of control dams (light grey bars). *$p < 0.01$; **$p < 0.001$. Adapted from Plagemann et al. (1999a).

14.3.3 Other animal models

Besides maternal STZ treatment, other models have been developed to induce materno-fetal hyperglycemia and/or perinatal hyperinsulinism in rodents. Bihoreau et al. (1986) induced maternal hyperglycemia by glucose infusions in pregnant rats, which is known to lead to fetal hyperinsulinism (Asplund, 1973). A further model used the spontaneously hyperglycemic Goto-Kakizaki (GK) rat to create a hyperglycemic intra-uterine environment. To separate the genetic component from the effects of exposure to maternal diabetes, these authors performed transfer of blastocysts from the genetically inconspicuous background strain into the uterus of GK rat dams (Gill-Randall et al., 2004). In a number of other studies, fetal or perinatal hyperinsulinism was induced by direct application of insulin to the rat fetus or neonate. Such a model of fetal insulin application has been described for the first time by Picon (1967). Besides further studies that used peripheral exogenous application during fetal (Catlin, Cha, and Oh, 1985) or neonatal life (Dörner and Götz, 1972; Plagemann et al., 1992b; Harder et al., 1998), intrahypothalamic insulin implantation has been performed to cause a selective intra-hypothalamic hyperinsulinism during a critical period of the development of central nervous structures that are decisively involved in the central nervous regulation of body weight and metabolism (Plagemann et al., 1992c; see chapter 14.3.4 below for further details). The common phenotypic feature in all of these models is the development of overweight and/or diabetogenic alterations in later life, including IGT and alterations of insulin secretion like hyperinsulinemia. Moreover, very similar to the STZ-based model of gestational diabetes, in models of exogenous perinatal hyperinsulinism also an increased type 1 diabetes susceptibility has been observed (Harder et al., 1999). Furthermore, the aforementioned alterations are not restricted to rodent models, as demonstrated by Susa and coworkers (1992) in rhesus monkeys, which also develop hyperinsulinemia in later life after exposure to fetal hyperinsulinism.

14.3.4 Pathophysiological mechanisms

Two major complexes of pathophysiological mechanisms have been proposed to be responsible for the increased risk of overweight and diabetogenic alterations in the off-spring of diabetic rat dams. The first one is related to peripheral mechanisms operating at the level of the pancreas and/or the skeletal muscle and liver. It has been proposed that, on one hand, exposure to maternal diabetes in utero leads to permanent alterations of insulin secretion. On the other hand, maternal diabetes has been suggested to be followed by insulin resistance in skeletal muscle and the liver (▶Fig. 14.3A; for review see Aerts, Holemans, and Van Assche, 1990).

Regarding alterations of insulin secretion during later life, both decreased and in-creased insulin levels can be observed in offspring of STZ-diabetic rat dams (Aerts and Van Assche, 1979; Aerts et al., 1990; Plagemann et al., 1999a). Initially, it was hypothe-sized that a reduced capacity of insulin secretion in later life might be the consequence of hyperactivity of fetal B-cells (for review see Van Assche, Holemans, and Aerts, 2001). In this context, in particular in the case of severe maternal diabetes during pregnancy, several signs of an altered ultrastructure of pancreatric B-cells, including disorganiza-tion of mitochondria and of the endoplasmatic reticulum, were observed (▶Fig. 14.4; Aerts and Van Assche, 1977; for review see Aerts and Van Assche, 2006).

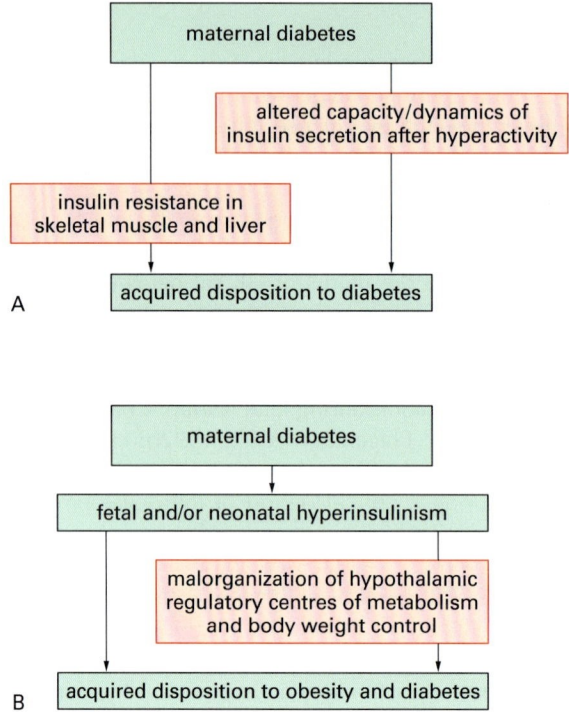

Fig. 14.3: Concepts of perinatal malprogramming of increased disposition to diabetes/obesity in offspring of diabetic mothers by (A) peripheral mechanisms and (B) central nervous mechanisms.

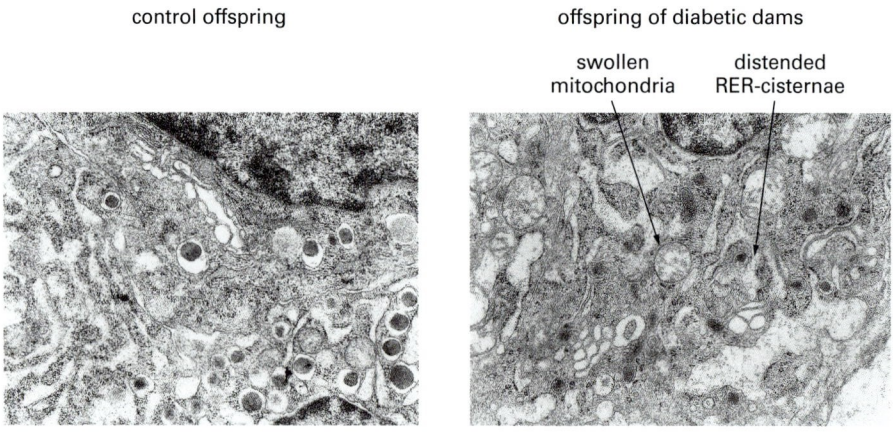

Fig. 14.4: Ultrastructural alterations of pancreatic B cells in offspring of diabetic rats dams (electron microscopy; magnification x 14,000). Adapted from Aerts and Van Assche (1977).

Increased insulin secretion in adult life in offspring of STZ-diabetic rat dams might have developed in the context of insulin resistance or might even have been causal for the latter. During euglycemic-hyperinsulinemic clamp experiments, offspring of diabetic dams needed lower glucose infusion rates to maintain euglycemia at a given level of plasma insulin, speaking for decreased insulin-dependent glucose uptake of skeletal muscle. Simultaneously, an impaired insulin-induced suppression of hepatic glucose production was observed in F1 offspring of diabetic rat dams (Holemans, Aerts, and Van Assche, 1991). Both the hepatic and the muscular component of insulin resistance have been suggested to be involved in the development of diabetogenic disturbances in ODM.

The second complex of potential pathophysiological mechanisms is related to the hypothalamic control of food intake, body weight, and glucose metabolism. It is long known that distinct nuclei in the mediobasal hypothalamus, such as the ventromedial hypothalamic nucleus (VMN), the lateral hypothalamic area (LHA), and the arcuate hypothalamic nucleus (ARC), play a decisive role in this context (for review see Kalra et al., 1999). In the rat, the critical perinatal developmental period of these hypothalamic structures lasts until the end of the third week of postnatal life (Dörner and Staudt, 1972; Pozzo-Miller and Aoki, 1992). It has therefore been suggested that perinatal hyperinsulinism resulting from exposure to maternal diabetes in utero leads to a malorganization and consecutive malfunctioning of such hypothalamic structures, thereby resulting in the perinatally acquired disposition to overweight and diabetes (▶Fig. 14.3B; Dörner and Plagemann, 1994; Plagemann, 2005, Plagemann, Harder, and Dudenhausen, 2008).

However, a necessary precondition for this hypothesis would be that peripheral hyperinsulinism of the fetus of the diabetic dam leads to increased levels of insulin within the hypothalamus. In fact, perinatally offspring of STZ-diabetic rat dams show not only peripheral hyperinsulinism, as measured by increased plasma insulin, but also an increased hypothalamic insulin content (Plagemann et al., 1998b). This central nervous hyperinsulinism during a critical window of perinatal development leads to an impaired organization of the VMN: studies showed that offspring of diabetic mother rats had a permanently decreased neuronal density/neuron number and a diminished neuronal size compared to control offspring, thereby showing a kind of hypotrophy and hypoplasia of this important satiety center (Plagemann et al., 1999b).

By contrast, the antagonistic LHA was morphologically unaltered (Plagemann et al., 1999b). These findings led to the conclusion that a perinatally acquired dysbalance between these two functionally antagonistic centers might contribute to the development of overweight and diabetogenic alterations induced by exposure to maternal diabetes in utero. Hypotrophy and hypoplasia of the VMN might result in a diminished function of this satiety center, thereby leading to a relative overactivity of the antagonistic LHA, which would stimulate appetite and subsequent weight gain as well as pancreatic insulin secretion (▶Fig. 14.5; Dörner and Plagemann, 1994; Plagemann, 2005; Plagemann et al., 2008).

However, the VMN is not the only hypothalamic structure that exhibits signs of malorganization and malfunction due to exposure to perinatal hyperinsulinism. During recent years, it has become clear that neuropeptides in the ARC play an important role in the regulation of food intake, body weight, and metabolism (for review see Kalra

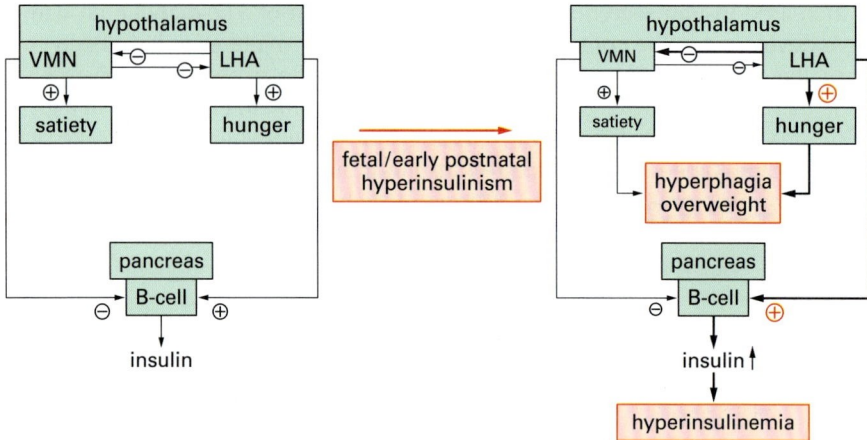

Fig. 14.5: A possible mechanism of hypothalamic malprogramming due to exposure to perinatal hyperinsulinism: the ventromedial hypothalamic nucleus (VMN) – lateral hypothalamic area (LHA) axis. Adapted from Dörner and Plagemann (1994); Plagemann (2005) and Plagemann et al. (2008).

et al., 1999). Among them, neuropeptide Y (NPY) is known to be the most potent orexigenic neuropeptide that is regulated via the circulating satiety factors leptin and insulin with both of them physiologically suppressing NPY expression. In offspring of diabetic rat dams, the expression of NPY in the ARC was found to be permanently increased and was positively correlated to increased food intake in adulthood, despite increased insulin levels (▶Fig. 14.2A). These data gave rise to a second pathophysiological concept: perinatal hyperinsulinism induces a resistance of the NPYergic system against the regulatory signals leptin and insulin, which leads to hyperphagia and consecutive overweight and its diabetogenic consequences (▶Fig. 14.6; Plagemann et al., 1998b, 1999a).

14.3.5 Malprogramming by maternal diabetes during the neonatal period

One important question with regard to the etiopathogenesis of long-term adipogenic and metabolic alterations in ODM is whether the impact of exposure to maternal diabetes is restricted to the prenatal period, or whether there might be an independent influence of exposure to breast milk from diabetic mothers in these processes. In fact, results from epidemiological studies suggest that neonatal exposure to breast milk from diabetic mothers might be coresponsible for the increased risk of obesity and diabetogenic disturbances observed in the offspring (Buinauskiene, Baliutaviciene, and Zalinkevivius, 2004; Kerssen et al., 2004; Plagemann et al., 2002). This appears to be biologically plausible because breast milk from mothers with diabetes shows considerable alterations in its composition compared to breast milk from nondiabetic women, such as increased levels of glucose and insulin (Jovanovic-Peterson et al., 1989; Neubauer, 1990). However, these issues are still a matter of intensive debate (Plagemann et al., 2007;

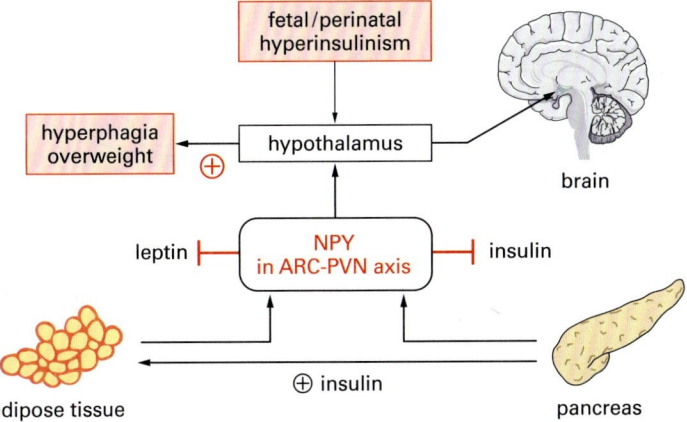

Fig. 14.6: A possible mechanism of hypothalamic malprogramming due to exposure to perinatal hyperinsulinism: the arcuate hypothalamic nucleus (ARC) – paraventricular hypothalamic nucleus (PVN) axis. Adapted from Plagemann (2005) and Plagemann et al. (2008).

Plagemann and Harder, 2011; Rodekamp et al., 2009) because contrary results also have been published (Hummel et al., 2009; Mayer-Davis et al., 2006).

Interestingly, Reifsnyder, Churchill, and Leiter (2000) demonstrated that pups of New Zealand obese mice (a genetic animal model for obesity and type 2 diabetes) suckled by their biological (diabetic) mothers became more obese and had higher insulin and leptin levels in adulthood than their littermates, who were reared by control dams, independent of their genetic background. Given these epidemiological and experimental findings, we hypothesized that the functional and hypothalamic alterations in the offspring of diabetic rat dams described previously might partly be a direct consequence of exposure to milk from diabetic rat dams. To investigate this, offspring of control rat dams were cross-fostered neonatally onto STZ-diabetic rat dams (CO-GD) and compared to their litter mates reared by normoglycemic control dams (CO-CO) (Fahrenkrog et al., 2004). At weaning, CO-GD rats showed signs of a structural and functional "malprogramming" of relevant hypothalamic structures. Immunopositivity of the main orexigenic neuropeptides NPY and agouti-related peptide (AgRP) was increased in the ARC, despite unchanged levels of the regulatory signals insulin and leptin. Simultaneously, CO-GD rats displayed decreased immunopositivity of the anorexigenic neuropeptide proopiomelanocortin (POMC) and its post-transcritional cleavage product alpha-melanocyte-stimulating hormone (alpha-MSH). Interestingly, in contrast to pups exposed to maternal diabetes prenatally, the structure of the VMN was not altered (Fahrenkrog et al., 2004).

Taken together, in the context of the aforementioned epidemiological and clinical studies, these animal data speak for an independent effect of exposure to "diabetic" breast milk for the development of long-term alterations of body weight and metabolism in ODM, which might be the result of a neonatal "malprogramming" of hypothalamic regulatory systems.

14.3.6 Prevention of neuroendocrine malprogramming

Given the aforementioned results and conclusions, one might hypothesize that normalization of maternal glycemia during pregnancy must be able to prevent these alterations. We tested this hypothesis using a novel model of therapeutic intervention in diabetic rat dams. As shown in ▶Fig. 14.7A, on day 15 of gestation diabetic rat dams were randomly assigned to either the treatment group (TxGD) or the placebo group (TsGD). In TxGD dams, an intraportal pancreatic islet transplantation was performed using 2,000 islets collected from newborn rats, whereas TsGD and CO dams only received a sham transplantation. Islet transplantation had a very fast effect on maternal blood glucose

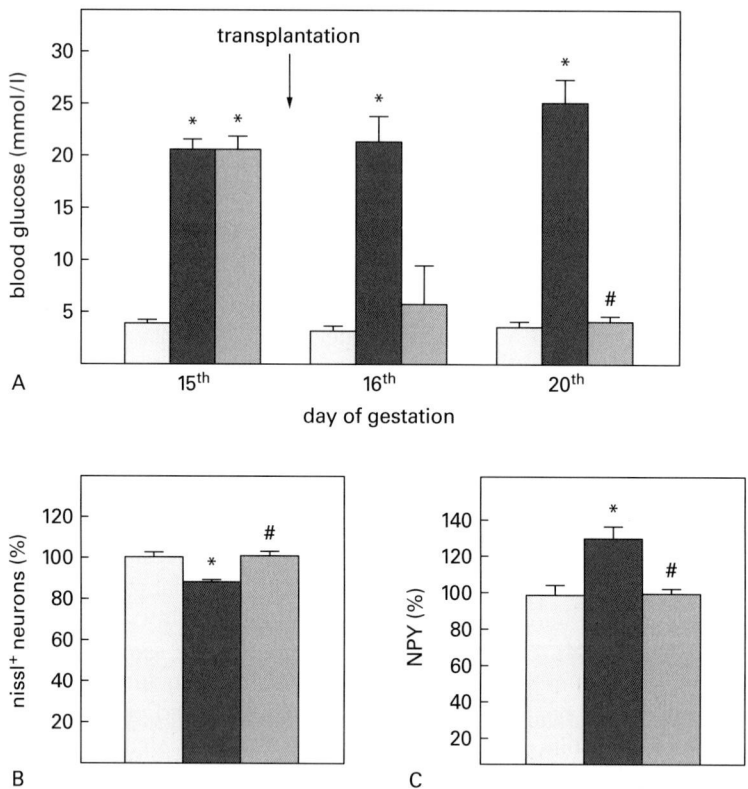

Fig. 14.7: Prevention of malprogramming of increased obesity and diabetes risk by treatment of maternal gestational hyperglycemia. (A) Maternal blood glucose during pregnancy before and after islet transplantation or sham transplantation on day 15 of gestation in control dams (light grey bars; n = 4) and diabetic dams with islet transplantation (dark grey bars; n = 3) or sham transplantation (black bars; n = 4); (B) number of Nissl-positive neurons in the ventromedial hypothalamic nucleus (VMN); and (C) immunopositivity of neuropeptide Y (NPY) in the arcuate hypothalamic nucleus in weanling offspring of control dams (light grey bars; n = 9) and diabetic dams with islet transplantation (dark grey bars; n = 10) or sham transplantation (black bars; n = 7). Neuronal data are shown as percentages of respective control group values. *$p < 0.05$ vs control; #$p < 0.05$ vs sham transplantation. Adapted from Harder et al. (2001, 2003) and Franke et al. (2005).

levels: already 24 hours after the operation, blood glucose in islet-transplanted TxGD dams was no longer significantly different from blood glucose of CO mothers, whereas glucose values were still increased in sham-transplanted TsGD dams (▶Fig. 14.7A) (Franke et al., 2005; Harder et al., 2001, 2003).

In a first experiment it was shown that this treatment regimen in the third trimester of pregnancy was able to prevent the development of impaired glucose tolerance and altered insulin secretion in the adult offspring (Aerts and Van Assche, 1992). Subsequent studies indicated that this effect might be due to prevention of malorganization of hypothalamic nuclei involved in the life-long regulation of body weight and metabolism. As shown in ▶Fig 14.7B, the number of neurons in the VMN from offspring of TxGD dams was not different from those from offspring of CO mother rats, whereas in the offspring of TsGD dams a significantly reduced number of VMN neurons was observed (Harder et al., 2001, 2003). Simultaneously, the increased orexigenic signaling in the ARC induced by exposure to maternal diabetes also was prevented: offspring of TxGD dams did not differ in NPY expression from CO offspring. By contrast, offspring of sham-transplanted TsGD dams had an increased NPY expression in the ARC (▶Fig. 14.7C) (Franke et al., 2005). Thereby, this series of experiments showed that malorganization and malprogramming of hypothalamic regulatory structures of body weight and metabolism in ODM can be prevented by timely correction of maternal hyperglycemia during pregnancy.

14.4 Conclusions and outlook

Taken together, experimental data support the results obtained in various epidemiological studies that exposure to maternal hyperglycemia during pregnancy has an independent impact on later risk of developing a wide spectrum of alterations, ranging from overweight, impaired glucose tolerance, insulin resistance, and alterations of insulin secretion to an increased type-1-diabetes – like beta-cell vulnerability. Remarkably, the majority of these alterations were observed not only in one single experimental approach, but also in a variety of different animal models of maternal diabetes and perinatal hyperinsulinism. The pathophysiological mechanisms elucidated in these studies and models include disorganization of pancreatic beta-cell ultrastructure as well as malorganization and consecutive malprogramming of hypothalamic structures that are decisively involved in the long-term regulation of food intake, body weight, and glucose metabolism. Thereby, these data strongly support the importance of detection and therapy of all kinds of maternal hyperglycemia during pregnancy as preventive measures with regard to long-term health of the offspring (▶Fig. 14.8).

Given this current "state of the art," the question of future research directions in this field arises. One topic will definitely relate to the consequences of obesity during pregnancy, related or not to the presence of gestational diabetes, as it is also in the focus in other chapters of this volume. A further highly promising field for the future relates to mitogenic effects of insulin as a possible causal factor for cancer (Draznin, 2010). In this context, one might expect that perinatal hyperinsulinism may put ODM at an increased risk of developing various types of cancer (Harder, Plagemann, and Harder, 2008, 2010; Van Assche, 1997; Van Assche et al., 2010). In fact, meta-analyses have shown that fetal macrosomia, as it is pathognomonic for ODM, leads to an increased

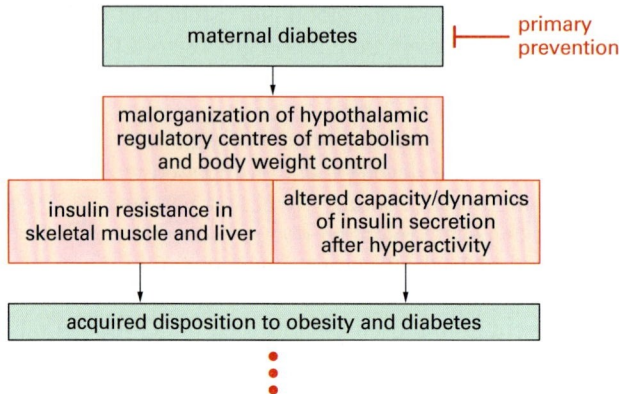

Fig. 14.8: Synopsis: Epigenetic perinatal programming of increased overweight and diabetes risk due to exposure to maternal diabetes and its prevention by detection and therapy of maternal hyperglycemia.

risk of breast cancer (Xue & Michels, 2007), astrocytoma and medulloblastoma (Harder et al., 2008), neuroblastoma (Harder et al., 2010), as well as nephroblastoma (Chu et al., 2010). It will be a challenge for the future to use appropriate animal models to verify these epidemiological findings and to develop pathophysiological concepts that might ultimately lead to the introduction of measures of primary prevention.

References

Aerts L, Van Assche FA. Rat foetal endocrine pancreas in experimental diabetes. *J Endocrinol* 1977;73: 339–46.

Aerts L, Van Assche FA. Is gestational diabetes an acquired condition? *J Dev Physiol* 1979;1: 219–25.

Aerts L, Van Assche FA. Endocrine pancreas in the offspring of rats with experimentally induced diabetes. *J Endocrinol* 1981;88: 81–8.

Aerts L, Holemans K, Van Assche FA. Maternal diabetes during pregnancy: consequences for the offspring. *Diab Metab Rev* 1990;6: 147–67.

Aerts L, Van Assche FA. Islet transplantation in diabetic pregnant rats normalizes glucose homeostasis in their offspring. *J Dev Physiol* 1992;17: 283–7.

Aerts L, Van Assche FA. Animal evidence for transgenerational development of diabetes mellitus. *Int J Biochem Cell Biol* 2006;38: 894–903.

Alcolado JC, Alcolado R. Importance of maternal history of non-insulin dependent diabetic patients. *BMJ* 1991;302: 1178–80.

Amendt P, Michaelis D, Hildmann W. Clinical and metabolic studies in children of diabetic mothers. *Endokrinologie* 1976;67: 351–61.

Asplund K. Effects of intermittent glucose infusions in pregnant rats on the functional development of the fetal pancreatic B-cells. *J Endocrinol* 1973;59: 285–93.

Bartelheimer H, Kloos K. Die Auswirkungen des experimentellen Diabetes auf Gravidität und Nachkommenschaft. *Z Ges Exp Med* 1952;119: 246–65.

Bihoreau MT, Ktorza A, Kinebanyan MF, Picon L. Impaired glucose homeostasis in adult rats from hyperglycaemic mothers. *Diabetes* 1986;35: 979–84.

Björntorp P, Enzi G, Karlsson K, Krotkiewski M, Sjöström L, Smith U. The effect of maternal diabetes on adipose tissue cellularity in man and rat. *Diabetologia* 1974;10: 205–9.

Buinauskiene J, Baliutaviciene D, Zalinkevivius R. Glucose tolerance of 2- to 5-yr-old offspring of diabetic mothers. *Pediatr Diabetes* 2004;5: 143–6.

Catlin EA, Cha CJ, Oh W. Postnatal growth and fatty acid synthesis in overgrown rat pups induced by fetal hyperinsulinism. *Metabolism* 1985;34: 1110–4.

Chu A, Heck JE, Ribeiro KB, et al. Wilms' tumour: a systematic review of risk factors and meta-analysis. *Paediatr Perinat Epidemiol* 2010;24: 449–69.

Claussen TD, Mathiesen ER, Hansen T, et al. High prevalence of type 2 diabetes and pre-diabetes in adult offspring of women with gestational diabetes mellitus or type 1 diabetes. *Diabetes Care* 2008;31: 340–6.

Dabelea D, Hanson RL, Lindsay RS, et al. Intrauterine exposure to diabetes conveys risks for type 2 diabetes and obesity: a study of discordant sibships. *Diabetes* 2000;49: 2208–11.

De Gasparo M, Milner RDG. The timing of fetal B cell hyperplasia in diabetic rat pregnancy. *Diabetologia* 1980;19: 54–7.

De Vlieger R, Casteels K, Van Assche FA. Reduced adaptation of the pancreatic B cells during pregnancy. *Acta Obs Gyn Scand* 2008;12: 1266–70.

Dörner G, Götz F. Hyperglykämie und Übergewicht bei neonatal insulinbehandelten erwachsenen Rattenmännchen. *Acta Biol Med Germ* 1972;29: 467–70.

Dörner G, Staudt J. Vergleichende morphologische Untersuchungen der Hypothalamusdifferenzierung bei Ratte und Mensch. *Endokrinologie* 1972;59: 152–5.

Dörner G, Mohnike A, Honigmann G, Singer P, Padelt H. Zur mögliche Bedeutung eines pränatalen Hyperinsulinismus für die postnatale Entwicklung eines Diabetes mellitus. *Endokrinologie* 1973;61: 430–2.

Dörner G, Steindel E, Thoelke H, Schliack V. Evidence for a decreasing prevalence of diabetes mellitus in childhood apparently produced by prevention of hyperinsulinism in the foetus and newborn. *Exp Clin Endocrinol* 1984;84: 134–42.

Dörner G, Steindel E, Kohlhoff R, et al. Further evidence for a preventive therapy of insulin- dependent diabetes mellitus in the offspring by avoiding maternal hyperglycaemia during pregnancy. *Exp Clin Endocrinol* 1985;86: 129–40.

Dörner G, Plagemann A, Reinagel H. Familial diabetes aggregation in type 1 diabetics: gestational diabetes an apparent risk factor for increased diabetes susceptibility in the offspring. *Exp Clin Endocrinol* 1987;89: 84–90.

Dörner G, Plagemann A, Rückert JC, et al. Teratogenetic maternofetal transmission and prevention of diabetes susceptibility. *Exp Clin Endocrinol* 1988;91: 247–58.

Dörner G, Plagemann A. Perinatal hyperinsulinism as possible predisposing factor for diabetes mellitus, obesity, and enhanced cardiovascular risk in later life. *Horm Metab Res* 1994;26: 213–21.

Dörner G, Plagemann A, Neu A, Rosenbauer J. Gestational diabetes as possible risk factor for type 1 childhood-onset diabetes in the offspring. *Neuroendocrinol Lett* 2000;21: 355–9.

Draznin B. Mitogenic action of insulin: friend, foe or "frenemy"? *Diabetologia* 2010;53: 229–33.

Dunn JS, McLetchie NGB. Experimental alloxan diabetes. *Lancet* 1943; 2: 384–5.

Eriksson U, Andersson A, Efendic S, Elde R, Hellerström C. Diabetes in pregnancy: effects on the foetal and newborn rat with particular regard to body weight, serum insulin concentration and pancreatic contents of insulin, glucagons and somatostatin. *Acta Endocrinol* 1980;94: 354–64.

Fahrenkrog S, Harder T, Stolaczyk E, et al. Effects of cross-fostering to diabetic rat dams on early development of hypothalamic nuclei regulating food intake, body weight and metabolism. *J Nutr* 2004;134: 648–54.

Farquhar JW. Prognosis für babies born to diabetic mothers in Edinburgh. *Arch Dis Child* 1969;44: 36–47.

Franke K, Harder T, Aerts L, et al. Programming of orexigenic and anorexigenic hypothalamic neurons in offspring of treated and untreated diabetic mother rats. *Brain Res* 2005;1031: 276–83.

Gill-Randall R, Adams D, Ollerton RL, Lewis M, Alcolado JC. Type 2 diabetes mellitus – genes or intrauterine environment? An embryo transfer paradigm in rats. *Diabetologia* 2004;47: 1354–9.

Goldner MG, Spergel G. On the transmission of alloxan diabetes and other diabetogenic influences. *Adv Metab Disord* 1972;60: 57–72.

Harder T, Plagemann A, Rohde W, Dörner G. Syndrome X-like alterations in adult female rats due to neonatal insulin treatment. *Metabolism* 1998;47: 855–62.

Harder T, Rake A, Rohde W, Dörner G, Plagemann A. Overweight and increased diabetes susceptibility in neonatally insulin-treated adult rats. *Endocrine Regulations* 1999;33: 25–31.

Harder T, Aerts L, Franke K, Van Bree R, Van Assche FA, Plagemann A. Pancreatic islet transplantation in diabetic pregnant rats prevents acquired malformation of the ventromedial hypothalamic nucleus in their offspring. *Neurosci Lett* 2001;299: 85–8.

Harder T, Franke K, Fahrenkrog S, et al. Prevention by maternal pancreatic islet transplantation of hypothalamic malformation in offspring of diabetic mother rats is already detectable at weaning. *Neurosci Lett* 2003;352: 163–6.

Harder T, Plagemann A, Harder A. Birth weight and subsequent risk of childhood primary brain tumors: a meta-analysis. *Am J Epidemiol* 2008;168: 366–73.

Harder T, Roepke K, Diller N, Stechling Y, Dudenhausen JW, Plagemann A. Birth weight, early weight gain and subsequent risk of type 1 diabetes: systematic review and meta-analysis. *Am J Epidemiol* 2009;169: 1428–36.

Harder T, Plagemann A, Harder A. Birth weight and risk of neuroblastoma: a meta-analysis. *Int J Epidemiol* 2010;39: 746–56.

Holemans K, Aerts L, Van Assche FA. Evidence for an insulin resistance in the adult offspring of pregnant streptozotocin-diabetic rats. *Diabetologia* 1991;34: 81–5.

Hultquist GT. An investigation on pregnancy in diabetic animals. *Acta Path Microbiol Scand* 1948;25: 131–40.

Hummel S, Pflüger M, Kreichauf S, Hummel M, Ziegler AG. Predictors of overweight during childhood in offspring of parents with type 1 diabetes. *Diabetes* 2009;32: 921–5.

Jovanovic-Peterson L, Fuhrmann K, Hidden K, Walker L, Peterson CM. Maternal milk and plasma glucose and insulin levels: studies in normal and diabetic subjects. *J Am Coll Nutr* 1989;8: 125–31.

Junod A, Lambert AE, Stauffacher W, Renold AE. Diabetogenic action of streptozotocin: relationship of dose to metabolic response. *J Clin Invest* 1969;48: 2129–39.

Kalra SP, Dube MG, Pu S, Xu B, FHorvath TL, Kalra PS. Interacting appetite-regulating pathways in the hypothalamic regulation of body weight. *Endocr Rev* 1999;20: 68–100.

Kerssen A, Evers IM, de Valk HW, Visser GH. Effect of breast milk of diabetic mothers on body-weight of the offspring in the first year of life. *Eur J Clin Nutr* 2004;58: 1429–31.

Kervran A, Guillaume M, Jost A. The endocrine pancreas of the fetus from diabetic pregnant rats. *Diabetologia* 1978;15: 387–93.

Mayer-Davis EJ, Rifes-Shiman SL, Zhou L, Hu FB, Colditz GA, Gillman MW. Breastfeeding and risk for childhood obesity. *Diabetes Care* 2006;29: 2231–7.

Mughal MZ, Eelloo J, Roberts SA, et al. Body composition and bone status of children born to mothers with type 1 diabetes mellitus. *Arch Dis Child* 2010;95: 281–5.

Neubauer SH. Lactation in insulin-dependent diabetes. *Prog Food Nutr Sci* 1990;14: 333–70.

Pedersen J, Bojsen-Moller B, Poulsen H. Blood sugar in newborn infants of diabetic mothers. *Acta Endocrinol* 1954;15: 33–52.

Pettitt DJ, Baird H, Aleck KA, Bennett PH, Knowler WC. Excessive obesity in offspring of Pima Indian women with diabetes during pregnancy. *N Engl J Med* 1983;308: 242–5.

Picon L. Effect of insulin on growth and biochemical composition of the rat fetus. *Endocrinology* 1967;81: 1419–21.

Plagemann A, Rückert JC, Friedrichs J, Götz F, Dörner G. Fetal and neonatal hyperinsulinism as risk factor of a lifelong enhanced diabetes susceptibility. In: Laron Z, Karp M, eds. *Genetic and Environmental Risk Factors for Type 1 Diabetes (IIDM) Including a Discussion on the Autoimmune Basis*. London: Freund Publishing House; 1992a: 73–78.

Plagemann A, Heidrich I, Rohde W, Götz F, Dörner G. Hyperinsulinism during differentiation of the hypothalamus is a diabetogenic and obesity risk factor. *Neuroendocrinol Lett* 1992b;14: 373–8.

Plagemann A, Heidrich I, Götz F, Rohde W, Dörner G. Lifelong enhanced diabetes susceptibility and obesity after temporary intrahypothalamic hyperinsulinism during brain organization. *Exp Clin Endocrinol* 1992c;99: 91–5.

Plagemann A, Harder T, Kohlhoff R, Rohde W, Dörner G. Overweight and obesity in infants of mothers with long-term insulin-dependent diabetes or gestational diabetes. *Int J Obes* 1997a;21: 451–6.

Plagemann A, Harder T, Kohlhoff R, Rohde W, Dörner G. Glucose tolerance and insulin secretion in children of mothers with pregestational insulin-dependent diabetes mellitus or gestational diabetes. *Diabetologia* 1997b;40: 1094–1100.

Plagemann A, Harder T, Lindner R, et al. Alterations of hypothalamic catecholamines in the newborn offspring of gestational diabetic mother rats. *Dev Brain Res* 1998a;109: 201–9.

Plagemann A, Harder T, Rake A, et al. Hypothalamic insulin and neuropeptide Y in the offspring of gestational diabetic mother rats. *NeuroReport* 1998b;9: 4069–73.

Plagemann A, Harder T, Melchior K, Rake A, Rohde W, Dörner G. Elevation of hypothalamic neuropeptide Y-neurons in adult offspring of diabetic mother rats. *NeuroReport* 1999a;10: 3211–6.

Plagemann A, Harder T, Janert U, et al. Malformations of hypothalamic nuclei in hyperinsulinaemic offspring of gestational diabetic mother rats. *Dev Neurosci* 1999b;21: 58–67.

Plagemann A, Harder T, Franke K, Kohlhoff R. Long-term impact of neonatal breast feeding on body weight and glucose tolerance in children of diabetic mothers. *Diabetes Care* 2002;25: 16–22.

Plagemann A. Perinatal programming and functional teratogenesis: impact on body weight regulation and obesity. *Physiol Behav* 2005;86: 661–8.

Plagemann A, Harder T, Rodekamp E, Dudenhausen JW. Breast-feeding and risk for childhood obesity (letter). *Diabetes Care* 2007;30: 451–2.

Plagemann A, Harder T, Dudenhausen JW. The diabetic pregnancy, macrosomia, and perinatal nutritional programming. In: Barker DJP, Bergmann RL, Ogra PL, eds. *The Window of Opportunity: Pre-pregnancy to 24 Months of Age*. Basel: Nestlé Nutr Workshop Ser Pediatr Program, Vol 61; 2008: 91–102.

Plagemann A, Harder T. Fuel-mediated teratogenesis and breastfeeding (editorial). *Diabetes Care* 2011;34: 779–81.

Pozzo-Miller LD, Aoki A. Postnatal development of the ventromedial hypothalamic nucleus: neurons and synapses. *Cell Mol Neurobiol* 1992;12: 121–9.

Rakieten N, Rakieten ML, Nadkarni MV. Studies on the diabetogenic action of streptozotocin (NSC-37917). *Cancer Chemother Rep* 1963;29: 91–5.

Reifsnyder PC, Churchill G, Leiter EH. Maternal environment and genotype interact to establish diabesity in mice. *Genome Res* 2000;10: 1568–78.

Reynolds WA, Chez RA, Bhuyan BK, Neil GL. Placental transfer of streptozotocin in the rhesus monkey. *Diabetes* 1974;23: 777–82.

Riley MD, Blizzard CL, McCarthy DJ, Senatro GB, Dwyer T, Zimmet P. Parental history of diabetes in an insulin-treated diabetes registry. *Diab Med* 1997;14: 35–41.

Rishi S, Golob EK, Becker KL. Streptozotocin diabetes in pregnant rats. *Fed Proc* 1969;28: 708–12.

Rizzo T, Metzger BE, Burn WJ, Burns K. Correlations between antepartum maternal metabolism and intelligence of offspring. *N Eng J Med* 1991;325: 911–6.

Rizzo TA, Dooley SL, Metzger BE, Cho NH, Ogata ES, Silverman BL. Prenatal and perinatal influences on long-term psychomotor development in offspring of diabetic mothers. *Am J Obstet Gynecol* 1995;173: 1753–8.

Rodekamp E, Harder T, Dudenhausen JW, Plagemann A. Predictors of overweight during child-hood in offspring of parents with type 1 diabetes (letter). *Diabetes Care* 2009;32: e140.

Sells CJ, Robinson NM, Brown Z, Knopp RH. Long-term developmental follow-up of infants of diabetic mothers. *J Pediatr* 1994;125: S9–17.

Silverman BL, Rizzo T, Green OC, et al. Long-term prospective evaluation of offspring of diabetic mothers. *Diabetes* 1991;40 Suppl 2: 121–5.

Silverman BL, Metzger BE, Cho NH, Loeb CA. Impaired glucose tolerance in adolescent offspring of diabetic mothers. *Diabetes Care* 1995;18: 611–7.

Susa JB, Boylan JM, Seghal P, Schwartz R. Persistence of impaired insulin secretion in infant rhesus monkeys that had been hyperinsulinemic in utero. *J Clin Endocrinol Metab* 1992;75: 265–9.

Tam WH, Ma RCW, Yang X, et al. Glucose intolerance and cardiometabolic risk in children ex-posed to maternal gestational diabetes mellitus in utero. *Pediatrics* 2008;122:1229–34.

Toeller M, Gries FA, Kuschak D, Potthoff S. Stoffwechselrisiko bei Kindern von Diabetikerinnen. *Arch Gynäkol* 1981;232: 548–9.

Van Assche FA, Gepts W. The cytological composition of the foetal endocrine pancreas in normal and pathological conditions. *Diabetologia* 1971;7: 434–44.

Van Assche FA, Gepts W, Aerts L. Immunocytochemical study of the endocrine pancreas in the rat during normal pregnancy and during experimental diabetic pregnancy. *Diabetologia* 1980;18: 487–91.

Van Assche FA. Birthweight as a risk factor for breast cancer. *Lancet* 1997;349:502.

Van Assche FA, Holemans K, Aerts L. Long-term consequences for offspring of diabetes during pregnancy. *Br Med Bull* 2001;60: 173–82.

Van Assche FA, Devlieger R, Harder T, Plagemann A. Mitogenic effect of insulin and developmen-tal programming (letter). *Diabetologia* 2010;53: 1243.

Weiss PAM, Scholz HS, Haas J, Tamussino KF, Seissler J, Borkenstein MH. Long-term follow-up of infants of mothers with type 1 diabetes. Evidence for hereditary and nonhereditary transmission of diabetes and precursors. *Diabetes Care* 2000;23: 905–11.

Xue F, Michels KB. Intrauterine factors and risk of breast cancer: a systematic review and meta-analysis of current evidence. *Lancet Oncol* 2007;8: 1088–1100.

15 Prenatal infections and long-term mental outcome: Modeling schizophrenia-related dysfunctions using the prenatal PolyI:C model in mice

Joram Feldon and Urs Meyer

Based on the epidemiological association between maternal infection during pregnancy and enhanced risk of neurodevelopmental brain disorders in the offspring, a number of in-vivo models have been established in rats and mice in order to study this link on an experimental basis. One such model is based on prenatal exposure to the viral mimic polyriboinosinic-polyribocytidilic acid (PolyI:C) in mice. This model has proven to be an excellent experimental tool to study the contribution of immune-mediated neurodevelopmental disturbances to complex behavioral and cognitive functions, which are especially known to be disrupted in schizophrenia and related psychotic disturbances. Since its initial establishment, the PolyI:C model has made a great impact on researchers concentrating on the neurodevelopmental and neuroimmunological basis of complex human brain disorders such as schizophrenia, and as a consequence, the model now enjoys wide recognition in the international scientific community. In this chapter, we summarize the features and methodology of the prenatal PolyI:C model with particular emphasis on its implementation in the mouse species. We highlight that the mouse PolyI:C model can successfully examine the influence of the precise timing of maternal immune activation, the role of pro- and anti-inflammatory cytokines, and the contribution of gene – environment interactions in the association between prenatal immune challenge and postnatal brain dysfunctions relevant to schizophrenia. Finally, we discuss how the PolyI:C model offers a unique opportunity to study the ontogeny of abnormal brain and behavioral functions and establish and evaluate early preventive interventions aiming to reduce the risk of long-lasting brain dysfunctions following prenatal exposure to infection.

15.1 Introduction

Disturbances directed at the maternal host during pregnancy can lead to direct physiological changes in the fetal environment and negatively affect the normal course of early brain development in the offspring (Rees and Harding, 2004; Rees and Inder, 2005). This can have long-lasting consequences for the development of postnatal brain dysfunctions, in which the primary cerebral insult or pathological process occurs during early brain development long before illness is clinically manifest. One prominent example of such neuropathological outcomes is schizophrenia. This disabling brain disorder seems to be associated with aberrations in early neurodevelopmental processes caused by a combination of environmental and genetic factors that predispose the organism to long-lasting neuropathology and psychopathology (Fatemi and Folsom, 2009; Rapoport et al., 2005).

Converging evidence suggests that maternal infection during pregnancy is one of the relevant environmental factors that can increase the risk of schizophrenia and related disorders in the offspring. Numerous (but not all) retrospective epidemiological studies have found a higher risk of schizophrenia in offspring born to mothers with viral or bacterial infections during early-to-middle stages of pregnancy (reviewed in Brown, 2006, 2008; Brown and Susser, 2002; Fatemi, 2005). Importantly, the establishment of prospective epidemiological approaches has provided clear serologic evidence for at least some of the infectious agents implicated in the prenatal infectious etiology of schizophrenia (Brown et al., 2004, 2005, 2009; Mortensen et al., 2007). Moreover, some of the reported effects identified by prospective epidemiological approaches appear to be relatively strong in magnitude (see, e.g., Brown et al., 2001). Even though all epidemiological studies are observational in nature (and thus cannot demonstrate causality), it is possible to comment on causal interferences from recent prospective epidemiological findings, which demonstrate markedly enhanced risk of schizophrenia and related disorders following serologically documented prenatal exposure to infection.

The epidemiological association between maternal infection during pregnancy and enhanced risk of schizophrenia in the offspring is not limited to a single viral or bacterial pathogen. Rather, a multitude of infectious agents is involved in this association, including influenza (Brown et al., 2004), rubella (Brown et al., 2001), toxoplasma gondii (Brown et al., 2005), measles (Torrey, Rawlings, and Waldman, 1988), polio (Suvisaari et al., 1999), herpes simplex (Buka et al., 2001), as well as infection with bacterial pathogens (Sørensen et al., 2009) and genital and/or reproductive infections (Babulas et al., 2006). Considering the wide variety of infectious agents involved, it has been suggested that factors common to the immune response to a multitude of pathogens may be the critical mediators of the association between prenatal infection and enhanced risk of schizophrenia. As discussed in detail elsewhere (Gilmore and Jarskog, 1997), abnormal expression of pro-inflammatory cytokines and other mediators of inflammation in the maternal host and eventually in the fetal brain may interfere with normal fetal brain development. However, there are several alternative (but not mutually exclusive) mechanisms whereby prenatal exposure to infection can bring about changes in brain and behavioral development (for a detailed discussion of such alternative mechanisms, see Fatemi, 2005; Meyer, Feldon, and Fatemi, 2009; Meyer, Feldon, and Yee, 2009). These include infection-induced stimulation of maternal/fetal stress response systems (Koenig, Kirkpatrick, and Lee, 2002), placental insufficiency and maternal/fetal nutritional deprivation (Brown and Susser, 2008; Susser, St Clair, and He, 2008), as well as penetration of viral pathogens and/or antibodies to the fetal brain (Aronsson et al., 2002; Whitley and Stagno, 1997). ▶Fig. 15.1 provides a schematic summary of putative neuroimmunological, developmental, and genetic factors involved in the association between prenatal exposure to infection and enhanced risk of neurodevelopmental brain disorders.

Based on the epidemiological association between maternal infection during pregnancy and enhanced risk of schizophrenia in the offspring, a number of in-vivo models have been established in rats and mice in order to study this link on experimental grounds (Meyer and Feldon, 2010; Meyer, Feldon, and Fatemi, 2009; Meyer, Feldon, and Yee, 2009). One such model is based on prenatal exposure to the viral mimic polyriboinosinic-polyribocytidilic acid (PolyI:C) in mice. This model has proven to be an excellent experimental tool to study the contribution of immune-mediated neurodevelopmental

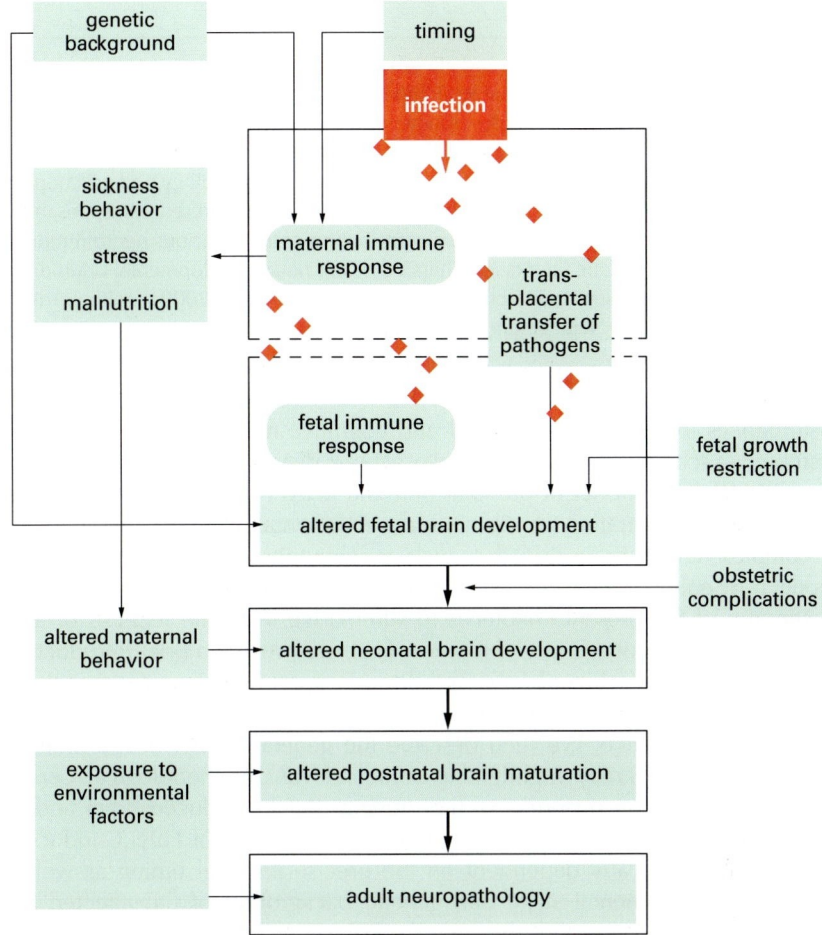

Fig. 15.1: Summary of putative neuroimmunological, developmental, and genetic factors involved in the association between prenatal exposure to infection and enhanced risk of neurodevelopmental brain disorders. Both the precise timing of maternal infection and the genetic background of the maternal host determine the specificity of the maternal immune response to infection, which in turn may significantly influence the specificity of inflammation-mediated neurodevelopmental disturbances in the fetus. Genetic abnormalities may directly induce mal-neurodevelopment and/or act synergistically with prenatal infection/inflammation to increase the risk of long-lasting alterations in brain and behavioral development. Activation of the fetal immune system may also participate in the induction of altered neurodevelopmental trajectories; however, this is critically influenced by the precise stage of prenatal development. In addition to stimulation of immunological factors in the maternal immune system, some infectious pathogens may cross the placenta and negatively affect fetal brain development directly upon penetration into fetal brain tissue. Furthermore, activation of the maternal immune system induces direct physiological changes in the maternal host, including sickness behavior and stress, which in turn may result in (temporary) undernutrition of the mother. Together with the maternal and/or fetal inflammatory responses, these additional physiological changes may lead to fetal growth

(Continued)

Fig. 15.1: (*Continued*)

---

restriction, obstetric complications, and alterations in postpartum maternal behavior, all of which may additionally affect normal fetal and/or neonatal brain development. Disturbances in early (prenatal and neonatal) brain development may predispose the offspring to alterations in subsequent postnatal brain maturation and may alter the offspring's sensitivity to environmental factors during this period, finally cumulating into adult neuropathology and psychopathology. In-vivo models of prenatal infection and/or immune activation represent indispensable experimental tools to elucidate the relative contribution of these various neuroimmunological, developmental, and genetic factors to enhanced risk of neurodevelopmental brain disorders following prenatal exposure to infection. Taken from Meyer et al. (2009a), with permission of the International Behavioral Neuroscience Society.

disturbances to complex behavioral and cognitive functions especially known to be disrupted in schizophrenia and related psychotic disturbances. Since its initial establishment, the PolyI:C model of prenatal immune activation has made a great impact on researchers concentrating on the neurodevelopmental and neuroimmunological basis of complex human brain disorders such as schizophrenia, and as a consequence, the model now enjoys wide recognition in the international scientific community.

The aim of the present chapter is to summarize the main features of and findings from the prenatal PolyI:C model in mice. First, we provide a brief introduction into the symptomatology of schizophrenia and discuss experimental approaches that allow the assessment of schizophrenia-like behavioral, cognitive, and psychopharmacological abnormalities in mice. We then describe the general design of the prenatal PolyI:C model in mice, thereby highlighting some relevant methodological considerations. Next, we provide an overview of the prenatal PolyI:C-induced brain and behavioral pathology and discuss how the long-term consequences of PolyI:C-induced immune challenge are critically dependent on the precise prenatal timing as well as on the postnatal developmental stage and genetic background of the affected individuals. Finally, we demonstrate that the prenatal PolyI:C model in mice offers a unique opportunity to study the relative contribution of specific neurochemical abnormalities to schizophrenia-related brain dysfunctions and to evaluate early preventive interventions aiming to reduce the risk of long-lasting brain dysfunctions following prenatal exposure to viral-like infection.

15.2 Schizophrenia and animal models

Schizophrenia is a major form of psychotic disorder that affects approximately 1% of the population worldwide (Tamminga and Holcomb, 2005). It is characterized by profound disturbances in mental functions, emotions, and behavior, and it disrupts many of the most basic human processes of perception and judgment. Typically, the psychotic symptoms in schizophrenia are divided into three main categories: positive, negative, and cognitive symptoms (Crow, 1980; Elvevag and Goldberg, 2000; Goldman-Rakic, 1991, 1994; McGlashan and Fenton, 1992; Nuechterlein and Dawson, 1984). Positive symptoms refer to features that are normally not present but appear as a result of the disease process. These include visual and/or auditory hallucinations, delusions, paranoia, and major thought disorders. On the other hand, negative symptoms refer to features that are normally present but are reduced or absent as a result of the disease process. This symptom category includes social withdrawal, apathy, anhedonia, alogia, and behavioral perseveration. Finally, the cognitive symptoms of schizophrenia involve disturbances in executive functions, working memory impairment, and inability to sustain attention.

Multiple lines of evidence suggest that the etiology of schizophrenia involves aberrant neurodevelopmental processes in which the primary cerebral insult or pathological process occurs during early brain development long before the illness is clinically expressed (Fatemi and Folsom, 2009; Rapoport et al., 2005). According to the neurodevelopmental hypothesis of schizophrenia, an interaction between early neurodevelopmental disturbances and periadolescent brain maturation seems to be necessary in order to trigger the onset of full-blown psychotic behavior, which typically emerges during adolescence or early adulthood. However, despite the growing consensus that schizophrenia is a brain disorder, a comprehensive neurobiological account of the disease (including the etiology, neuropathology, pathophysiology, psychopharmacology, and genetics) remains a considerable challenge to clinicians and scientists alike. Furthermore, the available symptomatic treatment of schizophrenia is only partially successful, and therefore, the development of novel therapeutic strategies is clearly warranted (Kapur and Remington, 2001; Tamminga, 1999). Together with direct exploration of these issues in human subjects, basic research in animals represents a fruitful approach to studying the neurobiological basis of brain and behavioral disturbances relevant to schizophrenia in order to establish and evaluate novel pharmacological therapies for their treatment. Indeed, the use of animal models allows a stringent experimental control of subjects in genetically homogenous populations and facilitates the identification of neurobiological factors contributing to distinct forms of schizophrenia-related brain and behavioral abnormalities. Furthermore, animal models provide indispensable tools for testing hypotheses that cannot be directly addressed in human subjects for technical and ethical reasons, including the verification of causal relationships in epidemiological studies.

The attempt to model any human psychiatric condition in animals has always been met with some skepticism, and schizophrenia is a particularly illustrative case (Boksa, 2007; Low and Hardy, 2007). The obvious reason for this is that the clinical manifestation of schizophrenia in humans includes symptoms such as hallucinations, delusions, and major thought disorders, which are specific to humans and impossible to ascertain without structured interviews. Hence, it is impossible to mimic a complex human brain disorder such as schizophrenia in animals. However, one fruitful experimental approach is to focus on individual behavioral, physiological, and neuroanatomical phenotypes of the disorder rather than to model the entire syndrome (Arguello and Gogos, 2006; Lipska and Weinberger, 2000).

In parallel with similar efforts in humans, behavioral neuroscience and related research fields have established a wide variety of sophisticated paradigms that allow the assessment of schizophrenia-related traits in experimental models and clinical trials. Such cross-species translational paradigms have been developed for the identification and characterization of neuropsychological, cognitive, and psychopharmacological core dysfunctions implicated in human psychotic disorders. ▶Tab. 15.1 provides a sample of the most commonly used paradigms for the phenotypic characterization

Tab. 15.1: A sample of behavioral and pharmacological paradigms used for evaluating schizophrenia-related neuropsychological and neurochemical abnormalities in rodents.

Neuropsychological and/or neurochemical domains	Experimental paradigm	Symptoms in schizophrenia
① Sensorimotor gating	Prepulse inhibition of the acoustic startle reflex	Impaired
② Attentional control of selective associative learning	Latent inhibition	Impaired in patients with acute positive symptoms; abnormally enhanced in patients with marked negative symptoms
	Kamin blocking	Reduced especially in acutely ill patients
③ Sustained attention and vigilance	5-choice serial reaction time test	Impaired in patients with schizophrenia and their nonpsychotic first-degree relatives
④ Working memory	Delayed nonmatch to sample/position	Impaired
	Radial arm maze	
	Morris watermaze	
	Y-maze	
⑤ Executive functions	Intradimensional/extradimensional shift	Impaired at impaired set-shifting and concept formation
	Discrimination reversal learning	Abnormally enhanced behavioral/cognitive flexibility in patients with marked positive symptoms (switching behavior); behavioral and/or cognitive inflexibility in patients with marked negative symptoms
⑥ Social behavior	Social interaction and recognition tests	Reduced especially in patients with negative symptoms
⑦ Stereotypy	Open field exploration test	Presence of stereotypic behavior
	Holeboard exploration test	
⑧ Dopamine-associated neurotransmission	Behavioral reaction to amphetamine	Increased sensitivity to dopamine-stimulating drugs; enhanced striatal dopamine release
	In-vivo microdialysis following systemic amphetamine challenge to assess the (striatal) release of dopamine and other neurotransmitters	

(Continued)

Tab. 15.1 (*Continued*)

Neuropsychological and/or neurochemical domains	Experimental paradigm	Symptoms in schizophrenia
⑨ Glutamate-associated neurotransmission	Behavioral reaction to ketamine, dizocilpine and phencyclidine	Increased sensitivity to NMDA-receptor-blocking drugs; reduced glutamatergic signaling at NMDA receptors
	In-vivo microdialysis following systemic treatment with ketamine, dizocilpine, and phencyclidine to assess the (striatal) release of dopamine and other neurotransmitters	

The table summarizes the most commonly used cross-species translational experimental paradigms used to assess schizophrenia-related functional brain abnormalities and outlines the corresponding psychopathological symptoms in the human clinical condition.

① Prepulse inhibition (PPI) of the acoustic startle reflex refers to the reduction of startle reaction to a startle-eliciting stimulus (pulse) when it is shortly preceded by a weak stimulus (prepulse). It is an operational measure of sensorimotor gating that reflects the ability to filter or gate intrusive sensory-motor information.

② Latent inhibition (LI) and Kamin blocking (KB) are forms of selective associative learning considered to index an organism's capacity to ignore irrelevant stimuli. LI is usually described as the retardation in learning about the significance of a stimulus as a result of its prior nonreinforced (nonconsequential) repeated pre-exposures. In associative conditioning, pre-exposure of the to-be-conditioned stimulus (CS) impedes the subsequent development of the conditioned response (CR) following pairings between the same CS and a significant event, the unconditioned stimulus (US). KB refers to the impediment of the development and/or expression of a CR when a target conditioned stimulus (CS2) is presented as part of a compound that includes another CS (CS1) that had been used previously to establish a CR.

③ Sustained attention and vigilance can be assessed using the 5-choice serial reaction time test (5-CSRTT), which tests the ability of a subject to sustain spatial attention divided among a number of locations over a large number of trials. This capacity is measured by the subject's accuracy of reporting the correct stimuli.

④ Working memory is a special short-term memory buffer with a limited temporal capacity and is used to hold relevant information active in order to guide on-going behavior, including comprehension, reasoning, and problem solving. Numerous experimental paradigms can be used for the assessment of working memory in experimental animals, including the delayed nonmatch to sample/position (DNMTS/P) task, the radial arm maze, the Morris watermaze, and the Y-maze. An important component of working memory as assessed in these paradigms is the short-term storage of trial-unique information, whereby unique information about specific stimuli (e.g., spatial location and object information) is retained briefly in a short-term memory buffer and discarded after an appropriate response is executed.

⑤ Executive functions are commonly referred to as a collection of brain processes that are crucial for planning, problem solving, maintenance of goal-directed behavior, and behavioral/cognitive flexibility. Two effective experimental procedures to study executive functions in rodents are the

(*Continued*)

Tab. 15.1 (*Continued*)

paradigms of intradimensional/extradimensional shifts and discrimination reversal learning. An intradimensional shift occurs when the subject is required to cease responding to one feature of a particular perceptual dimension (e.g., "red" for the dimension color) and begins responding to a new feature of the same dimension (e.g., "blue"). On the other hand, an extradimensional shift occurs when the subject is required to switch responding to a novel feature of a previously irrelevant perceptual dimension (e.g., from the color "blue" to "circles" from the dimension "shape"). In reversal learning, subjects first learn to respond differentially (typically approaching or avoiding) to two stimuli of opposing valence (S1+ vs S2−), and are then confronted with the same two stimuli but with the reversed valence (S1− vs S2+). The ability to recognize an unexpected consequence from a previously established associative learning rule and then to switch the response contingency accordingly is crucial to reversal learning.

⑥ Social behavior is commonly referred to as behavior that takes place in a social context and results from the interaction between and among individuals (of the same species). Because most of the commonly used experimental animals, including rats and mice, are highly social animals, social interaction and recognition tests can be efficiently used to study social behavior under experimental conditions.

⑦ Stereotypy is defined as uniform, repetitive, and compulsive actions within a restricted pattern that often have no obvious goals or end-points. Stereotype behavior can be assessed using open field or holeboard exploration tests, in which persistent repetitions of particular actions can be measured by observing the animal's behavior over a certain period of time.

⑧/⑨ One effective and informative way to assess the functional consequences of altered dopamine- and/or glutamate-associated neurotransmission is to measure a subject's behavioral sensitivity to acute treatment with dopamine receptor agonists such as amphetamine or NMDA-receptor antagonists such as ketamine, dizocilpine (MK-801), and phencyclidine (PCP). This can be coupled with in-vivo microdialysis in order to have a parallel measure of extracellular neurotransmitter release before, during, and after the drug challenge. Adapted from Meyer and Feldon (2010).

of schizophrenia-related neuropsychological, cognitive, and psychopharmacological core dysfunctions in rats and mice. These paradigms have been proven valuable and informative experimental tools for assessing psychosis-like traits in a variety of lesion-based, genetic, or psychopharmacological rodent models (for a review see Arguello and Gogos, 2006; Castner, Goldman-Rakic, and Williams, 2004; Meyer et al., 2005; Swerdlow and Geyer, 1998; Weiner 2003). It should be emphasized that the collection of paradigms summarized in ▶Tab. 15.1 is far from exhaustive. Theoretically, they are also not mutually exclusive of each other, even though they have been developed as tests of schizophrenia-related dysfunction largely independently of each other. Conversely, the neural substrate underlying performances on each of these behavioral, cognitive, and psychopharmacological tests share considerable common elements, and their identification is particularly crucial to the disease process of schizophrenia. Hence, the power of validation is magnified many fold when these tests are applied as a battery of tests for the phenotypic characterization of functional abnormalities relevant to complex neuropsychiatric disorders such as schizophrenia, especially when the experimental model system does not rely on any specific presumption of the disorder's neuronal substrates.

The extent to which it is possible to extrapolate from animal model systems to the clinical condition in humans, and consequently the value of the information that may be derived from animal models, depends on several validity criteria of the model. In general, there are three main criteria that should be applied for the validation of an animal model (Willner, 1984, 1986):

- *Face validity:* This refers to phenomenological and symptomatological similarities between the features of the model and the clinical condition. For example, face validity reflects the degree of descriptive similarity between the behavioral abnormalities seen in the model system and the human psychopathological condition. Face validity also includes the etiological and/or epidemiological significance of the experimental manipulation used for the induction of a particular phenotype that aims at mimicking the human condition.
- *Construct validity:* This refers to the degree of similarity between the mechanisms underlying the particular phenotype in the model and that underlying the phenotype in the condition that is being modeled. Hence, construct validity accounts for mechanistic similarities between the model and the clinical condition. In the context of animal models of human brain disorders, construct validity is a theory-driven, experimental substantiation of the behavioral, pathophysiological, and/or neuronal elements of the model. Hence, it reflects the degree of fitting of the theoretical rationale and of modeling the true nature of the symptoms to be mimicked by the animal model.
- *Predictive validity:* This implies that the model allows extrapolation of the effect of a particular experimental manipulation from one species to another (e.g., from rodents to humans) and from one condition to another (e.g., from the preclinical model in animals to the clinical condition in humans). A narrower concept of predictive validity is used in psychopharmacological contexts. Here, predictive validity usually implies that pharmacological compounds that are known to influence a clinical state in humans should have a similar effect in the animal model. Hence, this validity criterion refers to the sensitivity of the model system to clinically effective drugs. As a consequence, pharmacological treatments that precipitate or exacerbate a human pathological condition should exert a similar effect on the model, whereas those pharmacological treatments relieving the human pathological condition should have a similar beneficial effect on behavioral and/or cognitive abnormalities modeled in animals.

It should be emphasized that no animal model is likely to fulfill all validity criteria at the same time. In fact, validity criteria are often restricted to the specific purpose of the model, and there is no general consensus about how to weigh the different categories of validity in the model evaluation process.

15.3 Features and methodology of the mouse prenatal PolyI:C model

In the mouse prenatal PolyI:C model, pregnant dams are exposed to the viral mimic PolyI:C at a specific gestational stage, and the brain and behavioral consequences of the prenatal immunological manipulation are then compared in the resulting offspring relative to offspring born to vehicle-treated control mothers. PolyI:C is a commercially available synthetic analogue of double-stranded RNA. Double-stranded RNA is generated during viral infection as a replication intermediate for single-stranded RNA (ssRNA) or as a by-product of symmetrical transcription in DNA viruses. It is recognized as foreign by the mammalian immune system through the transmembrane protein toll-like receptor 3 (TLR3). TLRs are a class of pathogen recognition receptors that recognize invariant structures present on and/or associated with virulent pathogens. Upon binding to TLRs, double-stranded RNA or its synthetic analogue PolyI:C stimulates the production and release of many pro-inflammatory cytokines, including interleukin (IL)-1β, IL-6, and tumor necrosis factor (TNF)-α (Meyer et al., 2006b, 2008a). In addition, PolyI:C is a potent inducer of the type I interferons IFN-α and IFN-β (Takeuchi and Akira, 2007). Administration of PolyI:C can, therefore, efficiently mimic the acute phase response to viral infection.

There are several advantages to using viral-like immunogens such as PolyI:C instead of viral pathogens in in-vivo animal models of prenatal immune activation. Firstly, unlike viral pathogens, PolyI:C can be easily handled without stringent biosafety precautions. Secondly, the intensity of the cytokine-associated immune responses can be easily controlled by appropriate dose-response studies (Cunningham et al., 2007; Meyer et al., 2005; Shi et al., 2003). Thirdly, PolyI:C-induced immunological challenges in rodents are time-limited, ranging from 24 to 48 h depending on the precise dose used (Cunningham et al., 2007; Meyer et al., 2005). This facilitates the precise timing of the maternal immune activation corresponding to specific periods of fetal development. This aspect is particularly relevant when prenatal immune activation models are designed with the aim of exploring the impact of the precise timing in the association between prenatal immune challenge and postnatal brain dysfunctions. Finally, maternal exposure to PolyI:C can alter pro- and anti-inflammatory cytokine levels in the three relevant compartments of the maternal – fetal interface of rodents, namely the placenta, the amniotic fluid, and the fetus, including the fetal brain (Gilmore, Jarskog, and Vadlamudi, 2005; Meyer et al., 2006b, 2008a).

Compared to infection models using viral pathogens (Fatemi et al., 1999, 2002a, 2002b, 2008, 2009; Shi et al., 2003), one limitation of the PolyI:C model of immune activation is that it does not readily mimic the precise immunological insults occurring in the human environment. That is, it falls short in modeling the full spectrum of immune responses normally induced by viral exposure. Rather, it mimics especially the cytokine-associated viral-like acute phase responses in the maternal host and, thereafter, in the fetal environment. However, this aspect of the PolyI:C-based immune activation model is helpful in order to test specifically whether imbalances in maternal and/or fetal cytokine levels may be one of the crucial mediating factors in the link between maternal infection and the emergence of brain and behavioral pathology in the offspring.

Even though the principal design of the prenatal PolyI:C model in mice appears to be relatively simple and straightforward, several methodological considerations need to be taken into account to guarantee a successful realization. A detailed discussion of these considerations can be found elsewhere (see Meyer, Feldon, and Fatemi, 2009). Here, we would like to restrict our discussion to one of the most relevant methodological considerations, namely the species-specific timing of corresponding brain development in mice and humans.

Because prenatal development differs essentially between mice and humans, a careful extrapolation of the timing of brain development from mice to humans must be taken into account in the design and interpretation of translational neurodevelopmental studies. In terms of percentage of gestation and developmental biology, the gestational period in mice would only cover the first and early-to-middle second trimester of human pregnancy (Clancy, Darlington, and Finlay, 2001; Clancy et al., 2007a, 2007b; Kaufman, 2003). In the mouse species, development corresponding to the third trimester of human pregnancy would already be ex-utero, that is, during the first 10 days of postnatal development. One consequence is that in-vivo mouse models can only translate into experimental investigations of the long-term brain and behavioral effects of prenatal environmental insults during the first and early-to-middle second trimester of human pregnancy. Early neonatal immune activation and/or infections would thus be needed in experimental mouse (or rat) models in order to explore the long-term neurodevelopmental impact of immunological insults corresponding to late (third trimester) gestational infections in humans (see e.g., Hornig et al., 1999; Hornig and Lipkin, 2001; Pletnikov et al., 2000, 2002a, 2002b; Pletnikov, Moran, and Carbone, 2002).

It should also be noted that the exact correspondence of fetal developmental progression can also significantly differ between two closely related species such as rats and mice. Indeed, many key events in fetal development occur approximately 2 days later in rats as compared to mice (Clancy et al., 2001, 2007a, 2007b). A careful examination of the spatiotemporal events in prenatal brain development across different species is therefore indispensable for the delineation of the precise neurodevelopmental impact of prenatal environmental insults in humans as well as in rodents. The correspondence of fetal developmental progression in different species can be compared using database-driven Web sites. Such programs are based on statistical algorithms that integrate hundreds of empirically derived developing neural events in 10 mammalian species, including rats, mice, and humans (http://translatingtime.net/; see also Clancy et al., 2007a, 2007b).

15.4 Schizophrenia-related phenotypes in the mouse prenatal PolyI:C model

In the following sections, we review experimental findings derived from the prenatal PolyI:C model as applied primarily in the mouse species. Thereby, we focus on functional phenotypes relevant to schizophrenia and related psychotic disorders. A detailed review of the long-term neuroanatomical and neurochemical consequences of prenatal (PolyI:C-induced) immune challenge can be found elsewhere (Meyer and Feldon, 2009, 2010).

15.4.1 Dose-response studies

Based on the seminal work by Fatemi and colleagues, who studied the brain and behavioral consequences of prenatal exposure to human influenza in mice (Fatemi et al., 1999, 2002a, 2002b, 2008, 2009; Shi et al., 2003), our laboratory established a comprehensive dose-response study with the aim of exploring the effects of prenatal PolyI:C-induced immune challenge at low, middle, or high intensity on schizophrenia-related phenotypes in adulthood (Meyer et al., 2005). For this purpose, pregnant mice on gestation day (GD) 9 were subjected to a single injection of PolyI:C at a dose of 2.5, 5, or 10 mg/kg (i.v.), or were treated with corresponding vehicle (sterile pyrogen-free saline solution). The selected gestational window (i.e., GD 9) in mice corresponds roughly to the middle-to-late first trimester of human pregnancy, with respect to developmental biology and comparable percentage of gestation in mice and humans (see previous section). Behavioral, cognitive, and pharmacological phenotyping was conducted using a variety of paradigms summarized in ▶Tab. 15.1, including assessment of locomotor activity in a novel environment (open field), prepulse inhibition (PPI) of the acoustic startle reflex, latent inhibition (LI), US-pre-exposure effect (USPEE), working memory in the Morris water maze, left – right discrimination reversal learning in operant chambers, and locomotor response to acute treatment with a low dose (2.5 mg/kg, i.p.) of the indirect dopamine receptor agonist amphetamine (AMPH).

This initial dose response study confirmed that maternal immune activation by PolyI:C on GD 9 can lead to impairments in multiple neuropsychological, cognitive, and pharmacological domains, therefore mimicking a wide spectrum of psychopathology seen in schizophrenia patients (Meyer et al., 2005). Notably, some behavioral deficits showed a clear dose-dependent relationship across the three doses of PolyI:C examined, whereas some did not. The former includes PPI deficiency, attenuation of the USPEE, and enhanced reaction to systemic AMPH, which all emerged in adult mice subjected to prenatal treatment with 5 or 10 mg/kg PolyI:C (i.v.), but not so following PolyI:C exposure at a dose of 2.5 mg/kg (i.v.). On the other hand, all three doses examined led to the disruption of LI, spatial working memory impairment when the demand in temporal retention was high, and reduced spatial exploration as assessed in the open field test.

The identified dose-dependent effects of prenatal PolyI:C treatment given via the i.v. route are consistent with the dose-dependent nature of PPI disruption emerging following prenatal PolyI:C administration on GD 9 using i.p. routes in mice (Shi et al., 2003), as well as with the differential efficacy of PolyI:C treatment at low (~ 1 mg/kg, i.v.) versus middle (~ 4 mg/kg, i.v.) intensity to disrupt adult PPI in rats (Fortier, Luheshi, and Boksa, 2007; Wolff and Bilkey, 2008). Together, the apparent impact of the precise immune stimulus intensity in the prenatal PolyI:C model suggests that there is a threshold of (viral-like) immune activation that is required to induce long-term brain and behavioral pathology in the offspring. The dose-dependent nature of prenatal PolyI:C treatment parallels the findings derived from human epidemiological studies, suggesting that only a minority of offspring born to an infected mother eventually develop schizophrenia (Fatemi, 2005). According to the dose-response findings obtained in the prenatal PolyI:C model, maternal (viral-like) infection during pregnancy may enhance the risk of schizophrenia in the offspring only if the prenatal infectious process is associated with relatively strong immunological reactions in the maternal and/or fetal compartments.

15.4.2 Prenatal time-window studies

The strength of the association between maternal infection during pregnancy and enhanced risk of schizophrenia appears to be critically influenced by the precise prenatal timing. Many of the initial retrospective epidemiological studies found a significant association between maternal viral infection during pregnancy and a higher incidence of schizophrenia in the progeny only when the maternal host was infected in the second trimester of human pregnancy (e.g., Mednick et al., 1988; Stöber et al., 2002; Wright et al., 1995). However, recent findings from epidemiological studies using prospectively collected and quantifiable serologic samples indicate that there has been a somewhat excessive emphasis on second trimester infections. For example, there is serologic evidence that influenza infection in early gestation (i.e., in the first trimester of human pregnancy) is associated with the highest risk of schizophrenia in the offspring (Brown et al., 2004). This thereby challenges the prevailing view that influenza infection during the second trimester of pregnancy may confer the maximal risk for the offspring to develop schizophrenia and related disorders in adulthood. A similar conclusion can be drawn from recent epidemiological studies investigating the effects of maternal exposure to rubella infection (Brown et al., 2001), genital and reproductive infections (Babulas et al., 2006), and bacterial infections (Sørensen et al., 2009). The findings from these studies all point to more extensive effects on elevating the risk of schizophrenia if the maternal host is infected early in pregnancy, that is, from the periconceptional period to the end of the first trimester.

It follows that the vulnerability to infection-induced neurodevelopmental abnormalities associated with schizophrenia differs between distinct stages of fetal development. However, when comparing the epidemiological data derived from initial retrospective and recent prospective studies, it is still debatable whether there is a time window with maximal vulnerability in the prenatal infectious etiology of this disorder. Furthermore, the relevant neuroimmunological and developmental factors underlying the temporal dependency of the link between prenatal infection and risk of schizophrenia remain largely unidentified thus far.

Animal models of prenatal immune activation provide a powerful tool to examine the critical window hypothesis using prospective factorial research designs. This can be achieved by comparing the effects of prenatal immune challenge at distinct gestational stages, relative to prenatal control treatment, on the susceptibility to structural and functional brain abnormalities in postnatal life. Our laboratory has conducted a series of experiments designed to evaluate the influence of the timing of maternal PolyI:C-induced immune challenge on the emergence of brain and behavioral dysfunctions in the resulting offspring (Meyer et al., 2006a, 2006b, 2008c). These experiments demonstrated that the precise time of prenatal immune activation is a critical determinant of the specificity of both the structural and the functional brain abnormalities in later life. Indeed, we found that maternal PolyI:C-induced immunological stimulation at different gestational times precipitates distinct psychopathological and neuropathological symptom clusters in the offspring. More specifically, prenatal PolyI:C treatment (at 5 mg/kg, i.v.) on GD 9 leads to a pathological profile characterized by suppression in exploratory behavior, abnormalities in selective associative learning in the form of LI disruption and abolition of the US-pre-exposure effect, impairments in sensorimotor gating in the form of reduced PPI, enhanced sensitivity to the indirect dopamine receptor agonist AMPH, and deficiency in spatial working memory when the demand on temporal retention is high. On the other hand, identical PolyI:C treatment on GD 17 leads to a partially overlapping symptom profile involving the emergence of perseverative behavior in the form of impaired discrimination reversal learning, deficits in spatial working memory and recognition memory even when the demand on temporal retention is low, potentiated response to AMPH and to the noncompetitive *N*-methyl *D*-aspartate (NMDA)-receptor antagonist dizocilpine (MK-801), as well as abolition of the US-pre-exposure effect. Hence, some of the identified pathological traits are clearly restricted to the symptom cluster associated with prenatal PolyI:C-induced immune activation in early/middle or late gestation (e.g., loss of LI and impairments in reversal learning), whereas others are common to both symptom clusters (e.g., potentiation of AMPH sensitivity). Taken together, our prenatal time-window studies in the mouse PolyI:C model indicate that the developmental vulnerability of specific forms of postnatal brain dysfunction to prenatal exposure to immune-challenge varies across different gestational stages: maternal (viral-like) immune activation in early/middle (GD 9) and late (GD 17) pregnancy can lead to divergent behavioral and cognitive dysfunctions in the offspring. A similar conclusion can also be derived from analyses at the immunological and neuroanatomical levels (for a detailed discussion, see Meyer et al., 2006a, 2006b, 2008c; Meyer, Yee, and Feldon, 2007; Meyer, Feldon, and Yee, 2009).

Notably, the dissociation between the long-term functional effects of prenatal PolyI:C treatment in early/middle (GD 9) and late (GD 17) gestation may be related to differing symptom clusters of schizophrenia. It is known that schizophrenia is associated with myriad psychological and cognitive abnormalities. Symptoms tend to segregate into clusters (e.g., the positive–negative symptoms dichotomy in schizophrenia), which appear to follow separate developmental courses (Gross, 1997; Murray et al., 1992; Sporn et al., 2004). They also respond differentially to distinct classes of pharmacotherapy (Maguire, 2002) and are suggested to be associated with dysfunctions localized to discrete brain regions (Liddle et al., 1992). Based on genetic and epidemiological evidence the possibility has been suggested that these symptom clusters or even subtypes of schizophrenia may correspond to distinct neurodevelopmental disturbances (e.g., Cannon et al., 2003; Stöber et al., 2002).

One hypothesis emerging from our prenatal time-window studies in the mouse PolyI:C model postulates that the distinction between early/middle and late pregnancy immune challenge may capture the positive–negative dichotomy of schizophrenia (Sullivan et al., 2006). Experimental data available so far readily indicate that prenatal viral-like immune challenge at early/middle pregnancy in mice leads to a variety of abnormalities associated with positive symptoms of schizophrenia, including increased sensitivity to acute dopaminergic stimulation (Meyer et al., 2005, 2008b, 2008c), loss of the LI effect (Meyer et al., 2005, 2006a, 2006c), and abnormal sensorimotor gating, which is related to enhanced striatal dopaminergic activity (Meyer et al., 2005, 2008c; Vuillermot et al., 2010). On the other hand, viral-like immune activation on late gestation particularly leads to the emergence of behavioral, cognitive, and pharmacological dysfunctions associated primarily with (but not limited to) the negative symptoms, such as perseverative behavior (Meyer et al., 2006b) and strong potentiation of the sensitivity to NMDA-receptor antagonism (Meyer et al., 2008c). A follow-up characterization of the long-term consequences of GD 17 PolyI:C exposure in mice further supported our hypothesis that late prenatal immune challenge can lead to behavioral and neurochemical abnormalities relevant to the negative symptoms of schizophrenia. In a recent study, we found that prenatal PolyI:C treatment on GD 17 led to significant deficits in social interaction, anhedonic behavior, and alterations in the locomotor and stereotyped behavioral responses to acute apomorphine treatment in both male and female offspring (Bitanihirwe et al., 2010a, 2010b). In addition, male but not female offspring born to immune-challenged mothers displayed behavior/cognitive inflexibility as indexed by the presence of an abnormally enhanced LI effect (Bitanihirwe et al., 2010b). Prenatal immune activation in late gestation also led to numerous, partly sex-specific, changes in basal neurotransmitters levels, including reduced dopamine and glutamate contents in the prefrontal cortex and hippocampus, as well as reduced gamma-amino butyric acid (GABA) and glycine contents in the hippocampus and prefrontal cortex, respectively (Bitanihirwe et al., 2010b). Taken together, the constellation of behavioral and neurochemical abnormalities that emerges following early/middle (GD 9) and late (GD 17) prenatal PolyI:C exposure in mice leads us to conclude that these immune-based experimental model systems provide powerful neurodevelopmental animal models for the positive and negative/cognitive symptoms of schizophrenia, respectively.

Further examination and evaluation of the structural and functional consequences of in-utero immune challenge at different times of gestation may provide important insight into the fundamental neuroimmunological and neuropathological mechanisms underlying the segregation of positive and negative symptoms in schizophrenia from a neurodevelopmental point of view. Indeed, animal models are indispensable experimental tools in the study of possible causal links between specific neuronal dysfunctions and distinct forms of abnormal behavior. They are, therefore, valuable in the exploration of specific brain and behavioral relationships in complex neuropsychiatric disorders such as schizophrenia, which is characterized by multiple behavioral, cognitive, and pharmacological pathologies that are likely to involve neuronal disturbances beyond one single brain region and neurotransmitter system. Importantly, given that prenatal PolyI:C treatment in mice leads, at least in part, to differential behavioral and cognitive pathological outcomes depending on the precise prenatal timing and immune stimulus specificity, the mouse PolyI:C model provides a unique opportunity to link specific neuronal dysfunctions with distinct forms of psychosis-related behavior.

15.4.3 Gene-environment and environment-environment interaction studies

Maternal infection during pregnancy is relatively common (Laibl and Sheffield, 2005; Longman and Johnson, 2007). Yet, most offspring of mothers exposed to infection during pregnancy do not develop severe neurodevelopmental brain disorders such as schizophrenia. This suggests that if in-utero exposure to infection plays a role in the etiology of these brain disorders, then it probably does so by interacting with other factors, including genetic factors. Therefore, exploring the influence of the genetic background seems highly relevant in the association between prenatal immune challenge and risk of neurodevelopmental disorders.

In the experimental study of such gene – environment interactions, one may first consider the examination of genes that are directly involved in innate and acquired immunity. Some of the identified genetic risk factors of schizophrenia include promoter polymorphisms of pro-inflammatory (Boin et al., 2001) and anti-inflammatory cytokines (Chiavetto et al., 2002), as well as human leukocyte antigens and alleles (Wright et al., 2001). The precise immune-related genetic background of the maternal host may influence the liability to certain infections, or result in an excessive or inappropriate inflammatory response in the maternal periphery and thereafter in the fetal system. This may in turn determine the impact of prenatal infection on early neurodevelopmental processes and subsequent brain and behavioral development. We have recently obtained direct experimental evidence for this hypothesis by comparing the long-term functional consequences of prenatal PolyI:C exposure in wild-type mice and transgenic mice constitutively overexpressing the anti-inflammatory cytokine IL-10 in macrophages. The results show that enhanced IL-10-mediated anti-inflammatory signaling during prenatal development is sufficient to prevent the emergence of multiple behavioral and pharmacological abnormalities in the adult offspring after prenatal immune challenge by PolyI:C (Meyer et al., 2008a). In another study, Smith and colleagues (2007) have demonstrated that prenatal PolyI:C treatment is inefficient in inducing behavioral maldevelopment in animals with a genetic deletion of the pro-inflammatory cytokine IL-6 relative to wild-type animals. Hence, recent investigations in mice designed to examine immunological gene – environment interactions have successfully shown that the association between prenatal immune challenge and emergence of schizophrenia-like behavioral and pharmacological dysfunctions is critically influenced by the anti-inflammatory and pro-inflammatory genetic background of the infected host. These initial findings should be extended to the evaluation of other immune-associated genetic risk factors of neurodevelopmental disorders (Boin et al., 2001; Chiavetto et al., 2002; Wright et al., 2001).

An examination of the genes that have been identified as major genetic susceptibility factors of neuropsychiatric disorders of neurodevelopmental origin certainly also warrants consideration. For schizophrenia, this may include neuregulin-1 (NRG-1), catechol-O-methyltransferase (COMT), and/or disrupted in schizophrenia-1 (DISC-1) (Harrison and Weinberger, 2005). It is likely that many of these genes as such play only minor roles in infectious or inflammatory processes. Nevertheless, disruption of neurodevelopmental mechanisms by abnormal expression of these genes may act synergistically with prenatal infection/inflammation to increase the risk of long-lasting neurodevelopmental brain disorders (Ayhan et al., 2009). This scenario would be consistent with the hypothesis that the etiopathology of major neuropsychiatric disorders such as schizophrenia involves aberrations in neurodevelopmental processes that are caused by an interaction between environmental and genetic factors (Tsuang, 2000; van Os, Rutten, and Poulton, 2008). Therefore, the inclusion of genes beyond those involved in innate and acquired immunity is clearly warranted in experimental investigations of the role of gene – environment interactions in the association between prenatal infection and postnatal brain dysfunctions (Fatemi et al., 2008).

In addition to gene – environment interaction studies, the mouse prenatal PolyI:C model may also be an excellent experimental tool to study interactive effects between discreet environmental risk factors implicated in schizophrenia. Besides prenatal infection, exposure to stressful situations and/or drugs of abuse during periadolescent maturation have often been discussed as constituting significant postnatal environmental factors that can increase the risk and/or facilitate the expression of adult mental illness, especially schizophrenia (Corcoran et al., 2003; Henquet et al., 2008; Phillips et al., 2006). Importantly, the susceptibility to such postnatal environmental insults may be critically dependent on preceding vulnerability factors acting during early (fetal and early postnatal) brain development. In accordance with a "multiple-hit" hypothesis of mental illness (Keshavan, 1999; Keshavan and Hogarty, 1999), prenatal immune challenge may thus render the brain more vulnerable to periadolescent exposure to stress and/or drugs of abuse, thereby facilitating the development of full-blown brain abnormalities relevant to schizophrenia and related disorders. Experiments are currently underway in our laboratory to explore these issues directly using the prenatal PolyI:C model in mice.

15.4.4 Longitudinal studies

The onset of full-blown psychopathological symptoms in schizophrenia typically occurs in adolescence or early adulthood (Rapoport et al., 2005; Tamminga and Holcomb, 2005). One prevalent hypothesis suggests that this maturational dependency is related to the functional maturation of intracortical connectivity, especially within prefrontal – temporolimbic cortical pathways (Keshavan and Hogarty, 1999; Weinberger and Lipska, 1995). Other theoretical accounts of this maturational delay focus on the influence of (sex-dependent) hormonal refinements occurring during the periadolescent stage of life (Halbreich and Kahn, 2003) and/or interactions with exposure to stressful situations and associated changes in the stress-response system (Corcoran et al., 2003; Phillips et al., 2006).

Given the postpubertal onset of schizophrenia in the human clinical condition, longitudinal investigations that take into account both pre- and postpubertal stages of life are highly essential in attempts to model schizophrenia-like dysfunctions in animals. In many developmental rodent models, postnatal days 28–35 are typically chosen as prepubertal stages of development, whereas postnatal day 56 and beyond is typically regarded as the postpubertal life span (Koshibu, Levitt, and Ahrens, 2004; Spear, 2000). These developmental stages are defined based on the gradual attainment of sexual maturity and discontinuities in age-specific behavior from younger to older animals (for rats see Spear, 2000; for mice see Koshibu et al., 2004).

Consistent with the postpubertal onset of full-blown psychotic behavior in schizophrenia, most of the psychosis-related functional brain effects of prenatal PolyI:C-induced immune challenge appear to be dependent on postpubertal maturational processes. Our own experimental investigations in mice show that various behavioral, cognitive, and pharmacological abnormalities induced by prenatal PolyI:C treatment emerge only at postpubertal stages of life, not at prepubertal stages (Meyer et al., 2006c, 2008b; Vuillermot et al., 2010). For example, prenatal PolyI:C treatment on GD 9 leads to significant deficits in LI and PPI only when the offspring reach early adulthood (postnatal day 70) but not during their pubertal stages of development (postnatal day 35; Meyer et al., 2006c, 2008b; Vuillermot et al., 2010; see also Ozawa et al., 2006). A similar conclusion can be drawn from experimental investigations conducted in rats, showing that prenatal PolyI:C treatment on GD 15 leads to the postpubertal onset of LI disruption (Zuckerman and Weiner, 2003; Zuckerman et al., 2003). This maturational delay is indicative of a progression of pathological symptoms from prepubertal to adult life, which is consistent with the postpubertal onset of full-blown psychotic behavior in schizophrenia and related disorders (Fatemi and Folsom, 2009; Rapoport et al., 2005).

Against this background, the prenatal PolyI:C model provides a unique opportunity to identify the nature and developmental character of progressive brain changes relevant to schizophrenia, in general, and to psychosis-related disorders following exposure to prenatal and/or perinatal insults, in particular. Given that the PolyI:C model is characterized by a high degree of face and construct validity for schizophrenia-like pathologies, it is an excellent experimental tool to identify such progressive brain changes relevant to the onset of full-blown psychosis. For example, we have recently found a striking developmental correspondence between the onset of enhanced striatal dopamine D1 and D2 receptor expression and abnormalities in the behavioral sensitivity to the mixed dopamine D1/D2 receptor apomorphine as well as disruption of PPI in prenatally

PolyI:C-treated offspring, with both the neuroanatomical and behavioral effects emerging only in adult but not in peripubertal subjects (Vuillermot et al., 2010). This particular example demonstrates that the PolyI:C-based model of schizophrenia can be successfully used to study the developmental correspondence between specific brain and behavioral dysfunctions relevant to the onset of the disease in humans.

15.4.5 Symptomatic pharmacological treatment studies

An important feature of the PolyI:C model is that at least some of the behavioral and cognitive deficits induced by this immune-associated manipulation can be normalized by acute and/or chronic antipsychotic drug treatment, thus supporting the predictive validity of the model for schizophrenia-like dysfunctions. For example, Ozawa and colleagues (2006) have shown in mice that the prenatal PolyI:C-induced deficits in novel object recognition can be ameliorated by chronic treatment with the atypical antipsychotic drug clozapine. Similarly, we have recently found that chronic clozapine treatment can successfully improve spatial working memory deficits induced by prenatal PolyI:C exposure (Meyer et al., 2010). These beneficial effects are in accordance with numerous other studies conducted in rats or mice showing that schizophrenia-related behavioral dysfunctions induced by prenatal treatment with PolyI:C, the bacterial endotoxin lipopolysaccharide (LPS), or human influenza virus can be normalized by acute treatment with the atypical antipsychotic clozapine and/or the typical antipsychotic drug haloperidol (Borrell et al., 2002; Romero et al., 2007; Shi et al., 2003; Zuckerman and Weiner, 2003; Zuckerman et al., 2003). In addition, we found recent evidence that acute adult treatment with preferential dopamine D1 or D2 receptor antagonists is sufficient to normalize the prenatal PolyI:C-induced PPI deficits in mice (Vuillermot et al., 2010), emphasizing a critical role of dopaminergic abnormalities in the association between (viral-like) prenatal immune challenge and sensorimotor gating dysfunctions in adulthood.

One of the major difficulties in the pharmacotherapy of schizophrenia is that treatment with currently available antipsychotic medications can only partially normalize psychopathological symptoms (Kapur and Remington 2001; Tamminga, 1999). With respect to their treatment, different psychotic symptoms respond differentially to pharmacotherapy. Hence, there is still a need for the development and evaluation of novel compounds with antipsychotic properties that are effective in normalizing especially the negative and cognitive aspects of the disorder and that are accompanied by minimal side effects. Based on the solid face and construct validity, the prenatal PolyI:C model may be applied as a pharmacological screening test against different aspects of schizophrenia-related deficits. Indeed, the model provides important new avenues for the establishment and characterization of novel antipsychotic drugs because it accounts for the developmental nature of schizophrenia-like pathology and incorporates the etiological significance of the disorder. Furthermore, because the relevant experimental manipulation is carried out in prenatal life, the prenatal PolyI:C model is devoid of invasive manipulations in the adult animal. It is thus highly suitable for the screening of antipsychotic drugs in the absence of confounding pharmacological or surgical interventions in the adult animal.

Another unique feature of the prenatal PolyI:C model is that the precise timing of the specific environmental insult determines, at least in part, the specificity of the brain and behavioral dysfunctions emerging in adulthood (see previous sections). This offers the possibility to evaluate a compound's antipsychotic efficacy against specific symptom profiles or clusters. For example, prenatal PolyI:C exposure in early/middle gestation in mice may be a useful model to screen pharmacological compounds for their efficacy to correct positive-like symptoms, whereas prenatal PolyI:C exposure in late gestation may be a valuable tool to study compounds with potential therapeutic efficacy to normalize negative and cognitive symptoms.

15.4.6 Preventive pharmacological treatment studies

Therapeutic interventions during the offspring's periadolescent development may represent an effective strategy to reduce the incidence of, or even prevent the emergence of, multiple brain dysfunctions following maternal infection during pregnancy. As already mentioned, the full spectrum of behavioral, cognitive, and pharmacological abnormalities induced by prenatal immune challenge in rats and mice is dependent on postpubertal maturational processes and thus only emerges in adult, not prepubertal, subjects. This progression of pathological symptoms from periadolescent to adult life is remarkably similar to the progression of psychotic symptoms in individuals prodromally symptomatic for schizophrenia. The (initial) prodromal phase of schizophrenia refers to a muted form of psychosis-related behavior, which precedes the onset of full-blown schizophrenic disorder (Klosterkötter et al., 2001). It has been suggested that early pharmacological treatment during the prodromal phase may prevent the subsequent emergence of a full-blown psychotic episode by attenuating or even halting the progression of the underlying pathology (McGlashan, 1996). The underlying rationale is primarily based on the hypothesis that the longer a psychotic state is left untreated, the more severe the long-term psychopathological outcome is likely to be (Perkins et al., 2005). For this reason, chronic administration of antipsychotic or antidepressant drugs to periadolescent and/or adolescent subjects with prodromal symptoms has recently been introduced as preventive treatment of schizophrenia and other psychosis-related disorders in humans (Cornblatt et al., 2007; McGlashan et al., 2003, 2006; Woods et al., 2003).

In spite of the laudable rationale of this preventive approach, its implementation has provoked several ethical concerns and, therefore, still remains highly controversial (Haroun et al., 2006). One relative unknown is the conversion rate amongst individuals that have been identified as being at high risk for full-blown psychosis. With an estimation as low as 16% (Yung et al., 2008), one immediate implication of such preventive practice is that a substantial number of false-positive subjects (who otherwise would not progress into full psychosis) would be exposed to unnecessary antipsychotic and/or antidepressant drug treatment (Block, 2006), while the long-term side effects of such exposure in these individuals are unknown. Hence, the relative benefits (i.e., successful prevention) and costs (i.e., long-term side effects in false-positive subjects) of preventive pharmacological interventions targeting periadolescent subjects identified as being at high risk for schizophrenia in later life must be comprehensively evaluated.

Considering the apparent lack of knowledge about the long-term consequences of early preventive pharmacotherapy, along with the ethical concerns and technical difficulties in addressing these issues in humans, the explorative investigation of early preventive strategies in preclinical animal models is clearly warranted. Because a defined experimental manipulation allows the clear segregation of high-risk subjects from controls, the efficiency of preventive pharmacotherapy can be studied without potential confounds arising from treatment in false-positive subjects. The prenatal PolyI:C model in mice (and rats) is highly suitable for the experimental investigation of preventive pharmacological intervention in schizophrenia and related psychotic disorders because it mimics brain and behavioral abnormalities related to the full-blown schizophrenia phenotype in adult life, it incorporates etiological significance and the neurodevelopmental perspective of the disorder, and it captures the pathological progression from periadolescence to adulthood.

We have recently used the mouse PolyI:C model to study the efficacy of preventive antipsychotic or antidepressant drug treatment during the prodromal-like phase in the prenatal PolyI:C model of immune activation in mice (Meyer et al., 2008d; for a similar study in rats, see Piontkewitz, Assaf, and Weiner, 2009). The experimental data show that periadolescent treatment with reference antipsychotic and antidepressant drugs can successfully block at least some of the psychosis-related behavioral and pharmacological abnormalities in subjects predisposed to adult brain pathology by exposure to prenatal immune challenge (Meyer et al., 2008d; Piontkewitz et al., 2009). At the same time, however, this initial study has revealed numerous negative influences of the early pharmacological intervention on normal behavioral development in control (i.e., "false-positive") subjects (Meyer et al., 2008d). Hence, the PolyI:C-based prenatal immune activation model is sensitive for the detection of both beneficial and potentially harmful effects of chronic periadolescent pharmacological interventions designed for the preventive treatment of neuropsychiatric disorders, especially schizophrenia.

15.5 Concluding remarks

Over the last two decades, the neurodevelopmental hypothesis of schizophrenia has been highly influential in shaping our current thinking about modeling the disease in animals (Lipska and Weinberger, 2000; Meyer et al., 2005). The use of selective lesions in adult animals and the acute or chronic administration of psychotomimetic agents are indispensable tools in the elucidation of the contribution of specific brain regions or neurotransmitters to the genesis of a specific symptom or collection of symptoms and enjoy some degree of predictive validity, but they may be inaccurate, if not inadequate, in capturing the etiological mechanisms or ontology needed for a complete understanding of the disease (Lillrank, Lipska, and Weinberger, 1995; Lipska and Weinberger, 2000; Meyer et al., 2005). This has motivated the establishment of neurodevelopmental animal models that aim at identifying the etiological processes whereby the brain, following specific triggering events, develops into a "schizophrenia-like brain" over time. This approach not only is wider in its scope than conventional lesion and drug models, but also readily lends itself to addressing data and hypotheses concerning the subtle histopathological and neuroanatomical findings revealed in postmortem and imaging studies, as well as the contribution of genetic and environmental risk factors.

As a result of human epidemiological studies, a great deal of interest has been centered upon the establishment of neurodevelopmental animal models that are based on prenatal exposure to infection and/or immune activation. Unique to these models is their holistic appreciation of intricate interactions between the immune system and the development of the central nervous system. Besides other currently available models, the PolyI:C-based model of immune activation has achieved tremendous impact on researchers concentrating on the neurodevelopmental and neuroimmunological basis of complex human brain disorders such as schizophrenia. The constellation of the identified structural and functional brain abnormalities, and the fact that some of them show a developmental delay in their emergence, leads us to conclude that the PolyI:C model is a very powerful heuristic environmental – neurodevelopmental animal model of schizophrenia and related psychotic disorders. The heuristic value of this model rests on its ability to disrupt the development of the relevant brain circuitry and to mimic the diverse spectrum of neuroanatomical, neurochemical, and behavioral abnormalities in schizophrenia. Hence, it is characterized by a high level of face and construct validity, including intrinsic etiological significance to the disorder. Furthermore, even though the full potential of pharmacological screening tests against different aspects of psychotic-related deficits awaits further exploration, initial findings suggest the PolyI:C model also fulfils predictive validity for schizophrenia-like pathology.

The epidemiological literature reporting enhanced risk of schizophrenia following early-life exposure to environmental insults such as infection is still evolving, and so are the attempts to model these associations in experimental animals. As recently pointed out by McGrath and Richards (2009), there is a "need to build shared discovery platforms that encourage greater cross-fertilization between schizophrenia epidemiology and basic neuroscience research" (579). The establishment and application of the mouse (and rat) PolyI:C model represents an important step in this direction. At the same time, on-going epidemiological research is beginning to determine whether specific environmental insults such as prenatal infection may confer vulnerability to specific features of schizophrenia psychopathology and neuropathology (Brown et al., 2009). Hence, the continual integration of epidemiological and experimental work will significantly further our understanding of the developmental, cellular, and molecular mechanisms involved in the precipitation of enhanced risk of schizophrenia following early-life exposure to environmental insults and help to establish early preventive interventions that can successfully reduce the risk for exposed individuals to develop this disabling brain disorder.

Acknowledgements

The studies performed at the authors' institute were supported by the Swiss Federal Institute of Technology (ETH) Zurich (grant – 11 07/03) and the Swiss National Science Foundation (grant 3100AO-100309 and grant 3100A0–116719). JF received additional support from a 2009 NARSAD Distinguished Investigator Award.

JF dedicates this chapter to Michal Feldon, M.D.

References

Arguello PA, Gogos JA. Modeling madness in mice: one piece at a time. *Neuron* 2006;52: 179–96.
Aronsson F, Lannebo C, Paucar M, Brask J, Kristensson K, Karlsson H. Persistence of viral RNA in the brain of offspring to mice infected with influenza A/WSN/33 virus during pregnancy. *J Neurovirol* 2002;8: 353–7.

Ayhan Y, Sawa A, Ross CA, Pletnikov MV. Animal models of gene environment interactions in schizophrenia. *Behav Brain Res* 2009;204: 274–81.

Babulas V, Factor-Litvak P, Goetz R, Schaefer CA, Brown AS. Prenatal exposure to maternal genital and reproductive infections and adult schizophrenia. *Am J Psychiatry* 2006;163: 927–9.

Bitanihirwe BK, Peleg-Raibstein D, Mouttet F, Feldon J, Meyer U. Late prenatal immune activation in mice leads to behavioral and neurochemical abnormalities relevant to the negative symptoms of schizophrenia. *Neuropsychopharmacology* 2010a, August 25 (ahead of print).

Bitanihirwe BK, Weber L, Feldon J, Meyer U. Cognitive impairment following prenatal immune challenge in mice correlates with prefrontal cortical AKT1 deficiency. *Int J Neuropsychopharmacol* 2010b;13: 981–96.

Block JJ. Ethical concerns regarding olanzapine versus placebo in patients prodromally symptomatic for psychosis. *Am J Psychiatry* 2006;163: 1838.

Boin F, Zanardini R, Pioli R, Altamura CA, Maes M, Gennarelli M. Association between-G308A tumor necrosis factor alpha gene polymorphism and schizophrenia. *Mol Psychiatry* 2001;6: 79–82.

Boksa P. Of rats and schizophrenia. *J Psychiatry Neurosci* 2007;32: 8–10.

Borrell J, Vela JM, Arévalo-Martin A, Molina-Holgado E, Guaza C. Prenatal immune challenge disrupts sensorimotor gating in adult rats: implications for the etiopathogenesis of schizophrenia. *Neuropsychopharmacology* 2002;6: 204–221.

Brown AS, Cohen P, Harkavy-Friedman J, et al. Bennett Research Award. Prenatal rubella, premorbid abnormalities, and adult schizophrenia. *Biol Psychiatry* 2001;49: 473–86.

Brown AS, Susser ES. In utero infection and adult schizophrenia. *Ment Retard Dev Disabil Res Rev* 2002;8: 51–7.

Brown AS, Begg MD, Gravenstein S, et al. Serologic evidence of prenatal influenza in the etiology of schizophrenia. *Arch Gen Psychiatry* 2004;61: 774–80.

Brown AS, Schaefer CA, Quesenberry CP Jr, Liu L, Babulas VP, Susser ES. Maternal exposure to toxoplasmosis and risk of schizophrenia in adult offspring. *Am J Psychiatry* 2005;162: 767–73.

Brown AS. Prenatal infection as a risk factor for schizophrenia. *Schizophr Bull* 2006;32: 200–2.

Brown AS. The risk for schizophrenia from childhood and adult infections. *Am J Psychiatry* 2008;165: 7–10.

Brown AS, Susser ES. Prenatal nutritional deficiency and risk of adult schizophrenia. *Schizophr Bull* 2008;34: 1054–63.

Brown AS, Vinogradov S, Kremen WS, Poole JH, Deicken RF, Penner JD, McKeague IW, Kochetkova A, Kern D, Schaefer CA. Prenatal exposure to maternal infection and executive dysfunction in adult schizophrenia. *Am J Psychiatry* 2009;166: 683–90.

Buka SL, Tsuang MT, Torrey EF, Klebanoff MA, Bernstein D, Yolken RH. Maternal infections and subsequent psychosis among offspring. *Arch Gen Psychiatry* 2001;58: 1032–7.

Cannon TD, van Erp TG, Bearden CE, et al. Early and late neurodevelopmental influences in the prodrome to schizophrenia: Contributions of genes, environment, and their interactions. *Schizophr Bull* 2003;29: 653–69.

Castner SA, Goldman-Rakic PS, Williams GV. Animal models of working memory: insights for targeting cognitive dysfunction in schizophrenia. *Psychopharmacology* 2004;174: 111–25.

Chiavetto LB, Boin F, Zanardini R, et al. Association between promoter polymorphic haplotypes of interleukin-10 gene and schizophrenia. *Biol Psychiatry* 2002;51: 480–4.

Clancy B, Darlington RB, Finlay BL. Translating developmental time across mammalian species. *Neuroscience* 2001;105: 7–17.

Clancy B, Finlay, BL, Darlington RB, Anand KJ. Extrapolating brain development from experimental species to humans. *Neurotoxicology* 2007a;28: 931–7.

Clancy B, Kersh B, Hyde J, Darlington RB, Anand KJ, Finlay BL. Web-based method for translating neurodevelopment from laboratory species to humans. *Neuroinformatics* 2007b;5: 79–94.

Corcoran C, Walker E, Huot R, et al. The stress cascade and schizophrenia: etiology and onset. *Schizophr Bull* 2003;29: 671–92.

Cornblatt BA, Lencz T, Smith CW, et al. Can antidepressants be used to treat the schizophrenia prodrome? Results of a prospective, naturalistic treatment study of adolescents. *J Clin Psychiatry* 2007;68: 546–57.

Crow TJ. Positive and negative schizophrenic symptoms and the role of dopamine. *Br J Psychiatry* 1980;137: 383–6.

Cunningham C, Campion S, Teeling J, Felton L, Perry VH. The sickness behaviour and CNS inflammatory mediator profile induced by systemic challenge of mice with synthetic double-stranded RNA (poly I:C). *Brain Behav Immun* 2007;21: 490–502.

Elvevag B, Goldberg TE. Cognitive impairment in schizophrenia is the core of the disorder. *Crit Rev Neurobiol* 2000;14: 1–21.

Fatemi SH, Emamian ES, Kist D, et al. Defective corticogenesis and reduction in Reelin immunoreactivity in cortex and hippocampus of prenatally infected neonatal mice. *Mol Psychiatry* 1999;4: 145–54.

Fatemi SH, Earle J, Kanodia R, et al. Prenatal viral infection leads to pyramidal cell atrophy and macrocephaly in adulthood: implications for genesis of autism and schizophrenia. *Cell Mol Neurobiol* 2002a;22: 25–33.

Fatemi SH, Emamian ES, Sidwell RW, et a. Human influenza viral infection in utero alters glial fibrillary acidic protein immunoreactivity in the developing brains of neonatal mice. *Mol Psychiatry* 2002b;7: 633–40.

Fatemi SH. *Neuropsychiatric Disorders and Infection*. London: Martin Dunitz-Taylor & Francis Group; 2005.

Fatemi SH, Reutiman TJ, Folsom TD, et al. Maternal infection leads to abnormal gene regulation and brain atrophy in mouse offspring: implications for genesis of neurodevelopmental disorders. *Schizophr Res* 2008;99: 56–70.

Fatemi SH, Folsom TD. The neurodevelopmental hypothesis of schizophrenia, revisited. *Schizophr Bull* 2009;35: 528–48.

Fatemi SH, Folsom TD, Reutiman TJ, et al. Abnormal expression of myelination genes and alterations in white matter fractional anisotropy following prenatal viral influenza infection at E16 in mice. *Schizophr Res* 2009;112: 46–53.

Fortier ME, Luheshi GN, Boksa P. Effects of prenatal infection on prepulse inhibition in the rat depend on the nature of the infectious agent and the stage of pregnancy. *Behav Brain Res* 2007;181: 270–7.

Gilmore JH, Jarskog LF. Exposure to infection and brain development: cytokines in the pathogenesis of schizophrenia. Schizophr Res 1997;24: 365–7.

Gilmore JH, Jarskog LF, Vadlamudi S. Maternal poly I:C exposure during pregnancy regulates TNF alpha, BDNF, and NGF expression in neonatal brain and the maternal-fetal unit of the rat. *J Neuroimmunol* 2005;159: 106–12.

Goldman-Rakic PS. Prefrontal cortical dysfunction in working memory: the relevance of working memory. In: Caroll BJ, Barett JE, eds. *Psychopathology in the Brain*. New York, NY, USA: Raven; 1991.

Goldman-Rakic PS. Working memory dysfunction in schizophrenia. *J Neuropsychiatr Clin Neurosci* 1994;6: 348–57.

Gross G. The onset of schizophrenia. *Schizophr Res* 1997;28: 187–98.

Halbreich U, Kahn LS. Hormonal aspects of schizophrenias: an overview. *Psychoneuroendocrinology* 2003;28 Suppl 2: 1–16.

Haroun N, Dunn L, Haroun A, Cadenhead KS. Risk and protection in prodromal schizophrenia: ethical implications for clinical practice and future research. *Schizophr Bull* 2006;32: 166–78.

Harrison PJ, Weinberger DR. Schizophrenia genes, gene expression, and neuropathology: on the matter of their convergence. *Mol Psychiatry* 2005;10: 40–68.

Henquet C, di Forti M, Morrison P, Kuepper R, Murray RM. Gene-environment interplay between cannabis and psychosis. *Schizophr Bull* 2008;34: 1111–21.

Hornig M, Weissenböck H, Horscroft N, Lipkin WI. An infection-based model of neurodevelopmental damage. *Proc Natl Acad Sci USA* 1999;96: 12102–7.

Hornig M, Lipkin WI. Infectious and immune factors in the pathogenesis of neurodevelopmental disorders: epidemiology, hypotheses, and animal models. *Ment Retard Dev Disabil Res Rev* 2001;7: 200–10.

Kapur S, Remington G. Atypical antipsychotics: new directions and new challenges in the treatment of schizophrenia. *Annu Rev Med* 2001;52: 503–17.

Kaufman MH. *The Atlas of Mouse Development*. London: Academic Press; 2003.

Keshavan MS. Development, disease and degeneration in schizophrenia: a unitary pathophysiological model. *J Psychiatr Res* 1999;33: 513–21.

Keshavan MS, Hogarty GE. Brain maturational processes and delayed onset in schizophrenia. *Dev Psychopathol* 1999;11: 525–43.

Klosterkötter J, Hellmich M, Steinmeyer EM, Schultze-Lutter F. Diagnosing schizophrenia in the initial prodromal phase. *Arch Gen Psychiatry* 2001;58: 158–64.

Koenig JI, Kirkpatrick B, Lee P. Glucocorticoid hormones and early brain development in schizophrenia. *Neuropsychopharmacology* 2002;27: 309–18.

Koshibu K, Levitt P, Ahrens ET. Sex-specific, postpuberty changes in mouse brain structures revealed by three-dimensional magnetic resonance microscopy. *Neuroimage* 2004;22: 1636–45.

Laibl VR, Sheffield JS. Influenza and pneumonia in pregnancy. *Clin Perinatol* 2005;32: 727–38.

Liddle PF, Friston KJ, Frith CD, Hirsch SR, Jones T, Frackowiak RS. Patterns of cerebral blood flow in schizophrenia. *Br J Psychiatry* 1992;160: 179–86.

Lillrank SM, Lipska BK, Weinberger DR. Neurodevelopmental animal models of schizophrenia. *Clin Neurosci* 1995;3: 98–104.

Lipska BK, Weinberger DR. To model a psychiatric disorder in animals: Schizophrenia as a reality test. *Neuropsychopharmacology* 2000;23: 223–39.

Longman RE, Johnson TR. Viral respiratory disease in pregnancy. *Curr Opin Obstet Gynecol* 2007;19: 120–5.

Low NC, Hardy J. What is a schizophrenic mouse? *Neuron* 2007;54: 348–9.

Maguire GA. Comprehensive understanding of schizophrenia and its treatment. *Am J Health Syst Pharm* 2002;59: 4–11.

McGlashan TH, Fenton WS. The positive-negative distinction in schizophrenia. Review of natural history validators. *Arch Gen Psychiatry* 1992;49: 63–72.

McGlashan TH. Early detection and intervention in schizophrenia: research. *Schizophr Bull* 1996;22: 327–45.

McGlashan TH, Zipursky RB, Perkins D, et al. The PRIME North America randomized double-blind clinical trial of olanzapine versus placebo in patients at risk of being prodromally symptomatic for psychosis. I. Study rationale and design. *Schizophr Res* 2003;61: 7–18.

McGlashan TH, Zipursky RB, Perkins D, et al. Randomized, double-blind trial of olanzapine versus placebo in patients prodromally symptomatic for psychosis. *Am J Psychiatry* 2006;163: 790–9.

McGrath JJ, Richards LJ. Why schizophrenia epidemiology needs neurobiology – and vice versa. *Schizophr Bull* 2009;35: 577–81.

Mednick SA, Machon RA, Huttunen MO, Bonett D. Adult schizophrenia following prenatal exposure to an influenza epidemic. *Arch Gen Psychiatry* 1988;45: 189–92.

Meyer U, Feldon J, Schedlowski M, Yee BK. Towards an immuno-precipitated neurodevelopmental animal model of schizophrenia. *Neurosci Biobehav Rev* 2005;29: 913–47.

Meyer U, Feldon J, Schedlowski M, Yee BK. Immunological stress at the maternal-foetal interface: a link between neurodevelopment and adult psychopathology. *Brain Behav Immun* 2006a;20: 378–88.

Meyer U, Nyffeler M, Engler A, et al. The time of prenatal immune challenge determines the specificity of inflammation-mediated brain and behavioral pathology. *J Neurosci* 2006b;26: 4752–62.

Meyer U, Schwendener S, Feldon J, Yee BK. Prenatal and postnatal maternal contributions in the infection model of schizophrenia. *Exp Brain Res* 2006c;173: 243–57.

Meyer U, Yee BK, Feldon J. The neurodevelopmental impact of prenatal infections at different times of pregnancy: the earlier the worse? *Neuroscientist* 2007;13: 241–56.

Meyer U, Murray PJ, Urwyler A, Yee BK, Schedlowski M, Feldon J. Adult behavioral and pharmacological dysfunctions following disruption of the fetal brain balance between pro-inflammatory and IL-10-mediated anti-inflammatory signaling. *Mol Psychiatry* 2008a;13: 208–21.

Meyer U, Nyffeler M, Schwendener S, Knuesel I, Yee BK, Feldon J. Relative prenatal and postnatal maternal contributions to schizophrenia-related neurochemical dysfunction after in utero immune challenge. *Neuropsychopharmacology* 2008b;33: 441–56.

Meyer U, Nyffeler M, Yee BK, Knuesel I, Feldon J. Adult brain and behavioral pathological markers of prenatal immune challenge during early/middle and late fetal development in mice. *Brain Behav Immun* 2008c;22: 469–86.

Meyer U, Spoerri E, Yee BK, Schwarz MJ, Feldon J. Evaluating early preventive antipsychotic and antidepressant drug treatment in an infection-based neurodevelopmental mouse model of schizophrenia. *Schizophr Bull* 2008d, October 8 (ahead of print).

Meyer U, Feldon J. Neural basis of psychosis-related behaviour in the infection model of schizophrenia. *Behav Brain Res* 2009;204: 322–34.

Meyer U, Feldon J, Fatemi SH. In-vivo rodent models for the experimental investigation of prenatal immune activation effects in neurodevelopmental brain disorders. *Neurosci Biobehav Rev* 2009;33: 1061–79.

Meyer U, Feldon J, Yee BK. A review of the fetal brain cytokine imbalance hypothesis of schizophrenia. *Schizophr Bull* 2009;35: 959–72.

Meyer U, Feldon J. Epidemiology-driven neurodevelopmental animal models of schizophrenia. *Prog Neurobiol* 2010;90: 285–326.

Meyer U, Knuesel I, Nyffeler M, Feldon J. Chronic clozapine treatment improves prenatal infection-induced working memory deficits without influencing adult hippocampal neurogenesis. *Psychopharmacology* 2010;208: 531–43.

Mortensen PB, Nørgaard-Pedersen B, Waltoft BL, et al. Toxoplasma gondii as a risk factor for early-onset schizophrenia: analysis of filter paper blood samples obtained at birth. *Biol Psychiatry* 2007;61: 688–93.

Murray RM, O'Callaghan E, Castle DJ, Lewis SW. A neurodevelopmental approach to the classification of schizophrenia. *Schizophr Bull* 1992;18: 319–32.

Nuechterlein KH, Dawson ME. Information processing and attentional functioning in the developmental course of schizophrenic disorders. *Schizophr Bull* 1984;10: 160–203.

Ozawa K, Hashimoto K, Kishimoto T, Shimizu E, Ishikura H, Iyo M. Immune activation during pregnancy in mice leads to dopaminergic hyperfunction and cognitive impairment in the offspring: a neurodevelopmental animal model of schizophrenia. *Biol Psychiatry* 2006;59: 546–54.

Perkins DO, Gu H, Boteva K, Lieberman JA. Relationship between duration of untreated psychosis and outcome in first-episode schizophrenia: a critical review and meta-analysis. *Am J Psychiatry* 2005;162: 1785–1804.

Phillips LJ, McGorry PD, Garner B, et al. Stress, the hippocampus and the hypothalamic-pituitary-adrenal axis: implications for the development of psychotic disorders. *Aust N Z J Psychiatry* 2006;40: 725–41.

Piontkewitz Y, Assaf Y, Weiner I. Clozapine administration in adolescence prevents postpubertal emergence of brain structural pathology in an animal model of schizophrenia. *Biol Psychiatry* 2009;66: 1038–46.

Pletnikov MV, Rubin SA, Schwartz GJ, Carbone KM, Moran TH. Effects of neonatal rat Borna disease virus (BDV) infection on the postnatal development of the brain monoaminergic systems. *Dev Brain Res* 2000;119: 179–85.

Pletnikov MV, Moran TH, Carbone KM. Borna disease virus infection of the neonatal rat: developmental brain injury model of autism spectrum disorders. *Front Biosci* 2002;7: d593–607.

Pletnikov MV, Rubin SA, Vogel MW, Moran TH, Carbone KM. Effects of genetic background on neonatal Borna disease virus infection-induced neurodevelopmental damage. I. Brain pathology and behavioral deficits. *Brain Res* 2002a;944: 97–107.

Pletnikov MV, Rubin SA, Vogel MW, Moran TH, Carbone KM. Effects of genetic background on neonatal Borna disease virus infection-induced neurodevelopmental damage. II. Neurochemical alterations and responses to pharmacological treatments. *Brain Res* 2002b;944: 108–23.

Rapoport JL, Addington AM, Frangou S, Psych MR. The neurodevelopmental model of schizophrenia: update 2005. *Mol Psychiatry* 2005;10: 434–49.

Rees S, Harding R. Brain development during fetal life: influences of the intra-uterine environment. *Neurosci Lett* 2004;361: 111–4.

Rees S, Inder T. Fetal and neonatal origins of altered brain development. *Early Hum Dev* 2005;81: 753–61.

Romero E, Ali C, Molina-Holgado E, Castellano B, Guaza C, Borrell J. Neurobehavioral and immunological consequences of prenatal immune activation in rats. Influence of antipsychotics. *Neuropsychopharmacology* 2007;32: 1791–1804.

Shi L, Fatemi SH, Sidwell RW, Patterson PH. Maternal influenza infection causes marked behavioral and pharmacological changes in the offspring. *J Neurosci* 2003;23: 297–302.

Smith SE, Li J, Garbett K, Mirnics K, Patterson PH. Maternal immune activation alters fetal brain development through interleukin-6. *J Neurosci* 2007;27: 10695–702.

Sørensen HJ, Mortensen EL, Reinisch JM, Mednick SA. Association between prenatal exposure to bacterial infection and risk of schizophrenia. *Schizophr Bull* 2009;35: 631–7.

Spear LP. The adolescent brain and age-related behavioral manifestations. *Neurosci Biobehav Rev* 2000;24: 417–63.

Sporn AL, Addington AM, Gogtay N, et al. Pervasive developmental disorder and childhood-onset schizophrenia: Comorbid disorder or a phenotypic variant of a very early onset illness? *Biol Psychiatry* 2004; 55: 989–94.

Stöber G, Franzek E, Beckmann H, Schmidtke A. Exposure to prenatal infections, genetics and the risk of systematic and periodic catatonia. *J Neural Transm* 2002; 109: 921–9.

Sullivan R, Wilson DA, Feldon J, et al. The International Society for Developmental Psychobiology annual meeting symposium: Impact of early life experiences on brain and behavioral development. *Dev Psychobiol* 2006;48: 583–602.

Susser, E, St Clair D, He L. Latent effects of prenatal malnutrition on adult health: the example of schizophrenia. *Ann NY Acad Sci* 2008;1136: 85–92.

Suvisaari J, Haukka J, Tanskanen A, Hovi T, Lönnqvist J. Association between prenatal exposure to poliovirus infection and adult schizophrenia. *Am J Psychiatry* 1999;156: 1100–2.

Swerdlow NR, Geyer MA. Using an animal model of deficient sensorimotor gating to study the pathophysiology and new treatments of schizophrenia. *Schizophr Bull* 1998;24: 285–301.

Takeuchi O, Akira S. Recognition of viruses by innate immunity. *Immunol Rev* 2007;220: 214–24.

Tamminga CA. Principles of pharmacotherapy in schizophrenia. In: Charney DS, Nestler EJ, Bunney BS, eds. *Neurobiology of Mental Illness*. Oxford: Oxford University Press; 1999.

Tamminga CA, Holcomb HH. Phenotype of schizophrenia: a review and formulation. *Mol Psychiatry* 2005;10: 27–39.

Torrey EF, Rawlings R, Waldman IN. Schizophrenic births and viral diseases in two states. *Schizophr Res* 1988;1: 73–7.

Tsuang M. Schizophrenia: genes and environment. *Biol Psychiatry* 2000;47: 210–20.

van Os J, Rutten BP, Poulton R. Gene-environment interactions in schizophrenia: review of epidemiological findings and future directions. *Schizophr Bull* 2008;34: 1066–82.

Vuillermot S, Weber L, Feldon J, Meyer U. A longitudinal examination of the neurodevelopmental impact of prenatal immune activation in mice reveals primary defects in dopaminergic development relevant to schizophrenia. *J Neurosci* 2010;30: 1270–87.

Weinberger DR, Lipska BK. Cortical maldevelopment, anti-psychotic drugs, and schizophrenia: a search for common ground. *Schizophr Res* 1995;16: 87–110.

Weiner I. The "two-headed" latent inhibition model of schizophrenia: modeling positive and negative symptoms and their treatment. *Psychopharmacology* 2003;169: 257–97.

Whitley RJ, Stagno S. Perinatal infections. In: Scheld WM, Whitley RJ, Durack DT, eds. *Infections of the Central Nervous System*. New York, NY, USA: Lippincott-Raven Press; 1997.

Willner P. The validity of animal models of depression. *Psychopharmacology* 1984;83: 1–16.

Willner P. Validation criteria for animal models of human mental disorders: learned helplessness as a paradigm case. *Prog Neuropsychopharmacol Biol Psychiatry* 1986;10: 677–90.

Wolff AR, Bilkey DK. Immune activation during mid-gestation disrupts sensorimotor gating in rat offspring. *Behav Brain Res* 2008;190: 156–9.

Woods SW, Breier A, Zipursky RB, et al. Randomized trial of olanzapine versus placebo in the symptomatic acute treatment of the schizophrenic prodrome. *Biol Psychiatry* 2003;54: 453–64.

Wright P, Takei N, Rifkin L, Murray RM. Maternal influenza, obstetric complications, and schizophrenia. *Am J Psychiatry* 1995;152: 1714–20.

Wright P, Nimgaonkar VL, Donaldson PT, Murray RM. Schizophrenia and HLA: a review. *Schizophr Res* 2001;47: 1–12.

Yung AR, Nelson B, Stanford C, et al. Validation of "prodromal" criteria to detect individuals at ultra high risk of psychosis: 2 year follow-up. *Schizophr Res* 2008;105: 10–7.

Zuckerman L, Rehavi M, Nachman R, Weiner I. Immune activation during pregnancy in rats leads to a postpubertal emergence of disrupted latent inhibition, dopaminergic hyperfunction, and altered limbic morphology in the offspring: a novel neurodevelopmental model of schizophrenia. *Neuropsychopharmacology* 2003;28: 1778–89.

Zuckerman L, Weiner I. Post-pubertal emergence of disrupted latent inhibition following prenatal immune activation. *Psychopharmacology* 2003;169: 308–13.

16 Prenatal programming of cognition and emotion in humans: From birth to age 20

Bea R. H. Van den Bergh

While mediating and moderating factors and the long-lasting effect of exposure to prenatal maternal anxiety and stress (PMAS) on offspring behavior and (neuro)physiology are quite well-established in animal studies, in humans they are only beginning to be understood. In order to gain more insight in mechanisms underlying developmental (re)programming we examined emotion as well as cognition at both the behavioral and the (neuro)physiological level in the 15- to 20-year-old offspring of a cohort of pregnant women with varying degrees of anxiety ($n = 86$). In the 15-year-old offspring, HPA-axis function was measured through establishing a saliva diurnal cortisol profile, and depressive symptoms were measured with the Children's Depression Inventory. Maternal anxiety at 12–22 weeks of pregnancy was in female and male offspring associated with a diurnal cortisol profile that was attenuated due to elevated cortisol secretion in the evening. Moreover, in female adolescents this high-flattened cortisol profile mediated the link between PMAS and depressive symptoms. PMAS during week 12–22 of pregnancy was, at age 15 and 17, also associated with ADHD-related symptoms, lower intelligence scores, and impairments in endogenous cognitive control (i.e., the ability from within one self to control actions, strategies, and thoughts) as measured with neuropsychological tasks. Importantly, results of event-related potentials (ERPs) at age 17 and fMRI at age 20 confirmed a less optimal endogenous cognitive control function. Our results indicate that PMAS enhances neurobiological vulnerability and influences cognition and emotion, possibly by (re)programming) offspring (neuro)physiology and brain structure – function relationships.

16.1 Prenatal maternal anxiety and stress are associated with less favorable developmental outcomes

The developmental programming hypothesis encompasses the role of developmental plasticity in response to environmental cues, for example, to early life events. The fetus responds to the uterine environment and to changes and disturbance in this environment, for example, to maternal stress or undernutrition, and to placental dysfunction. The physiological and metabolic adaptations that enable the fetus to adapt to alteration in the early life environment may result in a permanent (re)programming of the developmental pattern within key tissues and organ systems (Gluckman et al., 2008).

Experimental animal research starting around 1950 demonstrated that exposure to adverse environmental factors in early life has several short- and long-term effects on offspring behavior, affects developing brain areas (i.e., the hippocampus, amygdala, and frontal lobes), and is associated with changes in neuronal circuits that are involved in cognitive and emotional processing and in modulating stress responses (De Kloet, Joëls, and Holsboer, 2005; Seckl and Meaney, 2004; Weinstock 2008). In humans, since 1990, an increasing number of prospective studies show that exposure to maternal anxiety or stress during pregnancy is associated with birth outcome and a range of less favorable child neurobehavioral outcomes. Most studies looked at emotional and behavioral problems (i.e., temperamental reactivity, externalizing behavior) measured with self-report questionnaires or assessed development with behavioral observation scales. A small number of studies examined specific aspects of cognitive function and found evidence for reduced attention, lowered IQ scores, and lowered linguistic competence. In fact, the pattern of results mirrors the results of animal studies, including inconsistent findings that probably result from genetic differences; differences in intensity/severity, duration/ chronicity, controllability/coping, and the developmental timing of prenatal maternal anxiety and stress (PMAS); and differences in postnatal environment (e.g., in adversity or in maternal caregiving style). In animal studies these variables can be experimentally manipulated, and their differential effects were clearly demonstrated (for reviews, see Glover, O'Connor, and O'Donnell, 2010; O'Donnell et al., 2009; Van den Bergh et al., 2005b; Weinstock, 2008) (see ▶Fig. 16.1).

While the mediating and moderating factors mentioned and the long-lasting effect of PMAS on offspring are quite well-established in animal studies, in humans they are only beginning to be understood. In studies focusing on offspring biological systems possibly altered by PMAS, some studies examined hypothalamo-pituitary-adrenocortical (HPA)-axis function; they found evidence for altered basal- or stress-related cortisol secretion (e.g., O'Connor et al., 2005; Yehuda et al., 2005). The few studies that focused on CNS structures or structure–function relationships found altered (brainstem) auditory evoked related potential (DiPietro et al., 2010; Harvison et al., 2009) and gray matter volume

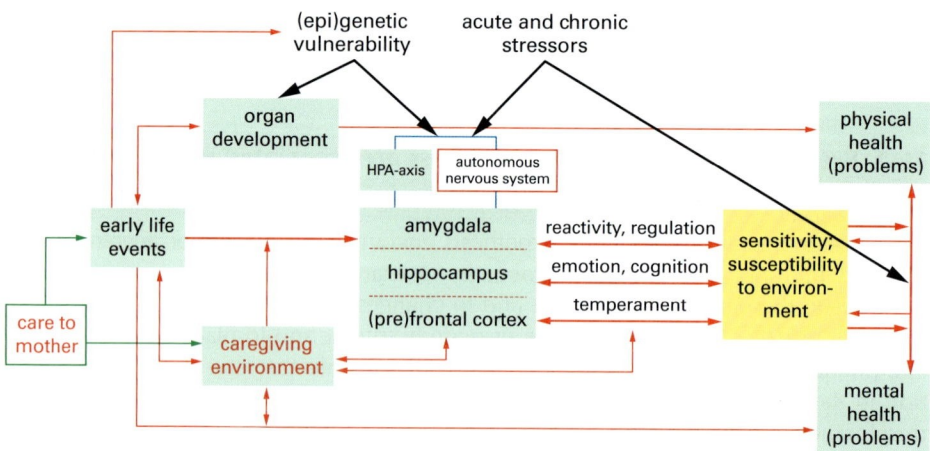

Fig. 16.1: Developmental programming of early brain and behavior development and mental health and physical health (problems) (Van den Bergh, 2011).

reductions in several parts of the brain, such as the prefrontal and premotor cortex, the medial temporal lobe, and the cerebellum (Buss et al., 2010).

Our study was aimed at a better understanding of developmental programming. Starting in 1986, we studied a cohort of pregnant women with varying degrees of anxiety from 12–22 weeks of gestation until their offspring were 20 years old. In the next three paragraphs we shortly describe the design of the study and the neurobehavioral effects of PMAS in the fetus, neonate, and child and continue with effects observed in the 14- to 17- and the 20-year-old adolescents. We examined the nature of some emotional and cognitive sequelae of PMAS at both the behavioral and the (neuro)physiological level in the following way:

1. Emotion- and stress-related emotional problems: to uncover biological mechanisms underlying depressed mood we examined whether an offspring's HPA-axis activity mediates the link between PMAS and offspring depressed mood.
2. Cognition: to uncover brain – behavior relationships we studied behavioral performance (reaction time and errors) on computerized cognitive tasks, and we simultaneously examined neural processes in the brain that are active while executing the tasks, namely with event-related brain potentials (ERPs) and functional magnetic resonance imaging (fMRI) measures.

16.2 PMAS is associated with altered fetal, infant, and child neurobehavioral development

Using a battery of standardized psychological questionnaires, anxiety and stress were measured in pregnant mothers during weeks 12–22, 23–31, and 32–40 of their pregnancy ($n = 86$). The main research variable, *anxiety,* was measured using the State Trait Anxiety Inventory (STAI). We had access to a full range of anxiety scores within our sample, including 25% women with high anxiety (i.e., mean state anxiety > 45). The same questionnaires were also completed by the mother at all postnatal research phases. This enabled us to control for the possible influence of maternal anxiety in infancy, childhood, and adolescence. An important finding was that although concurrent maternal anxiety had an influence on many outcome measures – but not on all, for example, not on the fMRI measures – it did not erase the influence of PMAS. Moreover, it is important to note that most of our findings have been shown to be (statistically) independent of potential confounding factors such as smoking and drinking during pregnancy and of birth weight.

In a first phase, we combined continuous ultrasound measurements (120 min) of body movements, eye movements and heart rhythm; this allowed us to identify behavioral states (i.e., sleep – wake cycles). It was shown that the state-dependent motor activity was significantly higher, and the percentage of time spent in quite (or deep) sleep was significantly lower in fetuses from pregnant women reporting high levels of anxiety compared to fetuses from pregnant women reporting low levels of anxiety. A mother's anxiety during pregnancy explained between 10% and 25% of the differences in irritability, excessive crying, irregularities in biological functions, and (difficult) temperament in the offspring during the first 7 months after birth. Clinical observations about the neurological condition, general cognitive and motor development, and feeding behavior revealed no significant differences between infants of high versus low anxiety pregnant women (Van den Bergh et al., 1989; Van den Bergh, 1990).

In a second phase the neurobehavioral development of the 8- or 9-year-old children ($n = 72$; 38 boys) was studied. The most important result showed that significantly more behavioral self-regulation problems were reported in children from highly anxious mothers (explained variance between 17% and 22%). Scores on clinical scales indicated problem behavior in the home situation and in class (as reported by mother and teacher) and during the test situations (as reported by a blind observer). They reflected impaired regulation of emotion and cognition, that is, attention deficit hyperactivity disorder (ADHD)-symptoms, externalizing behavior, and enhanced self-reported feelings of anxiety (Van den Bergh and Marcoen, 2004).

16.3 PMAS is associated with adolescent emotion and HPA activity: HPA mediates the link between PMAS and adolescent depressed mood

So far our study is the only one that tested whether offspring HPA-axis mediates the link between PMAS and offspring emotional problems. It was shown in the 15-year-old offspring ($n = 58$; 29 boys) that (1) in both, boys and girls, PMAS during week 12 to 22 of pregnancy is associated with a high, flattened diurnal cortisol profile that shows elevated cortisol secretion in the evening; and (2) only in girls, there is an effect of PMAS on depressed mood that can be explained, in part, by an effect of a flattened cortisol profile on depressed mood (Van den Bergh et al., 2008). These results may indicate that PMAS prenatally (re)programs the HPA-axis and induces a vulnerability phenotype in the offspring. Although we cannot prove it, *resetting* of the HPA-axis setpoints by antenatal exposure to maternal anxiety during critical periods leading to a hyperactive HPA-axis seems a plausible underlying mechanism (De Kloet et al., 2005; Seckl and Meaney, 2004).

However, not only the HPA-axis is supposed to be (re)programmed by PMAS. Animal research has shown that PMAS sequelae are also associated with alterations in neural circuits involved in emotional and cognitive processing. From the first month of gestation brain development proceeds as a continuous dialogue between the genome and the environment with the brain architecture of the fetus already established during the first two trimesters, and with most sensory organs already functional during the third trimester of pregnancy. Environmental factors that disturb the expression of genes involved in cellular proliferation, migration, and differentiation may have an impact on early brain development and constrain sensory and cognitive/emotional development even in the absence of structural brain alterations (Meaney, 2010; Van den Bergh et al., 2005b).

In the past, neurosciences have focused more on the neural base of cognition (i.e., cognitive neuroscience) than on the neural basis of emotion (i.e., affective neuroscience). Several computerized tasks measuring specific aspects of cognitive function have been developed. The prefrontal cortex is thought to have a central role in cognition, for instance, in the control of attention and in executive functions. It is, therefore, of interest to determine whether PMAS may affect the development of the PFC and of areas related to this region.

16.4 PMAS is associated with adolescent cognition: Neuropsychological, ERP, and fMRI measures reveal evidence for impaired endogenous cognitive control

We investigated cognition with IQ tests and with computerized neuropsychological tasks at age 15 (n = 64; 33 boys) and 17 (n = 49; 29 boys). Based on the type of problem behavior shown to be associated with PMAS in infancy and childhood, three tasks that assess different functions closely tied to aspects of self-regulation and that are related to the prefrontal cortex were used at age 15: (1) visual attention control and working memory (Encoding), (2) response control (Stop Task paradigm), and (3) sustained attention (Continuous Performance Task; CPT). At the age of 17 the battery of tasks was extended to five tasks, tapping five typical prefrontal functions: (1) the ability to orient attention (Cued Attention), (2) working memory (N-back), (3) external response inhibition (Go/NoGo), (4) the ability to perform two tasks simultaneously (Dual Tasks), and (5) the ability to switch between response sets (Response Shifting).

A specific pattern of cognitive deficits was shown in adolescents of mothers reporting high levels of anxiety during weeks 12–22 of their pregnancy. First, at both ages they were impaired in the CPT-task and Response shifting task, requiring the ability endogenously (i.e., autonomously, from within oneself and without external sources) to inhibit reactions to interfering and distracting stimuli or inhibit a learned response. Second, they had lowered scores on Vocabulary and Block Design, two subtests of the Wechsler Intelligence Scale for Children-Revised (WISC-R) at age 15. Third, they showed a decrease in performance when the cognitive load of the task was increased (e.g., in Dual Tasks) at age 17. Fourth, these adolescents performed adequately in tasks that triggered response inhibition in an exogenous manner and in tasks that measure working memory (Mennes et al., 2006; Van den Bergh et al., 2005a; Van den Bergh et al., 2006).

During some tasks, ERPs were measured. ERPs are small changes in the electrical activity of the brain caused by an internal or external event. Using small electrodes placed on the scalp this electrical activity can be measured. When measuring ERPs during cognitive tasks, one can make inferences about the cognitive processes underlying the changes seen in the electrical currents, and functional significance can be ascribed to the observed waveforms. We recorded ERPs with 19 scalp electrodes during four tasks, including a Go/Nogo paradigm assessing exogenous cognitive control and a newly developed (sixth) Gambling task requiring high levels of endogenous control. No effects of PMAS were observed on the behavioral and ERP data of the Go/Nogo paradigm, but PMAS had an effect on the pattern of decision making in the Gambling task. These differences were evident both in a less optimal behavioral performance of the high PMAS group and in their brain activity. Particularly, the early frontal P2a ERP component measured during endogenous cognitive trials was related to the level of PMAS. These results were the first to show an actual link between brain activity of the offspring and the level of anxiety experienced by their mother during pregnancy (Mennes, 2008; Mennes et al., 2009).

ERPs are measured with millisecond accuracy and have an excellent temporal resolution regarding the ongoing cognitive processes. To complement the ERP results with spatial information about which areas in the prefrontal cortex show differences in functionality related to prenatal maternal anxiety, we assessed endogenous cognitive control using fMRI at age 20. During fMRI scans the blood oxygenation level dependent (bold) response is measured while performing a (cognitive) task; this response can be coupled statistically to that performance, actually relating cognitive processes to certain areas of the brain. At the age of 20, all 10 boys of the high anxious groups were invited to participate, as well as 10 boys matched on IQ of the low-average anxious group (final $n = 18$). In line with previous results of this follow-up study, it was again found that high PMAS was related to a less optimal pattern of decision making in the Gambling task and to an altered brain activation pattern. The results indicated that areas in the prefrontal cortex, such as inferior frontal junction, and areas in middle frontal gyrus were related to the level of PMAS (Mennes, 2008).

16.5 Conclusion

While in behavioral studies it is well-established that PMAS is associated with offspring emotional and behavioral problems, our longitudinal study is the first to reveal evidence for (neuro)physiological consequences of PMAS. In our sample the period between 12 and 22 weeks of pregnancy clearly is the most critical in generating (neuro) physiological changes and associated unfavorable emotional and cognitive outcome, discernible even up to 20 years later. The finding of a specific time window makes it unlikely that the associations found can be explained by genetic mediations only. The results in the fetus and neonate show effects that must be independent of postnatal experience. The consistency in the results concerning cognitive function as measured with different methods from age 14–15 to age 20 is striking and shows the persistence of the effect. Although our results corroborate results from numerous preclinical studies, they need to be replicated before firm conclusions can be drawn. It is plausible that physiological events involved in high antenatal maternal anxiety changed gene regulatory mechanisms and, hence, the expression of specific genes in the placenta or fetus (Meaney, 2010). If this were the case, it would underline the importance of PMAS for offspring cognition and emotion.

References

Buss C, Davis EP, Muftuler LT, Head K, Sandman CA. High pregnancy anxiety during mid-gestation is associated with decreased greymatter density in 6–9-year-old children. *Psychoneuroendocrinology* 2010;35: 141–53.

De Kloet ER, Joëls M, Holsboer F. Stress and the brain: from adaptation to disease. *Nat Rev Neurosci* 2005;6: 463–75.

DiPietro JA, Kivlighan KT, Costigan KA, Rubin SE, Shiffler DE, Henderson JL, Pillion JP. Prenatal antecedents of newborn neurological maturation. *Child Dev* 2010;81: 115–30.

Glover V, O'Connor TG, O'Donnell K. Prenatal stress and the programming of the HPA axis. *Neurosci Biobehav Rev* 2010;35: 17–22.

Gluckman PD, Hanson MA, Cooper C, Thornburg KL. Effect of in utero and early-life conditions on adult health and disease. *N Engl J Med* 2008;359: 61–73.

Harvison KW, Molfese DL, Woodruff-Borden J, Weigel RA. Neonatal auditory evoked responses are related to perinatal maternal anxiety. *Brain Cogn* 2009;71: 369–74.

Meaney MJ. Epigenetics and the biological definition of gene x environment interactions. *Child Dev* 2010;81: 141–79.

Mennes M. Longitudinal study on the effects of maternal anxiety during pregnancy: Neuropsychological and neurophysiological examination of cognitive control in the adolescent offspring. Unpublished PhD Thesis, Katholieke Universiteit Leuven, 2008.

Mennes M, Stiers P, Lagae L, Van den Bergh B. Long-term cognitive sequelae of antenatal maternal anxiety: Involvement of the orbitofrontal cortex. *Neurosci Biobehav Rev* 2006;30: 1078–86.

Mennes M, Van den Bergh B, Lagae L, Stiers P. Developmental brain alterations in 17 year old boys are related to antenatal maternal anxiety. *Clin Neurophysiol* 2009;120: 1116–22.

O'Connor TG, Ben-Shlomo Y, Heron J, Golding J, Adams D, Glover V. Prenatal anxiety predicts individual differences in cortisol in pre-adolescent children. *Biol Psychiatry* 2005;58: 211–7.

O'Donnell K, O'Connor TG, Glover V. Prenatal stress and neurodevelopment of the child: Focus on the HPA axis and role of the placenta. *Dev Neurosci* 2009;31: 285–92.

Seckl JR, Meaney MJ. Glucocorticoid programming. *Ann NY Acad Sci* 2004;1032: 63–84.

Van den Bergh BRH, Mulder EJH, Poelman-Weesjes G, Bekedam DJ, Visser GHA, Prechtl HFR. The effect of (induced) maternal emotions on fetal behaviour: A controlled study. *Early Hum Dev* 1989;9: 9–19.

Van den Bergh BRH. The influence of maternal emotions during pregnancy on fetal and neonatal behavior. *Pre- and Perinatal Psycholog Journal* 1990;5: 119–30.

Van den Bergh BRH, Marcoen A. High antenatal maternal anxiety is related to ADHD symptoms, externalizing problems, and anxiety in 8- and 9-year-olds. *Child Dev* 2004;75: 1085–97.

Van den Bergh BRH, Mennes M, Oosterlaan J, et al. High antenatal maternal anxiety is related to impulsivity during performance on cognitive tasks in 14- and 15-year-olds. *Neurosci Biobehav Rev* 2005a;29: 259–69.

Van den Bergh BRH, Mulder EJH, Mennes M, Glover V. Antenatal maternal anxiety and stress and the neurobehavioural development of the fetus and child: Links and possible mechanisms. A review. *Neurosci Biobehav Rev* 2005b;29: 237–58.

Van den Bergh BRH, Mennes M, Stevens V, et al. ADHD deficit as measured in adolescent boys with a continuous performance task is related to antenatal maternal anxiety. *Pediatr Res* 2006;59: 78–82.

Van den Bergh BRH, Van Calster B, Smits T, Van Huffel S, Lagae L. Antenatal maternal anxiety is related to HPA-axis dysregulation and self-reported depressive symptoms in adolescence: A prospective study on the fetal origins of depressed mood. *Neuropsychopharmacology* 2008;33: 536–45.

Van den Bergh, BRH. Developmental programming of early brain and behaviour development and mental health: a conceptual framework. *Developmental Medicine and Child Neurology* 2011; DOI: 10.1111/j.1469-8749.2011.04057.x.

Weinstock M. The long-term behavioural consequences of prenatal stress. *Neurosci Biobehav Rev* 2008;32: 1073–86.

Yehuda R, Engel SM, Brand SR, Seckl J, Marcus SM, Berkowitz GS. Transgenerational effects of posttraumatic stress disorder in babies of mothers exposed to the world trade center attacks during pregnancy. *J Clin Endocrinol Metabol* 2005;90: 4115–8.

17 Perinatal programming of allergy

Renate L. Bergmann and Karl E. Bergmann

Critical windows in the development of the human immune system may start preconceptionally. In utero, allergen exposure occurs via maternal blood and via amniotic fluid. IgE synthesis was observed at 11 weeks gestation in fetal liver and lung. By 13–14 weeks fetal thymocytes respond to most mitogens, and in peripheral blood a response to inhalative and food allergens can be demonstrated at around 17 to 18 weeks. The intrauterine environment is different in atopic and nonatopic mothers. In addition to genetic factors in the fetus it may influence the developing immune system. Regulatory T-cells (T_{Reg}) play an important role in the fetal and postnatal development of tolerance, especially by the cytokine TGF-ß, which induces the development of T_{Reg}, and is produced by these cells. The capacity to generate T_{Reg} cells was impaired in neonates with a family history of allergy. Epigenetic programming translates the influences of the maternal, fetal, and postnatal environment by imprinting the immune system. During pregnancy, maternal stress and smoking, infestation with parasites, exposure to farm animals, microbes, and food- and aero-allergens, to vitamins, DHA, antioxidants, and medications have been shown to modulate the long-term immune response in the offspring. Likewise, the delivery method as well as the postnatal environment influence the development of allergies, for example, bacterial colonization, infant diet, and exposure to environmental allergens and pollutants. In conclusion, perinatal influences imprint long-term reactivity in peripheral organs and cells, suggesting an effective peripheral programming beside that in the central nervous system.

17.1 Allergy and atopy

Allergy is defined by Johansson et al. (2004) as

> a hypersensitivity reaction initiated by specific immunological mechanisms. Atopy is a personal and/or familial tendency usually in childhood or adolescence, to become sensitized and produce antibodies in response to ordinary exposures to allergens, usually proteins. As a consequence, these persons can develop typical symptoms of asthma, rhinoconjunctivitis or eczema. Atopy is a clinical definition of an IgE-antibody high responder. The term atopy can not be used until IgE-sensitization has been documented by IgE antibodies in the serum or by a positive skin prick test.

IgE antibodies are part of the *humoral* system of adaptive immunity. They are secreted by B lymphocytes, which, together with the T lymphocytes, belong to the *cellular* part of the adaptive immunity. In collaboration with the innate immunity, also made up by *humoral* and *cellular* elements, both functions are integrated into the total host defense

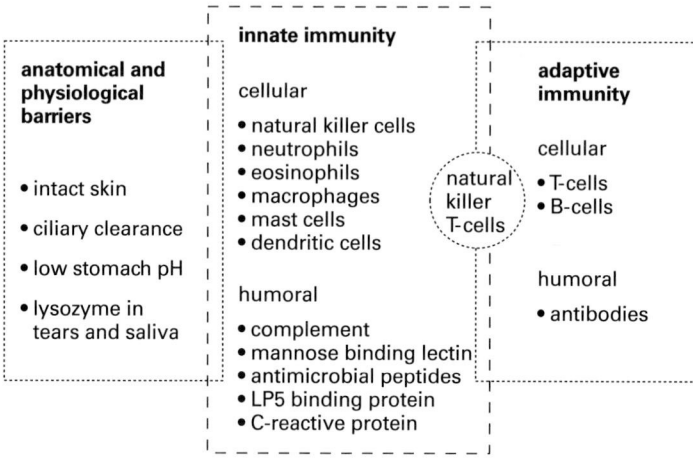

Fig. 17.1: The integrated human immune system (adapted from Turvey and Broide, 2010).

system (Turvey and Broide, 2010) (▶Fig. 17.1). Allergic or atopic diseases are complex genetic diseases resulting from multiple genetic and interacting environmental factors (Holloway, Yang, and Holgate, 2010). Epigenetic regulation is an important mechanism for the translation of environmental influences on the developing immune system during the perinatal period (Prescott and Clifton, 2009).

17.2 Early development of the immune system

Critical windows in the development of the human immune system may start even preconceptionally, especially for the oocyte (West, 2002). At approximately the seventh to eighth week after conception lymphocyte progenitors appear in fetal liver. T-cell progenitors begin migration from fetal liver to thymus during the 9th week. Peripheral lymphoid tissues are populated by T-cells as early as 10 gestational weeks (Haynes and Heinly, 1995). The thymus divides into cortex and medulla, and after 16 weeks the orderly development of the thymocytes progresses from cortex toward medulla. The T-cell receptors (TCR) and (among others) the coreceptors CD4 and CD8 are expressed (corresponding to the major histocompatability complex class I and II antigens [HLA]). "Thymic education" of T-lymphocytes with positive and then negative selection results in an export of single positive CD4 and CD8 T-lymphocytes after week 13. By 13–14 weeks gestation fetal thymocytes respond to most mitogens, and in peripheral blood a response to inhalative and food allergens can be demonstrated at around 17 to 18 weeks gestation (Jones et al., 1996; Stites, Carr, and Fudenberg, 1974). Most of the studies have used proliferative assays, but antigen-specific cytokine production, although poorer than in adults, has also been observed (Tang et al., 1994).

B cells are abundant in bone marrow at 16–20 weeks of gestation (Holt and Jones, 2000), but also, the liver is an important site of B-cell differentiation in mammals. B cells emerge into the circulation at 12 gestational weeks. Large amounts of IgG and IgM are produced by the spleen already at 10 weeks of gestation, but only IgG transverses the placenta. IgE synthesis was observed at 11 weeks in fetal liver and lung. Neonates have low levels of serum IgM, IgA, and IgE, and their IgG is generally of maternal origin. Neonatal B cells are mature in their capacity to switch to IgE producing cells if they are given IL-4. But the immature T-helper cell function was suggested to be responsible for a lack of IL-4 production and, thus, for a low production of IgE (Holt and Jones, 2000).

Allergen exposure in utero could occur via amniotic fluid and via maternal blood: in healthy women undergoing diagnostic amniocentesis at 16–17 weeks gestation the house-dust-mite allergen Der p1 was detectable in amniotic fluid if the concentration in the mother's plasma reached a threshold level (Holloway et al., 2000). With the progression of pregnancy a fetus swallows increasing volumes of amniotic fluid and is therefore even orally exposed to an aero-allergen. At term, higher Der p1 concentrations were found in cord blood than in maternal blood, implying that Der p1 can cross the placenta and challenge the fetus (Holloway et al., 2000).

17.3 Physiology and pathophysiology of early immune reactions

The two lymphocyte subpopulations of CD4 cells, namely Th1 and Th2 cells, are the source of important cytokines. The functional deviation from naïve Th0 cells into Th1 and Th2 cells is influenced by cytokines produced through the action of the innate immune system, involving the cytokines IL-12 and IFN-γ for the acquirement of the Th1 cell function, and IL-4 for the Th2 cell function (Akira, Takeda, and Kaisho, 2001). Th1 cells are mainly involved in cellular immune responses. They produce, for example, the interleukins IL-2, IL-12, and IFN-γ, while Th2 cells are engaged in the regulation of the humoral response and produce, for example, IL-4, IL-10, and IL-13.

The Th2 cytokine IL-4 plays an important role in the pathogenesis of allergy (Mosman and Sad, 1996). IL-4 activates B cells to produce IgE, and IFN-γ downregulates this effect (Tang et al., 1994). The balance of these cytokines during a successful pregnancy is shifted toward Th2 activity, which was considered to be important for the protection of fetal cells from Th1 cell – mediated destruction (Wegmann et al., 1993). But Th1 activity seems to have a role in the promotion of the Th2 response, the regulation of the placentation, and other important processes during pregnancy, therefore the term *Th1-Th2 cooperation* seems to be a more appropriate concept than the term *Th2 phenomenon* of pregnancy (Wilczynski, 2005).

Neonates with a familial atopy risk compared to nonatopy-prone neonates showed a significantly lower IFN-γ – production upon in vitro stimulation of their cord blood mononuclear cells (Rinas, Horneff, and Wahn, 1993). The low IFN-γ production at birth was a risk factor for the development of atopic disease during the first year of life (Tang et al., 1994). Additionally, to less IFN-γ producing cells a higher percentage of IL-4 producing cells was found in the cord blood of newborns who developed atopic dermatitis during the first 2 years of life (Herberth et al., 2009). IFN-γ production by pregnant women was lower in pregnancy than postpartum, and allergic women had an increased propensity to Th2 cell responses and failed to downregulate these responses in the latter half of pregnancy compared to nonallergic women (Breckler et al., 2008).

The intrauterine environment is therefore different in atopic and nonatopic mothers. Beside genetic factors it may influence the developing immune system of the fetus. This explanation is supported by the observations that an early onset atopy is much more common in infants born to mothers with atopic disease than those born to fathers with atopic disease (Moffat and Cookson, 1998; Warner et al., 2000).

17.4 Regulatory T cells

The adaptive immune system in the fetus has been regarded as functionally immature (see previous discussion). However, this has been challenged by the observation that regulatory Th cells (T_{Reg}), which are present at high frequency in fetal lymphoid tissue, actively suppress T cell proliferation and cytokine production in utero (Michaelsson et al., 2006). In the thymus of infants and adults, only a small number of Th cells are regulatory, recognized by the expression of their intracellular marker FOXP3, a nuclear transcription factor. In contrast, in the fetal lymph nodes and spleen, where mature T cells encounter antigen, 20%–25% of Th cells were T_{Reg} (Mold et al., 2008).

Substantial numbers of maternal cells cross the placenta to reside in fetal lymph nodes and induce the development of T_{Reg} cells, that suppress fetal antimaternal immunity and persist at least until early adulthood in the offspring (Mold et al., 2008). Fetal tolerance to maternal alloantigens can probably be used as a model for the response of the fetal immune system to other antigens encountered in utero, inducing, for example, a specific tolerance to food antigens. In cord blood of atopic mothers T_{Reg} cell numbers, expression, and function were impaired (Schaub et al., 2008). T_{Reg} cells were generated when cord blood mononuclear cells were stimulated with a food antigen in the presence of a lipopolysaccharide, which is recognized by toll-like receptors (TLR) of the innate immune system and supports the induction of an adaptive immune response. Maternal farm exposure increased cord blood T_{Reg} cell numbers and decreased Th2 cytokine levels (Schaub et al., 2009). An upregulation of genes of TLR2 and TLR4 of the innate immune system was still observed at school age when mothers had been exposed to stables during pregnancy (Ege et al., 2006). The capacity to generate T_{Reg} cells was impaired in neonates with a family history of allergy (Haddeland et al., 2005). Maternal smoking during pregnancy also inhibited neonatal immune responses to a variety of TLR ligands with the effect that the maturation of antigen presenting cells and T_{Reg} cells was delayed (Noakes et al., 2006).

17.5 The role of mucosal surfaces

Immune responses at mucosal surfaces are important in the development of allergy. The skin and gastrointestinal tract seem to be structurally mature already before birth, while the respiratory tract lags behind (Holt and Jones, 2000). Undamaged skin and mucosal membranes in the newborn and their secretions form an important mechanical defense against microbes. At delivery the sterile neonate meets microbes in the birth canal followed by a more pronounced exposure to the microflora of the mother's gut next to her anus. The mother's gut microflora consists nearly completely of anaerobic bacteria of very low virulence (Hanson and Silverdahl, 2009). This supports the establishment of a normal commensal microflora in the newborn, which protects from colonization with pathogenic microbes on mucosal surfaces of the gut and the respiratory tract, building up mucosal immunity in the newborn. At 1 month of age almost all newborns are colonized with anaerobic bifidobacteria, which outnumber all other bacteria (Penders et al., 2006), but a delayed fecal colonization and a disturbed gut microflora up to 6 months was observed in infants born by cesarean compared to vaginal deliveries (Grölund et al., 1999).

17.6 The role of early tolerance induction

Beside IgG antibodies that are transferred to the fetus via the placenta, breast-fed infants benefit from a high load of maternal SIgA via breast milk, antibodies directed against the mother's microflora and her surrounding and not producing an inflammatory response (Hanson and Silverdal, 2009). For the production of SIgA in the mother and in the developing infant intestinal dendritic cells (DCs) retain small numbers of live commensals for several days, which allows DCs to selectively induce IgA production (Mcpherson and Uhr, 2004). DCs may also play an important role in induction of tolerance, predominantly by induction of T_{Reg} cells (Frick, Grünebach, and Autenrieth, 2010). When human peripheral blood mononuclear cells (PBMC) were cocultivated in vitro with different (probiotic) lactic acid bacteria (e.g., bifidobacterium lactis), it could be shown that they can induce T_{Reg} cells, but some strains are potent inducers, while others are not (De Roock et al., 2010). T_{Reg} cells employ a broad range of suppressor factors, such as IL-10, and transforming growth factor (TGF)-ß, which play an important role in maintenance of intestinal homeostasis and tolerance induction (Palomares et al., 2010; Penttila, 2010). Two of the main functions of the TGF-ß-isoforms in the immune system are to promote and maintain tolerance to self, food, and environmental antigens and inhibit inflammatory responses (Penttila, 2010).

17.7 Murine models

In lactating mice it could be demonstrated that even an airborn allergen was efficiently transferred from the mother to the newborn through milk and that tolerance induction did not require the transfer of immunoglobulins (Verhasselt et al., 2008). Rather, breast-feeding-induced tolerance relied on the presence of TGF-ß during lactation and on breast milk – mediated transfer of an antigen leading to antigen-specific protection from allergic airway disease (Verhasselt et al., 2008). The dietary antigen in the milk of antigen-exposed mice was in the same range as that of antigens in human milk, that is, 180 µg/l.

But maternal tolerance against ovalbumin by oral antigen could be induced by application already in the last trimester of pregnancy, or even before pregnancy, and it was transferred from the mother to the offspring and protected them against the development of an asthma-like phenotype (Polte and Hansen, 2008; Polte, Henning, and Hansen, 2008). Prenatally initiated and postnatally sustained LPS exposure prevented allergen sensitization in offspring through an inhibition of the Th2 response (Gerhold et al., 2006). Prenatal stress not only reduced the corticotrophin-releasing hormone expression in the paraventricular nucleus of adult offspring, but triggered a higher Th2 response and higher IgE-levels in the offspring (Pincus-Knackstedt et al., 2006).

17.8 Human milk

Antigen concentrations in human milk of mothers vary considerably, and this is only partly explained by the atopic status of the mother, the infant, or the amount of allergenic food consumed (Palmer and Makrides, 2006). Additionally, it is well recognized that milk-allergic infants can have IgE mediated allergic symptoms to human milk due to cross sensitization or to genuine sensitization to human milk (Schulmeister et al., 2007). Other breast milk constituents could also play a role in the development of atopic symptoms. Breast milk from atopic mothers and breast milk given to atopic infants differed in the concentration of several ingredients, for example, fatty acids, cytokines, cow's milk – specific IgA antibodies, and TGF-ß (Böttcher et al., 2000; Duchen, Yu, and Björkstén, 1998; Järvinen et al., 2000; Österlund et al., 2004; Rothenbacher et al., 2005; Sidor et al., 2008).

17.9 Empirical results

The results of empirical studies support some of the discoveries in basic science and the pathophysiological findings, but in observational studies it is difficult to isolate the effect of a single risk factor among other factors influencing the outcome positively or negatively. Therefore, even despite statistical control for cofactors, studies often produced conflicting results.

Farmers' children in New Zealand aged 5–17 years had a lower prevalence of asthma and eczema than rural reference children (Douwes et al., 2008). Dose – response associations were demonstrated for maternal exposure to farm animals and grain or hay products during pregnancy and reduced rates of hay fever and eczema in their children. The risk for asthma was also significantly reduced, although it did not show a clear dose – response association. The strongest effect was observed for those children whose mothers had frequent exposure to farm animals during pregnancy and who were currently exposed.

In a longitudinal study in the United States it was observed that in the first 9 years children from allergic families had a higher risk for sensitization and allergic rhinitis if they had been delivered by cesarean section compared to vaginal birth (Pistiner et al., 2008). Repeat cesarean augmented the risk for allergic rhinoconjunctivitis but also for asthma in a large retrospective analysis of schoolchildren in the United States (Renz-Polster et al., 2005). Growth of pathogenic bacteria in amniotic fluid samples or swabs during a cesarean delivery were risk factors for asthma up to the age of 17 years (Keski-Nisula et al., 2009). In contrast, helminth infections of pregnant women in Uganda decreased the risk for atopic eczema in their children significantly, but Albendazol treatment resulted in higher eczema risk than placebo (Elliott et al., 2005).

Maternal smoking in pregnancy increased the risk of early wheezing (Lannerö et al., 2006). In the longitudinal cohort study MAS-90 in Germany, maternal smoking in pregnancy increased the odds for sensitization during the first 10 years twofold when children had one allergic parent and five-fold when both parents were allergic (Keil et al., 2009). In a randomized trial a high fish oil supplement in late pregnancy compared to olive oil significantly reduced the hazard rate of asthma up to 19 years of age (Olsen et al., 2008). This finding is supported by a German cohort study, observing a lower odds ratio for eczema in infants whose mothers had a high fish intake in the last weeks before delivery (Sausenthaler et al., 2007).

A meta-analysis of trials on maternal dietary antigen avoidance during pregnancy does not suggest a protective effect of antigen avoidance on the incidence of atopic eczema during the first 18 months of life (Kramer and Kakuma, 2006). Preliminary studies observed an association between gastric acid suppression during pregnancy and childhood asthma, a protective effect of a dietary antioxidant on early wheezing, or associations between anxiety during pregnancy and asthma in the child (Cookson et al., 2009; Dehlink et al., 2009; Litonjua et al., 2006). These observations are not easily explained by an influence of the specified risk factors on the immune development of the fetus. The same might be true for the influence of prematurity or of low birth weight: even after adjusting for smoking in pregnancy, gestational age, and familial and other confounders, the risk of low birth weight increased the asthma risk at school-age in a Swedish cohort of twins and within monocygotic twin pairs, probably by programming lung development (Örtquist et al., 2009). However, in a large population-based study in Alaska, preterm birth rather than intrauterine growth restriction had a higher impact for the asthma risk in the first 10 years (Gessner and Chimonas, 2007).

The "golden jubilee of controversy" on the protective role of breast-feeding against atopic diseases was acclaimed already in 1988 (Kramer, 1988), but the controversy still exists if the duration of any or of exclusive breast-feeding influences the development of atopic diseases. Even the best statistical adjustment for covariates, for example, for atopic family history, cannot exclude "reverse causality" related to exclusive breast-feeding and delayed introduction of other foods in infants with early symptoms of food allergy (Bergmann et al., 2002; Lowe et al. 2006).

The only randomized trial ever done in the area of human lactation is the PRO-BIT study, which studied 17,046 healthy breast-fed infants in 31 maternity hospitals/policlinics in Belarus, born in 1996–1997, which led to a large increase in exclusive breast-feeding at 3 months (44.3% vs 6.4%; $p < 0.001$) and a significantly higher prevalence of any breast-feeding up to and including 12 months. At the age of 6½ years, the experimental group had no reduction in risks of allergic symptoms or diagnoses or positive skin prick tests (Kramer et al., 2007).

Hypoallergenic formulas compared to conventional formulas given to infants from atopic families after weaning might offer some protection from allergic disease at least during the first years of life (Kneepkens and Brand, 2010; Szajewska and Horvath, 2010).

Probiotics during pregnancy, lactation, and early in infancy did not reduce the incidence of allergic rhinitis or asthma during childhood. A preventive effect on the development of atopic dermatitis could only be shown in some Finnish studies, so far (Kopp and Salfeld, 2009).

The timely introduction of complementary foods seems to play a role in tolerance induction. For instance, the prevalence of peanut allergy was 10 times higher in Jewish schoolchildren in the United Kingdom compared to those in Israel, although peanut is introduced earlier and is eaten more frequently and in larger quantities in Israeli than in UK infants after the first months of life (du Toit et al., 2008). A Swedish study found that the introduction of fish before the age of 9 months was associated with a lower risk of eczema (Alm et al., 2009).

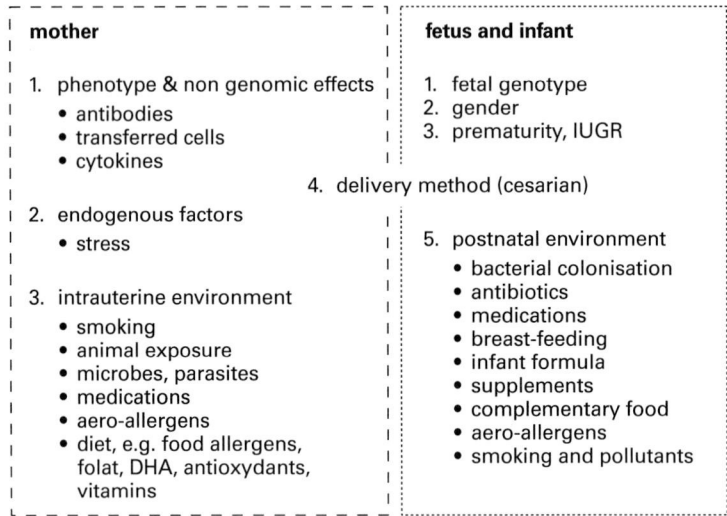

Fig. 17.2: Perinatal risk factor for allergy development (inspired by Prescott and Clifton, 2009).

In recent years the advice on the introduction of complementary food was changed by many academic societies (ESPGHAN, et al., 2008; Greer et al., 2008; Höst et al., 2008) and by the European Food Safety Authority (EFSA, 2009). They all agree that there is no convincing scientific evidence that avoidance or delayed introduction of potentially allergenic foods after the first 4–6 months of life reduces allergies in infants considered at increased risk for the development of allergy or in those not considered to be at increased risk. An Australian group even suggests that there is a window of tolerance from 3–4 months until 6–7 months (Prescott el al., 2008).

An overview of the perinatal risk factors is given in ▶Fig. 17.2.

17.10 DNA methylation and demethylation

FOXP3 gene appears to function as the master *regulator* in the development and function of *regulatory T cells*. RUNX transcription factors are a molecular link in TGF-ß induced FOXP3 gene expression (Klunker et al., 2009): because DNA methylation is a biologically and chemically stable epigenetic modification, locking long-term gene expression patterns, demethylation within the FOXP3 gene is used as a very specific marker for natural T_{Reg} cells (Wieczorek et al., 2009). In vitro hypomethylation induces FOXP3 expression and skewing toward a Th1 response, increasing the population of T_{reg} cells (Kim and Leonard, 2007). In mice an in utero exposure to a diet rich in methyl donors (compared to a diet containing methyldonors, e.g., folic acid, in an amount sufficient to prevent malformation) enhanced the severity of allergic airway disease in their offspring, and this predisposition appeared to be partially transmitted to subsequent generations (Hollingsworth et al., 2008). Methylation studies identified specific genes, including RUNX3, that may play a fundamental role in the development and severity of this condition. In an Australian prospective birth cohort study folic acid taken in supplement form in late pregnancy was associated with a small but significant increase in childhood asthma (RR 1.26) at 3.5 years (Whitrow et al., 2009). This is in line with the observation that FOX3 demethylation was increased in offspring of mothers with farm exposure (Schaub et al., 2009).

The proposed concept of a "maternally induced immunological imprinting phase à la Konrad Lorenz" seems to take shape (Lemke and Lange, 1999).

References

Akira S, Takeda K, Kaisho T. Toll-like receptors: critical proteins linking innate and acquired immunity. *Nature Immunol* 2001;2: 675–80.

Alm B, Åberg N, Erdes L, et al. Early introduction of fish decreases the risk of eczema in infants. *Arch Dis Child* 2009;94: 11–5.

Bergmann RL, Diepgen TL, Kuss O, et al. Breastfeeding duration is a risk factor for atopic eczema. *Clin Exp Allergy* 2002;32: 205–9.

Böttcher MF, Jenmalm MC, Garofalo RP, Björkstén B. Cytokines in breast milk from allergic and non allergic mothers. *Pediatr Res* 2000;47: 157–62.

Breckler LA, Hale J, Taylor A, Dunstan JA, Thornton CA, Prescott SL. Pregnancy interferon-gamma responses to foetal alloantigens are altered by maternal allergy and gravidity status. *Allergy* 2008;63: 1473–80.

Cookson H, Granell R, Joinson C, Ben-Shlomo Y, Henderson AJ. Mothers' anxiety during pregnancy is associated with asthma in their children. *J Allergy Clin Immunol* 2009;23: 847–53.

De Roock S, van Elk M, van Dijk MEA, et al. Lactic acid bacteria differ in their ability to induce functional regulatory T cells in humans. *Clin Exp Allergy* 2010;40: 103–10.

Dehlink E, Yen E, Leichtner AM, Hait EH, Fiebiger E. First evidence of a possible association between gastric acid suppression during pregnancy and childhood asthma: a population-based register study. *Clin Exp Allergy* 2009;39: 246–53.

Douwes J, Cheng S, Travier N, et al. Farm exposure in utero may protect against asthma, hay fever and eczema. *Eur Respir J* 2008;32: 603–11.

Duchen K, Yu G, Björkstén B. Atopic sensitization during the first year of life in relation to long chain polyunsaturated fatty acid levels in human milk. *Pediatr Res* 1998;44: 478–84.

Du Toit G, Katz Y, Sasieni P, et al. Early consumption of peanuts in infancy is associated with a low prevalence of peanut allergy. *J Allergy Clin Immunol* 2008;122: 984–91.

EFSA Panel on Dietetic Products NaAN. Scientific opinion on the appropriate age for introduction of complementary feeding of infants. *Eur Food Safety Authority J* 2009;7: 1423.

Ege MJ, Bieli C, Frei R, et al. Prenatal farm exposure is related to the expression of receptors of the innate immunity and to atopic sensitization in school-age children. *J Allergy Clin Immunol* 2006;117: 817–23.

Elliott AM, Mpairwe H, Quigley MA, et al. Helminth infection during pregnancy and development of infantile eczema. *JAMA* 2005;294: 2032–34.

ESPGHAN Committee on Nutrition, Agostoni C, Decsi T, et al. Complementary feeding: A commentary by the ESPGHAN Committee on Nutrition. *J Pediatr Gastroenterol Nutr* 2008;46: 99–110.

Frick JS, Grünebach F, Autenrieth IB. Immunmodulation by semimature dendtritic cells: A novel role of Toll-Like receptors and interleukin-6. *Int J Medical Microbiol* 2010;300: 19–24.

Gerhold K, Avagyan A, Seib C, et al. Prenatal initiation of endotoxin airway exposure prevents subsequent allergen-induced sensitization and airway inflammation in mice. *J Allergy Clin Immunol* 2006;118: 666–73.

Gessner BD, Chimonas MAR. Asthma is associated with preterm birth but not with small for gestational age status among a population-based cohort of Medicaid-enrolled children <10 years of age. *Thorax* 2007;62: 231–6.

Greer FR, Sicherer SH, Burks W, and the Committee on Nutrition, Section on Allergy and Immunology. Effects of early nutritional interventions on the development of atopic disease in infants and children: The role of maternal dietary restriction, breastfeeding, timing of introduction of complementary foods, and hydrolysed formulas. *Pediatrics* 2008;121: 183–91.

Grölund MM, Lehtonen OP, Eerola E, Kero P. Fecal microflora in healthy infants born by different methods of delivery: Permanent changes in intestinal flora after cesarian delivery. *J Pediatr Gastroent Nutr* 1999;28: 19–25.

Haddeland U, Karstensen AB, Farkas L, et al. Putative regulatory T cells are impaired in cord blood from neonates with hereditary allergy risk. *Pediatr Allergy Immunol* 2005;16: 104–12.

Hanson LA, Silverdal SA. The mother's immune system is a balanced threat to the foetus, turning to protection of the neonate. *Acta Paediatr* 2009;98: 221–8.

Haynes BF, Heinly CS. Early human T cell development: analysis of the human thymus at the time of initial entry of hematopoetic stem cells into fetal thymic microenvironment. *J Exp Med* 1995;181: 1445–58.

Herberth G, Heinrich J, Röder S, et al. Reduced interferon-y- and enhanced IL-4-producing CD4+ cord blood T-cells are associated with a higher risk for atopic dermatitis during the first 2 ys of life. *Pediatr Allergy Immunol* 2009;21: 5–13.

Hollingsworth JW, Maruoka S, Boon K, et al. In utero supplementation with methyl donors enhances allergic airway disease in mice. *J Clin Invest* 2008;118: 3462–9.

Holloway JA, Warner JO, Vance GHS, Diaper N, Warner G, Jones CA. Detection of house dust mite allergen in amniotic fluid and umbilical cord blood. *Lancet* 2000;356: 1900–2.

Holloway JW, Yang IA, Holgate ST. Genetics of allergic disease. *J Allergy Clin Immunol* 2010;125: S81–94.

Holt PG, Jones CA. The development of the immune system during pregnancy and early life. *Allergy* 2000;55: 688–97.

Höst A, Halken S, Muraro A, et al. Dietary prevention of allergic diseases in infants and small children. *Pediatr Allergy Immunol* 2008;19: 1–4.

Järvinen K-M, Laine ST, Järvenpää AL, Suomalainen HK. Does low IgA in human milk predispose the infant to development of cow's milk allergy? *Pediatr Res* 2000;47: 157–62.

Johansson SGO, Bieber T, Dahl R, et al. Revised nomenclature for allergy for global use; report of the nomenclature review committee of the World Allergy Organization, October 2003. *J Allergy Clin Immunol* 2004;113: 832–6.

Jones AC, Miles EA, Warner JO, Colwell BM, Bryant TN, Warner JA. Fetal blood mononuclear cell proliferative responses to mitogenic and allergenic stimuli during gestation. *Pediatr Allergy Immunol* 1996;7: 109–16.

Keil T, Lau S, Roll S, et al. Maternal smoking increases the risk of allergic sensitization and wheezing only in children with allergic predisposition: longitudinal analysis from birth to 10 years. *Allergy* 2009;64: 445–51.

Keski-Nisula L, Katila M-L, Remes S, Heinonen S, Pekkanen J. Intrauterine bacterial growth at birth and risk of asthma and allergic sensitization among offspring at the age of 15 to 17 years. *J Allergy Clin Immunol* 2009;123: 1305–11.

Kim H-P, Leonard WJ. CREB/ATF-dependent T cell receptor induced FoxP3 gene expression: a role for DNA methylation. *J Exp Med* 2007;204: 1543–51.

Klunker S, Chong MMW, Mantel PY, et al. Transcription factors RUNX1 and RUNX3 in the induction and suppressive function of Foxp3 inducible regulatory T cells. *J Exp Med* 2009;206: 2701–15.

Kneepkens CMF, Brand PLP. Clinical Practise: Breastfeeding and the prevention of allergy. *Eur J Pediatr* 2010;169:911–7.

Kopp MV, Salfeld P. Probiotics and the prevention of allergic disease. *Curr Opin Clin Nutr Metab Care* 2009;12: 298–303.

Kramer MS. Does breastfeeding help protect from atopic disease? Biology, methodology, and a golden jubilee of controversy. *J Pediatr* 1988;121: 181–90.

Kramer MS, Kakuma R. Maternal antigen avoidance during pregnancy or lactation, or both, for preventing or treating atopic disease in the child. *Cochrane Database of Systematic Reviews* 2006; Issue 3. Art. No.: CD000133.

Kramer MS, Matush L, Vanilovich I, et al. Effect of prolonged and exclusive breast feeding on risk of allergy and asthma: cluster randomised trial. *BMJ* 2007;335: 815–8.

Lannerö E, Wickman M, Pershagen G, Nordvall L. Maternal smoking during pregnancy increases the risk of recurrent wheezing during the first years of life (BAMSE). *Respir Res* 2006;7: 3.

Lemke H, Lange H. Is there a maternally induced immunological imprinting à la Konrad Lorenz? *Scand J Immunol* 1999;50: 348–54.

Litonjua AA, Rifas-Shiman SL, Ly NP, et al. Maternal antioxidant intake and wheezing illnesses in children at 2 years of age. *Am J Clin Nutr* 2006;84: 903–11.

Lowe AJ, Carlin JB, Bennett CM, et al. Atopic disease and breast-feeding-cause or consequence? *J Allergy Clin Immunol* 2006;117: 682–7.

Mcpherson AJ, Uhr T. Induction of protective IgA by intestinal dendritic cells carrying commensal bacteria. *Science* 2004;303: 1662–5.

Michaelsson J, Mold JE, Mc Cune JM, Nixon DF. Regulation of T cell responses in the developing human fetus. *J Immunol* 2006;176: 5741–8.

Moffat MF, Cookson WOCM. Maternal effects in atopic disease. *Clin Exp Allergy* 1998; S1: 58–61.

Mold JE, Michaelson J, Burt TD, et al. Maternal alloantigens promote the development of tolerogenic fetal regulatory T cells in utero. *Science* 2008;322: 1562–5.

Mosman TR, Sad S. The expanding evidence of T-cell subsets: Th1, Th2 and more. *Immunology Today* 1996;17: 138–46.

Noakes PS, Hale J, Thomas R, Lane C, Devadson SG, Prescott SL. Maternal smoking is associated with impaired neonatal toll-like-receptor-mediated immune responses. *Eur Respir J* 2006;28: 721–9.

Olsen SF, Österdal, ML, Salvig JD, et al. Fish oil intake compared with olive oil intake in late pregnancy and asthma in the offspring: 16 y of registry-based follow-up from a randomized controlled trial. *Am J Clin Nutr* 2008; 88: 167–175.

Örtquist AK, Lundholm C, Carlström E, Lichtenstein P, Cnattigius S, Almquist C. Familial doctors do not confound the association between birth weight and childhood asthma. *Pediatrics* 2009;124: e737–43.

Österlund P, Smedberg T, Hakulinene A, Heikkila H, Järvinen KM. Eosinophilic cationic protein in human milk is associated with development of cow's milk allergy and atopic eczema in breast-fed infants. *Pediatr Res* 2004;55: 296–301.

Palmer DJ, Makrides M. Diet of lactating women and allergic reaction in their infants. *Curr Opin Clin Nutr Metab Care* 2006;9: 284–8.

Palomares O, Yaman G, Azkur AK, Akkoc T, Akdis M, Akdis CA. Role of regulatory T cells in immune regulation of allergic diseases. *Eur J Immunol* 2010;40: 1232–40.

Penders J, Thijs C, Vink C, et al. Factors influencing the composition of the intestinal microbiota in early infancy. *Pediatrics* 2006;118: 511–21.

Penttila IA. Milk-derived transforming growth factor-ß and the infant immune response. *J Pediatr* 2010;156: S21–5.

Pincus-Knacksted MK, Joachim RA, Blois SM, et al. Prenatal stress enhances susceptibility of murine adult offspring toward airway inflammation. *J Immunol* 2006;177: 8484–92.

Pistiner M, Gold DR, Abdulkerim H, Hoffman E, Celedon JC. Birth by cesarian section, allergic rhinitis, and allergic sensitization among children with parental history of atopy. *J Allergy Clin Immunol* 2008;122: 274–9.

Polte T, Hansen G. Maternal tolerance achieved during pregnancy is transferred to the offspring via breast milk and persistently protects the offspring from allergic asthma. *Clin Exp Allergy* 2008;38: 1950–8.

Polte T, Henning C, Hansen G. Allergy prevention starts before conception: maternofetal transfer of tolerance protects against the development of asthma. *J Allergy Clin Immunol* 2008;122: 1022–30.

Prescott SL, Noakes P, Chow BWY, et al. Presymptomatic differences in Toll-like receptor function in infants who have allergy. *J Allergy Clin Immunol* 2008;122: 391–9.

Prescott SL, Clifton V. Asthma and pregnancy: emerging evidence of epigenetic interactions in utero. *Curr Opinion Allergy Clin Immunol* 2009;9: 417–26.

Renz-Polster H, David MR, Buist AS, et al. Caesarian section delivery and the risk of allergic disorders in childhood. *Clin Exper Allergy* 2005;35: 1466–72.

Rinas U, Horneff G, Wahn V. Interferon-γ production by cord-blood mononuclear cells is reduced in newborns with a family history of atopic disease and is independent from cord blood IgE-levels. *Pediatr Allergy Immunol* 1993;4: 60–4.

Rothenbacher D, Weyerman M, Beerman C, Brenner H. Breastfeeding, soluble CD14 concentration in breast milk and risk of atopic dermatitis and asthma in early childhood: birth cohort study. *Clin Exp Allergy* 2005;35: 1014–21.

Sausenthaler S, Koletzko S, Schaaf B, et al. Maternal diet during pregnancy in relation to eczema and allergic sensitization in the offspring at 2 year of age. *Am J Clin Nutr* 2007;85: 530–7.

Schaub B, Liu J, Höppler S, et al. Impairment of T-regulatory cells in cord blood of atopic mothers. *J Allergy Clin Immunol* 2008;121: 1491–9.

Schaub B, Liu J, Höppler S, et al. Maternal farm exposure modulates neonatal immune mechanisms through regulatory T cells. *J Allergy Clin Immunol* 2009;23: 774–8.

Schulmeister U, Swoboda I, Quirce S, et al. Sensitization to human milk. *Clin Exp Allergy* 2007;38: 60–8.

Sidor K, Jarmotlovka B, Kaczmarski M, Kostyra E, Iwan M, Kostyra H. Content of casomorphin in milk of women with a history of allergy. *Pediatr Allergy Immunol* 2008;19: 587–91.

Stites DP, Carr MC, Fudenberg HH. Ontogeny of cellular immunity in the human fetus. *Cell Immunol* 1974;11: 257–71.

Szajewska H, Horvath A. Meta-analysis of the evidence for a partially hydrolysed 100% whey formula for the prevention of allergic diseases. *Curr Med Res Opin* 2010;26: 423–37.

Tang MLK, Kemp AS, Thorburn J, Hill DJ. Reduced interferon-γ-secretion in neonates and subsequent atopy. *Lancet* 1994;344: 983–5.

Turvey SE, Broide DH. Innate immunity. *J Allergy Clin Immunol* 2010; 125: S24–32.

Verhasselt V, Milcent V, Cazareth J, et al. Breast milk-mediated transfer of an antigen induces tolerance and protection from allergic asthma. *Nat Med* 2008;14: 170–5.

Warner JO, Jones CA, Kilburn SA, Vance GHS, Warner JA. Prenatal sensitization in humans. *Pediatr Allergy Immunol* 2000;13: 6–8.

Wegmann TG, Lin H, Guilbert H, Mosman TR. Bidirectional cytokine interactions in the maternal-fetal relationship: is successful pregnancy a TH2 phenomenon? *Immunology Today* 1993;14: 353–6.

West LJ. Defining critical windows in the development of the human immune system. *Hum Exp Toxicol* 2002;21: 499–505.

Whitrow M, Moore VM, Rumboldt AR, Davies MJ. Effect of supplemental folic acid in pregnancy on childhood asthma: a prospective birth cohort study. *Am J Epidemiol* 2009;170: 1486–93.

Wieczorek G, Asemissen A, Model F, et al. Quantitative DNA methylation analysis of FOXP3 as a new method for counting regulatory T cells in peripheral blood and solid tissue. *Cancer Res* 2009;69: 599–608.

Wilczynski JR. Th1/Th2 cytokines balance-yin and yang of reproductive immunology. *Eur J Obstet Gyecol* 2005;122: 136–43.

18 Perinatal origin of testicular germ cell cancer: Possible involvement of developmental reprogramming

Kristian Almstrup, Ewa Rajpert-De Meyts, and Niels E. Skakkebæk

Testicular dysgenesis syndrome is manifested as poor semen quality, undescended testes, hypospadias, or testicular germ cell cancer. The current hypothesis on the pathogenic events leading to testicular dysgenesis involves improper development of somatic nurse cells and consequently delayed germ cell development. Most evidence comes from testicular germ cell cancer, which is the most common cancer in young men. It develops through a pre-invasive carcinoma *in situ* (CIS) stage. Much data indicate that the CIS cell is a neoplastic and pluripotent counterpart of a primordial germ cell (PGC) or gonocyte that has failed to differentiate. During their development both PGC and gonocytes undergo extensive epigenetic modifications, including erasure and reestablishment of genome-wide DNA methylation and exchange of histone modifications. This chapter reviews the current knowledge on the perinatal reprogramming of fetal germ cells and its possible involvement in testicular cancer pathogenesis.

18.1 Introduction

Testicular cancer is today the most frequent cancer among young males and accounts for approximately 1% of all cancers in men. Worldwide, testicular cancer has more than doubled in the last 40 years, but the incidence varies considerably in different geographical areas and also between ethnic groups (Huyghe, Matsuda, and Thonneau, 2003). Testicular cancer is 4.5 times more common among white men than black men in the United States (Moul et al., 1994) and twice more frequent in Denmark than Sweden (Chia et al., 2010). Interestingly, analysis of incidence rates in second-generation immigrants to Sweden has revealed that these acquire the Swedish risk irrespectively of the parental geographical origin (Hemminki and Li, 2002a, 2002b; Hemminki, Li, and Czene, 2002), indicating that the place of birth determines the risk. Clinical risk factors include male infertility (RR = 3) (Mancini et al., 2007; Walsh et al., 2009) and a history of cryptorchidism (RR = 2–8) (Dieckmann and Pichlmeier, 2004; Wood and Elder, 2009).

Despite the observed increase in incidence, there has been a dramatic decrease in mortality as a result of new and effective treatments regimes. In particular cis-platin based therapies have proven effective (Einhorn, 2002; Peckham et al., 1983). Testicular cancer nevertheless causes a significant amount of posttreatment complications as survivors have a 2-fold higher standardized mortality rate (Fosså et al., 2004), a 2-fold higher risk of developing a secondary tumor, and up to 10-times increased risk of developing metabolic syndrome (Feldman et al., 2008).

The vast majority of human testicular tumors are derived from germ cells. Testicular cancer manifests either as a seminoma or nonseminoma, which are very different tumors, both in terms of histology and treatment regimes. Seminoma is a homogeneous tumor composed of mitotically dividing germ cells, whereas nonseminomas are heterogeneous tumors that may contain varying proportions of undifferentiated embryonal carcinoma, partially differentiated somatic tissues (teratoma), and extra-embryonic elements, such as choriocarcinoma and yolk sac tumor (Ulbright, Amin, and Young, 1999). Both of these very different tumor types are preceded by a symptomless preinvasive stage, where the common precursor cell of germ cell tumors, the carcinoma *in situ* (CIS) cell (Skakkebaek, 1972), can be found in usually normally arranged seminiferous tubules (►Fig. 18.1). CIS is also known as intratubular germ cell neoplasia unclassified (ITGCN) or testicular intraepithelial neoplasia (TIN).

According to our hypothesis, understimulation or disarrangement of germ cells (primordial germ cells or gonocytes) during early development is a key event leading to disorders of germ cell differentiation. CIS cells, in similarity to early fetal germ cells, retain a high expression of pluripotency genes (Almstrup et al., 2004), and hormonal stimulation of these cells in pubertal testis is thought to increase proliferation and at some point triggers a malignant phenotype. During early fetal development migrating primordial germ cells as well as gonocytes undergo extensive epigenetic modifications, which include erasure and reestablishment of genome-wide DNA methylation and exchange of histone modifications. These sequential epigenetic modifications seem to be a prerequisite of normal germ cell development. This chapter focuses on the current knowledge on the early perinatal reprogramming of germ cells and possible implications in testicular cancer pathogenesis.

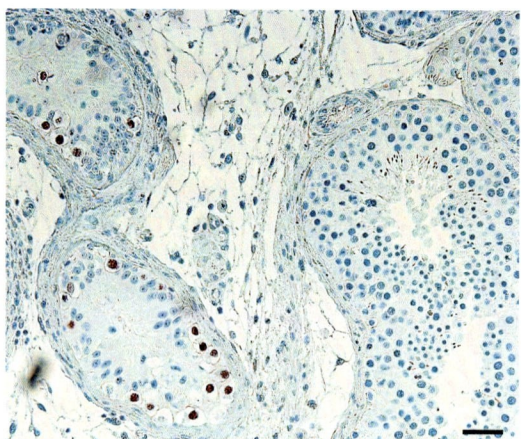

Fig. 18.1: Immunohistochemistry with an antibody against the CIS marker transcription factor AP-2γ (TFAP2C). AP-2γ is almost exclusively found in fetal and cancerous cells (Hoei-Hansen et al., 2004). On the left are tubules containing CIS cells (AP-2γ positive, dark), and on the right a tubule with normal spermatogenesis is shown. Bar represents 50 microns.

18.2 Carcinoma *in situ* testis

Carcinoma *in situ* was first described in 1972 (Skakkebaek, 1972) and already a few years later, morphological studies indicated that the CIS cell was very similar to fetal germ cells (Albrechtsen et al., 1982; Nielsen, Nielsen, and Skakkebaek, 1974; Skakkebaek et al., 1987). Comparative studies of protein markers (reviewed in Rajpert-De Meyts et al., 2003) and global gene expression profiles of CIS cells (Almstrup et al., 2004, 2007; Sonne et al., 2009) later substantiated that indeed CIS cells are very similar to gonocytes. Most likely the CIS cell in fact is a gonocyte, which failed to mature during perinatal development and later underwent malignant transformation. Further transformation of CIS cells, however, most likely occurs during adaptation to the changed endocrine environment of the peri- and postpubertal testis. CIS cells undergo polyploidization (Oosterhuis et al., 1989) and acquire a characteristic pattern of genomic aberrations, including gain of chromosome 12p (Ottesen et al., 2003; Rosenberg et al., 2000), often seen as the isochromosome 12p (Atkin and Baker, 1982). Interestingly, embryonic stem cell lineages apparently gain chromosomal amplifications in similar areas upon prolonged culturing, suggesting that chromosomal gains in these areas lead to survival advantages (Almstrup et al., 2004; Draper et al., 2004). In analogy to primordial germ cells and gonocytes, CIS cells highly express transcription factors associated with embryonic stem cell pluripotency and somatic tissue-specific stem cell lineages, including, for example, POU5F1/OCT-3/4, NANOG, GDF3, KIT, and AP-2γ (Almstrup et al., 2004; Biermann et al., 2007; Hoei-Hansen et al., 2004, 2005; Looijenga et al., 2003; Skotheim et al., 2005; Sperger et al., 2003).

Our current hypothesis is that developmental arrest of gonocytes is caused by disruption of the endocrine environment in the testis (niche). The niche comprises somatic cells (mainly Sertoli and Leydig cells), which secrete hormones and paracrine factors that stimulate male-specific germ cell maturation into spermatogonia (Rajpert-De Meyts, 2006). Indeed, evidence from animal models indicates that perinatally administered endocrine disrupters like phthalates can induce dysgenic lesions in the testes of rats and rabbits (Fisher et al., 2003; Foster et al., 2001; Higuchi et al., 2003), similar to those frequently observed in patients with testicular germ cell cancer (Hoei-Hansen et al., 2003; Skakkebaek et al., 2003). Interestingly, these dysgenic patterns seem to be affecting primarily somatic cells, in particular Leydig cells, and not directly germ cells (Mahood et al., 2005). The effect on germ cells thus seems to be secondary but nevertheless adversely affects their perinatal development. Increased and widespread use of industrial products that act like endocrine disrupters (e.g., phthalates) combined with an increase in endocrine-related diseases, which may cause dysgenesis of the testis, for example, obesity, have thus raised growing concerns of possible association between exposure of endocrine disrupting chemicals and human adverse effects. Indeed, elevated levels of chemicals, such as polychlorinated biphenyls, hexachlorobenzene, and chlordanes, have been detected in blood from the mothers of men with testicular cancer (Hardell et al., 2003).

18.3 Testicular dysgenesis

Clinical observations of patients with various kinds of disorders related to endocrine and reproductive function in 2001 lead to the hypothesis of the testicular dysgenesis syndrome (TDS) (Skakkebaek, Rajpert-De Meyts, and Main, 2001). It was suggested

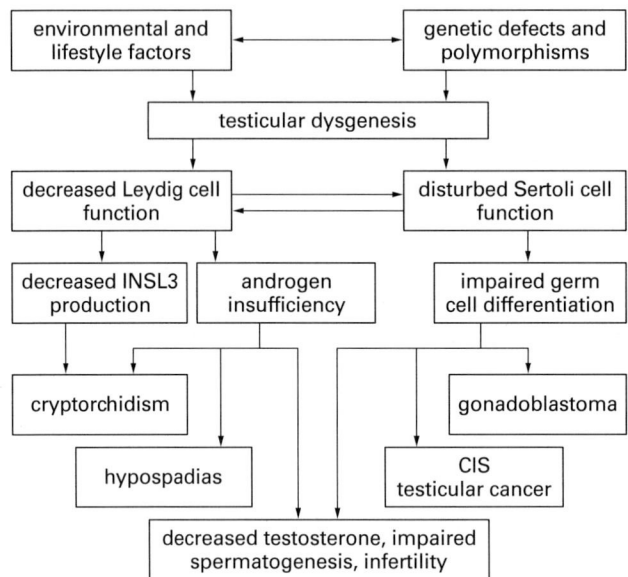

Fig. 18.2: Outline of the TDS concept. Genetic factors increase sensitivity toward yet unknown environmental or lifestyle factors that cause testicular dysgenesis. Effects are probably induced primarily in the somatic nurse cells surrounding the germ cells. This in turn leads to a delayed germ cell maturation and decreased secretion of reproductive hormones. Probably depending on the susceptibility and how severe the effects are, fetal dysgenesis is manifested by several clinical outcomes, including impairment of testicular descent, hypospadias, neoplastic transformation of germ cells (CIS in testes or gonadoblastoma in intersex gonads), or some forms of impaired testicular function and spermatogenesis later in life. Adapted from Skakkebæk et al. (2007).

that many cases of poor semen quality, hypospadias, and cryptorchidism (undescended testis) may share the same etiological origin with testicular cancer, namely improper development of the testes. The hypothesis was based on observations of common risk factors, which in all cases seem to operate *in utero* or early infancy and that the trends in incidence follow each other within geographical regions (Boisen et al., 2004; Hemminki and Li, 2002b; Hemminki et al., 2002). However, not all of the symptoms may be present in an individual with TDS; that happens very rarely in patients with genetic disorders of sex differentiation, for example, *AR* or *SRY* mutations with only partial loss of the gene function (Isidor et al., 2009). Obviously, factors other than TDS may cause poor semen quality and genital malformations (see ▶Fig. 18.2).

Of disorders regarded as part of the TDS, testicular cancer offers the best clinical, epidemiological, and biological evidence, and most of the knowledge related to TDS has been gained from testicular cancer.

18.4 Perinatal reprogramming of germ cells

In order to deduce possible effects of endocrine disruption on germ cells leading to development of CIS, it is a prerequisite to understand the perinatal reprogramming of normal fetal germ cells. Most of our current knowledge on fetal germ cell development comes from studies in mice, probably due to difficulties in obtaining sufficient material for human studies. During embryonic development, embryonic ectoderm gives rise to somatic germ layers and primordial germ cells (PGC), which are first observed at embryonic day E7.25 (mice) in the posterior end of the primitive streak. BLIMP1 positive cells are, however, already seen at E6.25 and mark pre-PGCs (Ohinata et al., 2005). BLIMP1 is crucial for normal germ cell specification and is thought to be engaged in suppression of somatic programs by *Hox* genes (i.e., *HoxA1* and *HoxB1*) (Ohinata et al., 2005). Approximately at embryonic day E8 (mice) PGC start to migrate toward the genital ridge and colonize the primitive gonad, which is tightly associated with the mesonephros. This primitive gonad is still sexually bipotential, and sex-determination first takes place between E10.5 and E11.5. Female germ cells are bound to subsequently enter meiosis, but male germ cells, gonocytes, continue to proliferate and later differentiate to prespermatogonia, which are locked in mitotic arrest. Expression of the gene *Sry* in precursors of Sertoli cells is thought to be one of the most important switches involved in sex-determination. If *Sry* is expressed, this subsequently triggers expression of *Sox9* and several other masculinizing genes that are essential for proper differentiation of Sertoli cells (recently reviewed in Koopman, 2010). Sertoli cells are stimulated, embedding PGC/gonocytes and form cord structures, which in mice are seen at E12. Migration of human PGCs takes place during gestational week (GW) 4–6, and after GW 6 germ cells are found in the gonadal anlage and begin to be surrounded by immature Sertoli cells. From that point of time, the term *gonocyte* is used to describe the germ cells in the male gonad (Fujimoto, Miyayama, and Fuyuta, 1977).

During specification and migration mice PGCs undergo specific epigenetic reprogramming, which includes genome-wide DNA demethylation (starting at E8), progressive erasure of histone H3 K9 demethylation (H3K9me2; starting at E7.5), and subsequently establishment of H3K27me3 (starting at E8.25) in a progressive, cell-by-cell manner (Seki et al., 2005, 2007). Around the time of gonadal colonization (E11.5) further modifications of the chromatin occur. Such epigenetic programs of PGCs presumably are tightly regulated during development and are a prerequisite for proper maturation of germ cells.

Both H3K9me2 and H3K27me3 are repressive modifications, and in the period during exchange of these modifications (E7.5 and E8.25) the PGC is free of repressing chromatin leading to hypertranscription. Transcriptional activity dependent on RNA polymerase II is, however, transiently repressed in PGC during this period (Seki et al., 2007). Accordingly, the histone methyltransferase, GLP, which methylates H3 at K9, is downregulated prior to H3K9 demethylation (Tachibana et al., 2008).

In early pre-PGC and migrating PGCs BLIMP1 (expressed from E6.25) is found in the nucleus complexed with PRMT5, where the complex mediates symmetrical methylation of histones H4 and H2A at arginine 3 (H4/H2AR3me2). When murine PGC arrive in the genital ridge this complex is translocated to the cytoplasm, leading to reduced levels of H4/H2AR3me2 (Ancelin et al., 2006). Translocation of Blimp1/Prmt5 to the cytoplasm leads to downregulation of Blimp1, which in turn coincides with re-expression of pluripotency-associated genes such as *Nanog* and *Sox2* (Ohinata et al., 2005; Yabuta et al., 2006). In this particular stage, there is a significant difference between species: human PGCs do not express SOX2 while retaining high expression of NANOG and POU5F1 (Perrett et al., 2008).

When mice PGCs colonize the genital ridge (E11.5) extensive chromatin and epigenetic reprogramming occurs. These include linker histone H1, H3K9ac, H3K9me3, H3K27me2, DAPI chromocenters, and H4/H2A R3me2 (Hajkova et al., 2008) and a second wave of DNA demethylation, where parental imprints are erased (Hajkova et al., 2002). Some parental imprints are already set again starting at E14.5, while others first are acquired at the newborn stage (Li et al., 2004). By FACS analysis of dissected urogenital ridges of an *Oct4-GFP* transgenic mouse, Hajkova et al. (2008) identified two Oct4+ (GFP) populations of PGCs at E11.5. These two populations were shown to reflect a developmentally primitive and a more advanced PGC population. The advanced population showed low levels of H2A.Z, linker H1, H3K9ac, H3K9me3, and H3K27me3, as well as H2A/H4R3me2, when compared to the primitive population showing higher levels of these marks. Accordingly, the primitive population showed variations in the levels of DNA methylation (5-methyl-cytosine levels), whereas the advanced population was practically devoid of DNA methylation (Hajkova et al., 2008).

After colonization PGC proliferate and when a sufficient amount is reached female germ cells enter meiotic prophase, while male germ cells (gonocytes) arrest in the G0/G1-phase of the cell cycle until after birth. After birth, gonocytes give rise to primitive spermatogonia (spermatogonial stem cells) that start to proliferate and develop into spermatocytes at days 10–14 postnatal in mice.

PGC in the genital ridge are virtually devoid of DNA methylation (Reik and Walter, 2001), but *de novo* methylation is initiated in male germ cells at E14.5 and thereafter in female germ cells, and mature gametes of both sexes will eventually become highly methylated. Additional DNA demethylation and histone modifications take place in pubertal and adult male germ cells after meiosis during spermatogenesis (Bernardino et al., 2000; del Mazo et al., 1994; Norris et al., 1994). Histones are exchanged with transition proteins and finally with protamines. Additionally, it has been suggested that remethylation and possible further chromatin modifications may occur when spermatozoa undergo final maturation in the epididymis (Xie et al., 2002).

18.5 Involvement of perinatal reprogramming in the CIS phenotype?

It has never been possible to cultivate CIS cells, nor does an appropriate animal model for CIS and testicular germ cell cancer exist. Investigations of CIS cells are thus limited to archived material from human testicular tissue, and very little is known about the epigenetic status of CIS cells. So far it is only known that CIS cells show H4/H2AR3me2 modifications (Eckert et al., 2008) and that CIS have very low levels of DNA methylation (Netto et al., 2008). Most seminomas show H4/H2A R3me2, while low levels are found in nonseminomas (Eckert et al., 2008). DNA methylation levels in seminomas are variable but mainly low, while high levels are found in nonseminomas (Netto et al., 2008; Smiraglia et al., 2002). This pattern of DNA methylation coincides very well with our findings of high expression of the DNA methylation enzymes DNMT3A and DNMT3L in the undifferentiated component of nonseminoma, embryonal carcinoma (EC), when compared to seminoma and CIS (Almstrup et al., 2005).

From the limited knowledge of epigenetic patterns in CIS cells, these patterns seem to be retained in seminomas, while nonseminomas (EC) show a different and more "somatic-like" pattern. Similar relations have earlier been suggested from studies of histology and gene expression (Rajpert-De Meyts et al., 2003).

In recent years, studies of the mechanistic pathways affected by some environmental chemicals have suggested a possibility of heritable changes in epigenetic patterns in fetal germ cells (Anway et al., 2005, 2006). It is, therefore, a pertinent scientific question whether dysregulation of epigenetic patterns in fetal germ cells is involved in the pathogenesis of testicular cancer.

18.6 Concluding remarks

Both biological and epidemiological data indicate that testicular germ cell cancer has a fetal origin. Dysgenetic patterns similar to those frequently observed in human testes of testicular cancer patients can be mimicked by perinatal exposure to, for example, phthalates in rats. We do not have any direct human evidence, but the animal studies raise the likelihood of such environmental perinatal exposures in the pathogenesis of testicular cancer and testicular dysgenesis. Probably exposure in an early time-window during pregnancy is critical, but further reprogramming and genomic changes during subsequent development are likely. Further investigations in humans are needed, however, in order to prove direct effects of perinatal environmental exposure.

References

Albrechtsen R, Nielsen MH, Skakkebaek NE, Wewer U. Carcinoma in situ of the testis. Some ultrastructural characteristics of germ cells. *Acta Pathol Microbiol Immunol Scand A* 1982;90: 301–3.

Almstrup K, Hoei-Hansen CE, Wirkner U, et al. Embryonic stem cell-like features of testicular carcinoma in situ revealed by genome-wide gene expression profiling. *Cancer Res* 2004;64: 4736–43.

Almstrup K, Hoei-Hansen CE, Nielsen JE, et al. Genome-wide gene expression profiling of testicular carcinoma in situ progression into overt tumours. *Br J Cancer* 2005;92: 1934–41.

Almstrup K, Leffers H, Lothe RA, et al. Improved gene expression signature of testicular carcinoma in situ. *Int J Androl* 2007;30: 292–302; discussion 303.

Ancelin K, Lange UC, Hajkova P, et al. Blimp1 associates with Prmt5 and directs histone arginine methylation in mouse germ cells. *Nat Cell Biol* 2006;8: 623–30.

Anway MD, Cupp AS, Uzumcu M, Skinner MK. Epigenetic transgenerational actions of endocrine disruptors and male fertility. *Science* 2005;308: 1466–9.

Anway MD, Leathers C, Skinner MK. Endocrine disruptor vinclozolin induced epigenetic transgenerational adult-onset disease. *Endocrinology* 2006;147: 5515–23.

Atkin NB, Baker MC. Specific chromosome change, i(12p), in testicular tumours? *Lancet* 1982;2: 1349.

Bernardino J, Lombard M, Niveleau A, Dutrillaux B. Common methylation characteristics of sex chromosomes in somatic and germ cells from mouse, lemur and human. *Chromosome Res* 2000;8: 513–25.

Biermann K, Heukamp LC, Steger K, et al. Gene expression profiling identifies new biological markers of neoplastic germ cells. *Anticancer Res* 2007;27: 3091–100.

Boisen KA, Kaleva M, Main KM, et al. Difference in prevalence of congenital cryptorchidism in infants between two Nordic countries. *Lancet* 2004;363: 1264–9.

Chia VM, Quraishi SM, Devesa SS, Purdue MP, Cook MB, McGlynn KA. International trends in the incidence of testicular cancer, 1973–2002. *Cancer Epidemiol Biomarkers Prev* 2010;19: 1151–9.

Del Mazo J, Prantera G, Torres M, Ferraro M. DNA methylation changes during mouse spermatogenesis. *Chromosome Res* 1994;2:147–52.

Dieckmann KP, Pichlmeier U. Clinical epidemiology of testicular germ cell tumors. *World J Urol* 2004;22: 2–14.

Draper JS, Smith K, Gokhale P, et al. Recurrent gain of chromosomes 17q and 12 in cultured human embryonic stem cells. *Nat Biotechnol* 2004;22: 53–4.

Eckert D, Biermann K, Nettersheim D, et al. Expression of BLIMP1/PRMT5 and concurrent histone H2A/H4 arginine 3 dimethylation in fetal germ cells, CIS/IGCNU and germ cell tumors. *BMC Dev Biol* 2008;8: 106.

Einhorn LH. Chemotherapeutic and surgical strategies for germ cell tumors. *Chest Surg Clin N Am* 2002;12: 695–706.

Feldman DR, Bosl GJ, Sheinfeld J, Motzer RJ. Medical treatment of advanced testicular cancer. *JAMA* 2008;299: 672–84.

Fisher JS, Macpherson S, Marchetti N, Sharpe RM. Human "testicular dysgenesis syndrome": a possible model using in-utero exposure of the rat to dibutyl phthalate. *Hum Reprod* 2003;18: 1383–94.

Fosså SD, Aass N, Harvei S, Tretli S. Increased mortality rates in young and middle-aged patients with malignant germ cell tumours. *Br J Cancer* 2004;90: 607–12.

Foster PM, Mylchreest E, Gaido KW, Sar M. Effects of phthalate esters on the developing reproductive tract of male rats. *Hum Reprod Update* 2001;7: 231–5.

Fujimoto T, Miyayama Y, Fuyuta M. The origin, migration and fine morphology of human primordial germ cells. *Anat Rec* 1977;188: 315–30.

Hajkova P, Erhardt S, Lane N, et al. Epigenetic reprogramming in mouse primordial germ cells. *Mech Dev* 2002;117: 15–23.

Hajkova P, Ancelin K, Waldmann T, et al. Chromatin dynamics during epigenetic reprogramming in the mouse germ line. *Nature* 2008;452: 877–81.

Hardell L, van Bavel B, Lindström G, et al. Increased concentrations of polychlorinated biphenyls, hexachlorobenzene, and chlordanes in mothers of men with testicular cancer. *Environ Health Perspect* 2003;111: 930–4.

Hemminki K, Li X. Cancer risks in childhood and adolescence among the offspring of immigrants to Sweden. *Br J Cancer* 2002a;86: 1414–8.

Hemminki K, Li X. Cancer risks in second-generation immigrants to Sweden. *Int J Cancer* 2002b;99: 229–37.

Hemminki K, Li X, Czene K. Cancer risks in first-generation immigrants to Sweden. *Int J Cancer* 2002;99: 218–28.

Higuchi TT, Palmer JS, Gray LE Jr, Veeramachaneni DN. Effects of dibutyl phthalate in male rabbits following in utero, adolescent, or postpubertal exposure. *Toxicol Sci* 2003;72: 301–13.

Hoei-Hansen CE, Holm M, Rajpert-De Meyts E, Skakkebaek NE. Histological evidence of testicular dysgenesis in contralateral biopsies from 218 patients with testicular germ cell cancer. *J Pathol* 2003;200: 370–4.

Hoei-Hansen CE, Nielsen JE, Almstrup K, et al. Transcription factor AP-2gamma is a developmentally regulated marker of testicular carcinoma in situ and germ cell tumors. *Clin Cancer Res* 2004;10: 8521–30.

Hoei-Hansen CE, Almstrup K, Nielsen JE, et al. Stem cell pluripotency factor NANOG is expressed in human fetal gonocytes, testicular carcinoma in situ and germ cell tumours. *Histopathology* 2005;47: 48–56.

Huyghe E, Matsuda T, Thonneau P. Increasing incidence of testicular cancer worldwide: a review. *J Urol* 2003;170: 5–11.

Isidor B, Capito C, Paris F, et al. Familial frameshift SRY mutation inherited from a mosaic father with testicular dysgenesis syndrome. *J Clin Endocrinol Metab* 2009;94: 3467–71.

Koopman P. The delicate balance between male and female sex determining pathways: potential for disruption of early steps in sexual development. *Int J Androl* 2010;33: 252–8.

Li JY, Lees-Murdock DJ, Xu GL, Walsh CP. Timing of establishment of paternal methylation imprints in the mouse. *Genomics* 2004;84: 952–60.

Looijenga LH, Stoop H, de Leeuw HP, et al. POU5F1 (OCT3/4) identifies cells with pluripotent potential in human germ cell tumors. *Cancer Res* 2003;63: 2244–50.

Mahood IK, Hallmark N, McKinnell C, Walker M, Fisher JS, Sharpe RM. Abnormal Leydig Cell aggregation in the fetal testis of rats exposed to di (n-butyl) phthalate and its possible role in testicular dysgenesis. *Endocrinology* 2005;146: 613–23.

Mancini M, Carmignani L, Gazzano G, et al. High prevalence of testicular cancer in azoospermic men without spermatogenesis. *Hum Reprod* 2007;22: 1042–6.

Moul JW, Schanne FJ, Thompson IM, et al. Testicular cancer in blacks. A multicenter experience. *Cancer* 1994;73: 388–93.

Netto GJ, Nakai Y, Nakayama M, et al. Global DNA hypomethylation in intratubular germ cell neoplasia and seminoma, but not in nonseminomatous male germ cell tumors. *Mod Pathol* 2008;21: 1337–44.

Nielsen H, Nielsen M, Skakkebaek NE. The fine structure of possible carcinoma-in-situ in the seminiferous tubules in the testis of four infertile men. *Acta Pathol Microbiol Scand A* 1974; 82: 235–48.

Norris DP, Patel D, Kay GF, et al. Evidence that random and imprinted Xist expression is controlled by preemptive methylation. *Cell* 1994;77: 41–51.

Ohinata Y, Payer B, O'Carroll D, et al. Blimp1 is a critical determinant of the germ cell lineage in mice. *Nature* 2005;436: 207–13.

Oosterhuis JW, Castedo SM, de Jong B, et al. Ploidy of primary germ cell tumors of the testis. Pathogenetic and clinical relevance. *Lab Invest* 1989;60: 14–21.

Ottesen AM, Skakkebaek NE, Lundsteen C, Leffers H, Larsen J, Rajpert-De Meyts E. High-resolution comparative genomic hybridization detects extra chromosome arm 12p material in most cases of carcinoma in situ adjacent to overt germ cell tumors, but not before the invasive tumor development. *Genes Chromosomes Cancer* 2003;38: 117–25.

Peckham MJ, Barrett A, Liew KH, et al. The treatment of metastatic germ-cell testicular tumours with bleomycin, etoposide and cis-platin (BEP). *Br J Cancer* 1983;47: 613–9.

Perrett RM, Turnpenny L, Eckert JJ, et al. The early human germ cell lineage does not express SOX2 during in vivo development or upon in vitro culture. *Biol Reprod* 2008;78: 852–8.

Rajpert-De Meyts E, Bartkova J, Samson M, et al. The emerging phenotype of the testicular carcinoma in situ germ cell. *APMIS* 2003;111: 267–78; discussion 278–9.

Rajpert-De Meyts E. Developmental model for the pathogenesis of testicular carcinoma in situ: genetic and environmental aspects. *Hum Reprod Update* 2006;12: 303–23.

Reik W, Walter J. Genomic imprinting: parental influence on the genome. *Nat Rev Genet* 2001;2: 21–32.

Rosenberg C, Van Gurp RJ, Geelen E, Oosterhuis JW, Looijenga LH. Overrepresentation of the short arm of chromosome 12 is related to invasive growth of human testicular seminomas and nonseminomas. *Oncogene* 2000;19: 5858–62.

Seki Y, Hayashi K, Itoh K, Mizugaki M, Saitou M, Matsui Y. Extensive and orderly reprogramming of genome-wide chromatin modifications associated with specification and early development of germ cells in mice. *Dev Biol* 2005;278: 440–58.

Seki Y, Yamaji M, Yabuta Y, etal. Cellular dynamics associated with the genome-wide epigenetic reprogramming in migrating primordial germ cells in mice. *Development* 2007;134: 2627–38.

Skakkebaek NE. Possible carcinoma-in-situ of the testis. *Lancet* 1972;2: 516–7.

Skakkebaek NE, Berthelsen JG, Giwercman A, Müller J. Carcinoma-in-situ of the testis: possible origin from gonocytes and precursor of all types of germ cell tumours except spermatocytoma. *Int J Androl* 1987;10: 19–28.

Skakkebaek NE, Rajpert-De Meyts E, Main KM. Testicular dysgenesis syndrome: an increasingly common developmental disorder with environmental aspects. *Human Reproduction* 2001;16: 972–8.

Skakkebaek NE, Holm M, Hoei-Hansen C, Jorgensen N, Rajpert-De Meyts E. Association between testicular dysgenesis syndrome (TDS) and testicular neoplasia: Evidence from 20 adult patients with signs of maldevelopment of the testis. *APMIS* 2003;111: 1–11.

Skakkebaek NE, Rajpert-De Meyts E, Jørgensen N, et al. Testicular cancer trends as 'whistle blowers' of testicular developmental problems in populations. *Int J Androl* 2007;30: 198–204; discussion 204–5.

Skotheim RI, Lind GE, Monni O, et al. Differentiation of human embryonal carcinomas in vitro and in vivo reveals expression profiles relevant to normal development. *Cancer Res* 2005;65: 5588–98.

Smiraglia DJ, Szymanska J, Kraggerud SM, Lothe RA, Peltomäki P, Plass C. Distinct epigenetic phenotypes in seminomatous and nonseminomatous testicular germ cell tumors. *Oncogene* 2002;21: 3909–16.

Sonne SB, Almstrup K, Dalgaard M, et al. Analysis of Gene Expression Profiles of Microdissected Cell Populations Indicates that Testicular Carcinoma In situ Is an Arrested Gonocyte. *Cancer Res* 2009;69: 5241–50.

Sperger JM, Chen X, Draper JS, et al. Gene expression patterns in human embryonic stem cells and human pluripotent germ cell tumors. *Proc Natl Acad Sci USA* 2003;100: 13350–5.

Tachibana M, Matsumura Y, Fukuda M, Kimura H, Shinkai Y. G9a/GLP complexes independently mediate H3K9 and DNA methylation to silence transcription. *EMBO J* 2008;27: 2681–90.

Ulbright TM, Amin MB, Young RH. *Atlas of Tumor Pathology. Tumors of the Testis, Adnexa, Spermatic Cord, and Scrotum.* Washington DC: Armed Forces Institute of Pathology; 1999.

Walsh TJ, Croughan MS, Schembri M, Chan JM, Turek PJ. Increased risk of testicular germ cell cancer among infertile men. *Arch Intern Med* 2009;169: 351–6.

Wood HM, Elder JS. Cryptorchidism and testicular cancer: separating fact from fiction. *J Urol* 2009;181: 452–61.

Xie W, Han S, Khan M, DeJong J. Regulation of ALF gene expression in somatic and male germ line tissues involves partial and site-specific patterns of methylation. *J Biol Chem* 2002;277: 17765–74.

Yabuta Y, Kurimoto K, Ohinata Y, Seki Y, Saitou M. Gene expression dynamics during germline specification in mice identified by quantitative single-cell gene expression profiling. *Biol Reprod* 2006;75: 705–16.

19 Epigenetic adaptation during early life

Moshe Szyf

Adaptation of the genome through sequence alterations to changing environments is a slow process that requires selection. However, the DNA molecule itself bears an additional level of information: the pattern of distribution of methyl groups that are covalently bound to cytosine bases in DNA. DNA methylation is an important regulator of gene function and serves as part of the mechanism that allows one genome to express multiple phenotypes in a multicellular organism. DNA methylation was originally proposed to serve as a marker of cellular identity that was generated during cellular differentiation. Recent data that will be discussed here supports the hypothesis that DNA methylation is a reversible biological signal and could therefore potentially serve in genome adaptation beyond cellular differentiation. DNA methylation is proposed to act as a genomic response to both physical and social signals from the environment at different time points in life and to serve as a genomic memory of these exposures at different time scales, stably altering gene expression programming and thus modulating the physical and behavioral phenotypes to respond to these environments.

19.1 DNA methylation patterns and cellular identity

DNA from bacteria to humans contains in addition to the 4 bases that are replicated by strict Watson and Crick rules modified bases such as 5-methylcytosine, 6-methyladenine and 5-hydroxymethylcytosine. A two-step process generates these modified bases. First, the DNA is copied and in the second step enzymes termed DNA methyltransferases (DNMT) catalyze the transfer of methyl moieties to cytosines or adenines bases in DNA from the donor molecule S-adenosylmethionine (Adams, 1995; Bestor and Verdine, 1994). DNA methyltransferases exhibit different levels of specificity for the sequence context and this creates information in the DNA molecule. In vertebrates, the most commonly methylated cytosine is found in the CG dinucleotide (Gruenbaum et al., 1981; Gruenbaum et al., 1982). In bacteria species-specific DNA methylation patterns serve to differentiate self versus non-self and protect the bacteria from bacteriophage and foreign DNA invasion by restricting it with DNA methylation resistant enzymes. What makes DNA methylation a unique set of information in multicellular organisms, particularly vertebrates, is the fact that it is differentially methylated in different cell types. DNA methylation was therefore proposed to confer cellular identity to the genome and thus explain the mystery of how could one genome encode multiple phenotypes in a multicellular organism as predicted by Waddington (Waddington, 1959).

In contrast to the situation in unicellular bacteria where the DNA methylation pattern is strictly sequence specific, the presence of a differential methylation patterns in different cell types in the same organism bearing the same genome implies that during embryogenesis, this pattern is differentially carved and sculpted (Razin and Riggs, 1980). Since cellular differentiation is extremely tight and highly conserved across individuals it implies that an innate process that is highly conserved across individuals generates DNA methylation patterns. As differentiation has been believed to be terminal, the DNA methylation pattern was believed to be terminal as well. It has been therefore the belief that DNA methylation patterns once generated are strictly conserved during the entire life course.

Two principles were believed to be responsible for the faithful maintenance of the DNA methylation patterns throughout life. First, DNA methylation patterns are faithfully copied during cell division by a semiconservative maintenance DNA methyltransferase DNMT1. The CG dinucleotide sequence is a principal target of DNA methylation (Gruenbaum et al., 1981) since it is preferentially recognized by vertebrate DNA methyltransferases (Gruenbaum et al., 1982). CG is the only dinucleotide sequence that contains a cytosine that is a palindrome and could be copied during cell division by a semiconservative DNA methyltransferase from the parental strand onto the daughter strand (Razin and Riggs, 1980). It was shown that DNMT1 prefers hemimethylated substrates that are generated during cell division when a methylated CG on the parental strand is replicated. Restricting DNA methylation to CG dinucleotides is essential for the heritability of the DNA methylation mark. Second, it was believed that no de novo methyltransferases or demethylases are present in cells after cellular differentiation is completed thus the pattern could be copied accurately but not altered (▶Fig. 19.1).

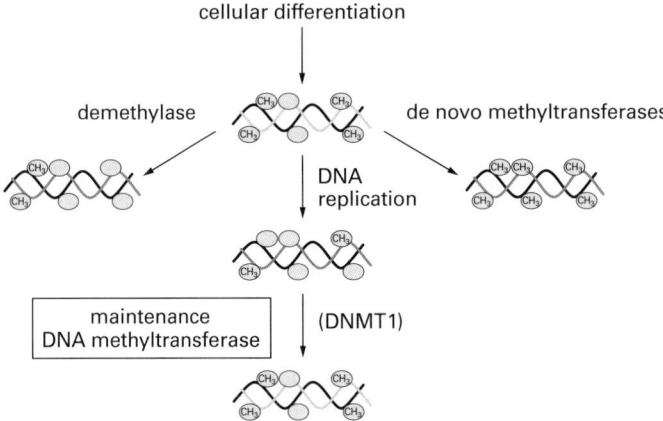

Fig. 19.1: Maintenance of DNA methylation pattern in somatic cells. It has been generally believed that in somatic cells the DNA methylation pattern is faithfully preserved because it is copied from the parental strand to the daughter strand by the semi-conservative DNA methyltransferase 1 (DNMT1). De novo methyltransferases that add methyl groups to new sites or demethylase activities that remove methyl groups from DNA were believed to be absent in somatic cells. Recent data suggest that de novo methylation and demethylase activity are present in postmitotic fully differentiated cells such as neurons.

19.2 Early life environment and DNA methylation

The DOHAD hypothesis claims that the origin of late onset disease is in events that occur early in life and program gene expression in a manner that increases susceptibility to disease later in life (Hanson and Gluckman, 2008). Although the classic model of DNA methylation postulated high fidelity of maintenance DNA methylation, stochastic changes in DNA methylation could still occur during gestation when the embryo is exposed to chemicals that interfere with DNA methylation enzymes during the critical time when these patterns are generated. Such stochastic changes could possibly result in altered gene expression leading to susceptibility to disease (Sinclair et al., 2007). Examples are nutritional restriction during pregnancy (Unterberger et al., 2009) and low folic acid/vitamin B12 diets during the periconception period (Bistulfi et al., 2010; Herbert, 1986). An elegant illustration of how the dietary environment affects the supply of methyl donors and alters DNA methylation in the embryo resulting in changes in the coat color phenotype of the offspring comes from Randy Jirtle's work with the Agouti mouse model (Dolinoy et al., 2007a; Dolinoy et al., 2007b; Jirtle and Skinner, 2007; Waterland and Jirtle, 2003). Stochastic drifts in DNA methylation patterns could occur in sperm DNA (Flanagan et al., 2006) and some of these that escape erasure could be maintained and propagated in the embryo and result in polymorphisms in DNA methylation pattern that might affect gene expression and the phenotype.

19.3 Reversibility of DNA methylation; adaptive responsivity of the methylome

The big question is whether the involvement of DNA methylation in adult disease is a result of accidental stochastic drift as predicted by the classic and well-accepted models of DNA methylation or whether these differences in DNA methylation reflect an adaptive response of the methylome (genome wide DNA methylation pattern) to the environment. Moreover, the postnatal nutritional and social environment is critical for health trajectories later in life. An attractive hypothesis is that DNA methylation could adapt to changing environments by a truly physiologically adaptive response rather than a collection of accidents. If DNA methylation is adaptive to the environment it must be dynamic after birth and in postmitotic tissues as well. For DNA methylation to function as a biological signal that is responsive to the environment it must be reversible (Ramchandani et al., 1999). However the general focus in the field was on DNA methyltransferases since it was believed that true active demethylation is energetically unfeasible. The great mystery in the field is the identity of the enzymatic processes that reverse the DNA methylation reaction.

We have previously shown that DNA demethylation could be induced using drugs that inhibit histone deacetylation and increase histone acetylation in a replication independent manner (Cervoni and Szyf, 2001; Szyf et al., 1985). Since these agents are not demethylating the DNA, these results imply that there must be enzymatic processes that remove methyl groups from DNA that are facilitated by increased histone acetylation. The most remarkable observations illustrating dynamic methylation-demethylation come from the brain where several studies have already shown demethylation in postmitotic neurons (Feng et al., 2010; Levenson et al., 2006; Miller et al., 2007; Weaver et al., 2004). Conditional knock out of DNMT1 in postmitotic neurons results in DNA demethylation (Feng et al., 2010).

The main open question is mechanism. The most widely accepted mechanisms for active DNA demethylation involve DNA repair and replacement of the methylated cytosine nucleotide by an unmethylated cytosine nucleotide. One possible mechanism is removal of the methylated cytosine by a glycosylase activity, the abasic site is then repaired and replaced with an unmethylated cytosine (Razin et al., 1986). A study proposed that DNMTs participate in demethylation by deaminating the methyl cytosine to thymidine creating a C/T mismatch repair, which is then corrected by a mismatch-repair mechanism (Kangaspeska et al., 2008). DNMTs were previously shown to deaminate 5-methylcytosines (Shen et al., 1992; Zingg et al., 1998) under conditions of low SAM. Growth arrest and DNA-damage-inducible protein 45 alpha (GADD45A), a DNA repair protein was proposed to participate in catalysis of active DNA demethylation by an unknown DNA repair based mechanism (Barreto et al., 2007). However, this was disputed (Jin et al., 2008). A very recent study suggested that demethylation in zebra fish embryos involves a complex sequence of coupled enzymatic reactions; activation-induced cytidine deaminase (AID, which converts 5-meC to thymine) and a G:T mismatch-specific thymine glycosylase methyl-CpG binding domain protein 4 (MBD4) and repair promoted by GADD45A (Rai et al., 2008). AID has been implicated in the global demethylation in mouse primordial germ cells (Popp et al., 2010).

In contrast to these repair based mechanisms we have previously proposed that demethylation is truly a reversible reaction that involves removal of the methyl moiety rather than breaking the DNA and fixing it with an unmethylated cytosine (Ramchandani et al., 1999). We proposed that the methylated DNA binding protein MBD2 was a bona fide demethylase that removed methyl groups from DNA and truly reversed the DNA methylation reaction. This is to date the only described bona fide demethylase. MBD2 has been implicated in the activation of both methylated and unmethylated genes (Angrisano et al., 2006; Fujita et al., 2003). Several groups (Ng et al., 1999; Wade et al., 1999) have contested the demethylase and transcriptional activating properties of MBD2. Studies by Detich et al. have demonstrated, however, MBD2 demethylase activity in vitro (Detich et al., 2002). Hamm et al. (2008) have proposed an oxidative mechanism of 5-cytosine DNA demethylation by MBD2. According to this mechanism, oxidation of the methyl moiety generates 5-hydroxymethylcytosine by oxidation, which is followed by release of the methyl residue in formaldehyde. Interestingly, 5-hydroxymethylcytosine was recently discovered in mammalian DNA (Pelizzola et al., 2008). A recent study has shown that TET1, an enzyme that converts methylcytosine to hydroxymethylcytosine, is required for maintaining the demethylated state of nanog in mouse ES cells supporting a possible role for TET1 and 5-hydroxymethylcysoine as an intermediary in the demethylation reaction (Ito et al., 2010). In summary, although there is no agreement as of yet on the mechanism of DNA demethylation, the presence of active demethylation in somatic cells is widely acknowledged (▶Fig. 19.2).

The fact that DNA methylation is reversible allows us to postulate that it could function as a mechanism for genome adaptation to the environment (▶Fig. 19.3). It is possible that in addition to the well-established role of DNA methylation in conferring cellular identity to the same genome, DNA methylation provides "environmental exposure" identity to similar genomes. Whereas cell type differential DNA methylation

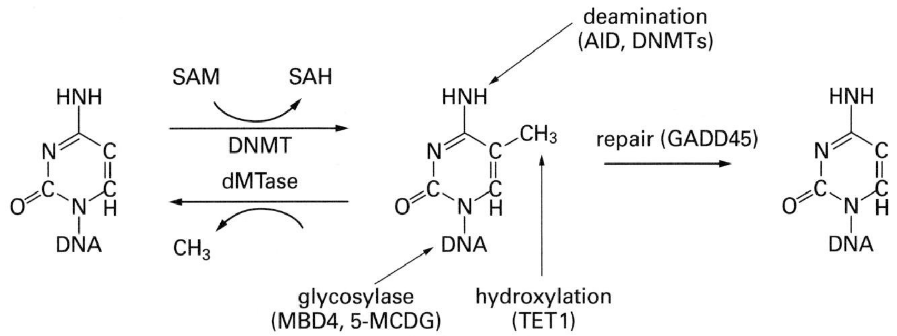

Fig. 19.2: The DNA methylation equilibrium and mechanisms of demethylation of DNA. DNA is methylated by a transfer of a methyl moiety from the methyl donor S-adenosyl-L-methionine (SAM) to the 5′ position on a cytosine ring by DNA methyltransferases (DNMT) releasing S-adenosyl-homocysteine (SAH). Several demethylation reactions were suggested. Direct demethylation by a demethylase enzyme (dMTase) would release a methyl moiety (CH3) in the form of either methanol or formaldehyde reversing the DNA methylation reaction. Alternatively, the methyl cytosine ring could be modified by either deamination catalyzed for example by AID or by the DNA methyltransferases (DNMT) which were shown to catalyze deamination of 5-methylcytidine in the absence of SAM or hydroxylation of the methyl moiety catalyzed by TET1. The modified base is then excised and repaired. Alternatively, the bond between the sugar and the base is cleaved (by glycosylases such as MBD4 or 5-methylcytosine glycosylase 5-MCDG) followed by repair. Repair proteins were shown to be associated with demethylation. An example is GADD45 (a and b).

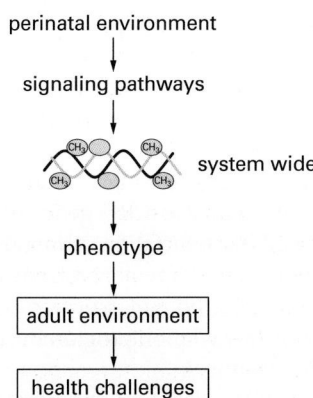

Fig. 19.3: Genome adaptation by DNA methylation in response to the perinatal environment; a model. Signals from the perinatal environment act on cellular signaling pathways in the brain, immune system and other tissues to modulate DNA methylation and thus stably adapt gene expression and the phenotype system-wide to the anticipated life-long environment. When there is a misfit between the anticipated environment during the perinatal period and the real environment during adulthood the methylation pattern programming becomes maladaptive and would lead to health challenges.

patterns enable the same genome express multiple phenotypes in the same individuals, environmental methylome programming would allow similar genomes express different phenotypes in different individuals that bear otherwise similar genes. Whereas innate processes that are highly conserved must define the origination of differential DNA methylation patterns during development, modulation of these patterns in response to environmental cues requires dynamic DNA methylation machinery.

19.4 Adaptation of the methylome early in life

We propose that DNA methylation serves as an adaptive mechanism of the genome to changing environments. Although stochastic polymorphisms in DNA methylation might in certain instances result in late onset disease (Feinberg and Irizarry, 2010), we propose that the response of the methylome to the environment is fundamentally a physiological response that is driven by signaling pathways. If indeed changes in DNA methylation are a physiological response to the environment, it has immediate implications on the frequency of such responses in the population and therefore on the size of the population that needs to be examined to unravel informative DNA methylation studies. Stochastic polymorphisms in DNA methylation such as genetic polymorphisms will clearly require larger numbers than physiological responses. Although the evidence for such a "DNA methylation adaptive" mechanism is still sparse, there is emerging evidence for programming of behavior and metabolic state by early life environment in rodents and association studies in humans.

The most widely accepted definitions of "epigenetics" include heritability either mitotically or meiotically as a basic component. However, if indeed DNA methylation is dynamic in non-dividing cells then DNA methylation could potentially act at different time scales from rapid transient time scales (Kangaspeska et al., 2008; Métivier et al., 2008) to evolutionary time scales. Long-term adaptations in DNA methylation do not necessarily require mitotic stability. DNA methylation changes could occur in postmitotic cells such as neurons early in life and affect the life-long phenotype. These DNA methylation responses should not be limited to early-life. An interesting example of a DNA methylation change occurring in postmitotic neurons in adult rodents that has a long-term impact was recently reported; exposure of adult mice to chronic social stress induced demethylation of the corticotropin release factor (CRF) gene (Elliott et al., 2010). We will focus here on examples of life-long DNA methylation "adaptations" that occur early in life in response to exposure to the social environment and have a life-long impact on the phenotype. These sparse but nevertheless thought-provoking examples could serve as a model for exploring the role of DNA methylation programming early in life in other late-onset disease including metabolic disorders.

The overall hypothesis that is proposed here is that the perinatal and postnatal early life environments which include the physical sphere, the biosphere and the social sphere modulate the methylome system-wide to adapt genome functions to the anticipated life long environments. Any misfit between the anticipated and the real environments could turn this DNA methylation pattern from adaptive to "maladaptive" leading to health disorders. There are a few examples from rodents, primates and humans that are consistent with this hypothesis.

19.5 Epigenetic programming by maternal care in the rat

There are several models that measure the impact of the early life social environment on behavior and other health phenotypes later in life. Models of maternal deprivation in primates and rodents and natural variation in maternal care in rodents were used to demonstrate the profound impact of maternal care and "nurture" on a panel of phenotypes in the offspring that last into adulthood (Ruppenthal et al., 1976; Suomi et al., 1976).

In rodents a model of natural variation in maternal care was originally used to study the impact of maternal care on stress behavior and stress responsivity in the offspring. The major response mediating adaptation to stress is activation of the hypothalamic-pituitary-adrenal axis (HPA), with stimulation of corticotropin releasing factor (CRF) and vasopressin (VP) from parvocellular neurons of the hypothalamic paraventricular nucleus, stimulating pituitary ACTH secretion, which in turn triggers glucocorticoid secretion from the adrenal cortex. Hippocampal glucocorticoid receptor controls the negative feedback of the axis by glucocorticoids thus attenuating the stress response. In the rat, the adult offspring of mothers that exhibit increased levels of pup licking/grooming (i.e., high LG mothers) over the first week of life show increased hippocampal (GR) expression, enhanced glucocorticoid feedback sensitivity, decreased hypothalamic CRF expression and more modest HPA stress responses compared to animals reared by low LG mothers (Francis et al., 1999; Liu et al., 1997). A genetic explanation was ruled out by cross-fostering studies that demonstrated that the behavior of the fostering mother and not the genetic mother defined the stress responsivity of the offspring (Francis et al., 1999; Liu et al., 1997). We therefore tested the possibility that maternal behavior resulted in differential DNA methylation in the offspring hippocampus that mediated the change in the phenotype in response to the environment. Differences in DNA methylation and histone acetylation in the regulatory regions of the glucocorticoid receptor (GR exon 17 promoter) gene were observed in the hippocampus of the offspring of high and low LG mothers early in life and remained stable into adulthood (Weaver et al., 2004).

The implications of this early study are supported by recent studies in other models of early life social adversity. Exposure of infant rats to stressed caretakers that displayed abusive behaviour produced persisting changes in methylation of BDNF gene promoter in the adult prefrontal cortex (Roth et al., 2009). Early-life stress (ELS) in mice caused sustained DNA hypomethylation of an important regulatory region of the arginine vasopressin (AVP) gene (Murgatroyd et al., 2009). Interestingly, stressful environments such as chronic social stress could induce stable DNA methylation changes in adult mice as well (Elliott et al., 2010). This further illustrates that the brain has life-long mechanisms to adapt to changing social environments. This has implications on the possibility of therapeutics by either pharmacological or behavioral interventions aiming at altering adverse DNA methylation patterns later in life. Thus, although epidemiological and animal data suggests that the early life environment is critical, and there might be critical windows for DNA methylation programming early in life, these results suggest that the methylome continues to be responsive to stressful signals throughout life and that theses alter DNA methylation as well as the phenotype.

19.6 Signaling cascades leading from maternal care to epigenetic programming

An important question that remains to be answered is what are the mechanisms that link exposure to an environmental exposure early in life to a persistent differential DNA methylation in one or several tissues. A reasonable hypothesis is that exposure to environmental cues results in firing of a signaling cascade that activates transacting factors that deliver DNA and chromatin modifying enzymes to specific regulatory sequences of genes. Evidence for such a mechanism comes from the rat maternal care model. Maternal behavior triggers a signaling pathway that involves the serotonin receptor, increase in cAMP, recruitment of the transcription factor nerve growth factor-induced protein A (NGFI-A), (Weaver et al., 2007) which in turn recruits the histone acetyltransferase CBP, and the methylated DNA binding protein and candidate DNA demethylase MBD2 to the GR promoter unpublished data. Our hypothesis is that the increased histone acetylation triggered by CREB binding protein (CBP) or by other recruited histone acetyltransferases (HATs) facilitates the demethylation of the gene by MBD2 or other DNA demethylases (unpublished data). These data chart a possible conduit through which exposure to a social behavior such as maternal behavior results in epigenetic modification of a specific gene in the brain. Although it is certain that there are other molecular pathways that link social exposure and changes in DNA methylation, in particular positions in the genome, this example provides evidence for the feasibility of transducing a social signal into a DNA methylation mark. Similar mechanism can transduce other critical environmental exposures such as nutritional or oxygen restriction.

A different signaling cascade linking social exposure to DNA demethylation was proposed more recently to explain how early life stress results in persistent life-long hypomethylation of the arginine vasopressin (AVP) gene. The AVP promoter is methylated and bound by the methyl CpG binding protein MECP2. Depolarization of hypothalamic neurons triggers phosphorylation of MeCp2 at Ser438 by calcium dependent CamKII (calmodulin kinase II; Murgatroyd et al., 2009). This phosphorylation converts MeCp2 from a transcriptional silencer with high affinity to methylated DNA into a transcriptional activator with low affinity to methylated DNA that facilitates demethylation of the AVP gene (Zhou et al., 2006). The change in MeCp2 affinity to methylated DNA by phosphorylation in response to neuronal activation was shown before to facilitate demethylation of the BDNF promoter (Chen et al., 2003). This signaling pathway delineates a direct link between neuronal activation and the phosphorylation state of a protein interacting with methylated genes in the brain. Neuronal activation resulting in signaling through phosphorylation of proteins interacting with methylated DNA might be a general pathway that links social exposure and the activation of neurons.

19.7 Reversibility of early life DNA methylation programming by maternal care

The changes in DNA methylation in response to early life stress remain into adulthood and they could possibly explain how early life experience would shape the phenotype. However, since DNA methylation is potentially dynamic as discussed above the critical question is whether patterns of epigenetic modification programmed early in life are final states or whether they are potentially reversible. The idea that epigenetic states might be reversible even in adult brain as well as other tissues has immense implications on the potential for interventions to override the effects of early life adversity.

Our previous studies have shown that increasing histone acetylation using the HDAC inhibitor trichostatin A (TSA) facilitates replication-independent demethylation of non-replicating plasmid DNA in human cells (Cervoni and Szyf, 2001; Cervoni et al., 2002). This experiment demonstrated that human somatic cells contained the enzymatic machinery required to demethylate DNA in the absence of DNA replication and that it was possible to alter the DNA methylation pattern using pharmacological agents that change histone acetylation. We tested whether a similar strategy would reverse epigenetic states established through maternal care and whether they would reside in a change in the phenotype. Injection of the HDAC inhibitor TSA into the brains of adult offspring of low LG maternal care reversed the epigenetic programming of the GR exon 17 promoter and reestablished stress responsivity and open field behavior that was indistinguishable from the offspring of high LG maternal care (Cervoni and Szyf, 2001; Cervoni et al., 2002).

We have previously shown that it is possible to alter the state of methylation of a non-replicating plasmid in the opposite way by treating cells with the methyl donor SAM which inhibits the DNA demethylation reaction (Detich et al., 2003.). Injection of the amino acid methionine, the precursor of SAM, into the brains of adult offspring of high maternal LG resulted in increased DNA methylation and downregulation of GR as well as heightened stress responsivity and an open field behavior that was indistinguishable from the adult offspring of low maternal LG (Weaver et al., 2004; Weaver et al., 2005). These data suggest that both the methylating and demethylating enzyme are present in the adult neuron and are amenable to pharmacological modulation.

19.8 Epigenetic programming by early life events in humans

An extremely important question is whether the results in rodents could be translated to humans? We therefore took advantage of a well phenotyped – brain bank to address the question of whether early life adversity leaves its mark in the DNA methylation pattern of the adult human brain hippocampus.

The first study looked at the promoter of the ribosomal RNA (rRNA) genes. rRNA forms the skeleton of the ribosome, the protein synthesis machinery. Protein synthesis is essential for building new memories and creating new synapses in the brain. Our genome contains around 400 copies of the genes encoding rRNA. One possible way to control the protein synthesis capacity of a cell is through changing the fraction of active rRNA alleles in a cell (Brown and Szyf, 2007). We have previously shown that the fraction of rRNA genes that is active and is associated with the RNA Pol1 transcription machinery is unmethylated while the fraction that is inactive is methylated (Brown and Szyf, 2007). Our results showed that the suicide victims who experienced childhood abuse had higher overall methylation in their rRNA genes and expressed less rRNA. This difference in methylation was region specific: it was specific to the hippocampus and was not observed in the cerebellum. Moreover, although significant methylation differences were observed between the controls and the suicide victims, no sequence differences were observed. The fact that the difference in methylation was brain-region specific and that no sequence differences were observed further strengthens the conclusion that this difference in methylation is driven by an environmental rather than genetic variation (McGowan et al., 2008). RRNA genes are ubiquitously expressed and encode a ubiquitous function protein synthesis that seems to be an unlikely candidate to be affected by early-life adversity. However, protein synthesis is required for learning and memory in the brain. These data point to the possibility that the effects of early life adversity might not be limited to the usual suspects of highly tissue specific genes whose specific physiological function is well documented but that ubiquitously expressed genes might be involved as well.

In our second study, we examined whether epigenetic differences were driven by early childhood adversity or by other processes leading to suicide. We compared suicide completers who were abused as children to suicide completers who were not. This time we looked at the GR exon 1f promoter that is homologous to the promoter affected by maternal care in the rat. Individuals with treatment-resistant forms of major depression show decreased GR expression and increased HPA activity. Site-specific differences in DNA methylation in the GR exon 1f promoter between suicide completers who had reported social adversity early in life and suicide completers who did not experience social adversity early in life were detected. These differences in DNA methylation were associated with reduced expression of the GR gene. The site-specific methylation interfered with binding of the transcription factor NGFI-A to the human GR exon 1f promoter. Reporter-activity transfection assays indicated that this site-specific methylation inhibited GR promoter activity (McGowan et al., 2009). These data are a first demonstration that it is possible to identify the epigenetic imprints of early life exposure in the methylome in the adult brain. These epigenetic differences have functional consequences resulting in reduced expression of a key regulator of the HPA axis.

Recently, this line of studies was extended to peripheral blood cell; the GR promoter was more methylated in lymphocytes in newborns exposed prenatally to maternal depression than control newborns (Oberlander et al., 2008).

Epigenetic modulation of other candidate genes was implicated in suicide; the Gamma-aminobutyric acid A receptor alpha 1 subunit (GABRA1) promoter (Linthorst et al., 1995) within the frontopolar cortex (Poulter et al., 2008) and Tropomyosin-related kinase B (TRKB) in the frontal cortex of suicide completers (Ernst et al., 2009). It is unknown yet whether these changes in DNA are also associated with early life adversity.

19.9 Genome-wide and system-wide effects of early life adversity

The first studies examining DNA methylation in the brain focused on a few gene suspects that were very well known to mediate stress behavior as well as other dedicated brain functions. Most of our studies were biased toward the candidate gene approach assuming that phenotype associated with early life adversity would involve a few critical brain-specific genes. In addition, unsurprisingly the first line of studies examining the impact of early life adversity focused on specific brain regions. However, it is becoming clear that genes work in networks and that the total output of a network could be significantly affected by a combination of subtle changes in several nodes of a network. The fact that methylation differences in suicide victims were found in rRNA genes (McGowan et al., 2008) supports the idea that genes outside the usual brain specific suspects are involved. Preliminary data from our lab supports both the idea that changes in DNA methylation associated with early life adversity are genome-wide and that they are not limited to the brain.

We recently performed a detailed mapping of 6.5 megabases of DNA spanning the locus of the GR gene from both directions and identified numerous differences in DNA methylation between the suicide and the control groups. Recent high density-epigenome mapping of chromosome 18 in the adult rat offspring of high and low maternal care reveals broad differences in DNA methylation and histone acetylation that cover wide regions of chromosome 18. We also started looking at association between early life adversity and DNA methylation differences in white blood cells. Our unpublished data indicates associations between DNA methylation patterns in 45 year adults and social adversity early in life (Borghol et al., unpublished).

19.10 Prospects

DNA methylation is a stable mark that is part of the covalent structure of DNA. As such it is predicted to serve as a persistent epigenetic mark. On the other hand DNA methylation is laid down by enzymatic machinery that is potentially reversible. This bimodal nature of the methylome leaves us with important questions that are critical for both understanding how DNA methylation serves as a mediator of the link between perinatal environments and late-onset disease and how and when could we intervene to either protect or prevent the emergence of diseases driven by early life DNA methylation programming.

Are there critical periods for DNA methylation programming and if there are critical periods are they reversible later in life? A related question is whether the DNA methylation pattern continues to be responsive during adulthood and what is the relative contribution of the later-life exposures to the phenotype?

We propose that there are two time-scales of adaptations involving DNA methylation; those that occur in early life as well as life-long responses and that they have evolved to address different challenges of adaptation to the dynamic environment. There must be mechanisms that protect perinatal DNA methylation programming from environmental noise later in life and maintain it persistent during the life-course. This might imply that interventions should be preferably limited to this time zone. However, if mechanisms for DNA methylation changes during adulthood exist they could be harnessed for other interventional strategies later in life.

In any case the potential for DNA methylation changes later in life and during adulthood has important implications on the feasibility of either behavioral or pharmacological interventions to reverse the trajectories of late onset disease. The critical challenges that need to be addressed are to define the timing and nature of efficacious interventions.

References

Adams RL. Eukaryotic DNA methyltransferases – structure and function. *Bioessays* 1995;17: 139–45.

Angrisano T, Lembo F, Pero R, Natale F, Fusco A, Avvedimento VE, Bruni CB, Chiariotti L. TACC3 mediates the association of MBD2 with histone acetyltransferases and relieves transcriptional repression of methylated promoters. *Nucleic Acids Res* 2006;34: 364–72.

Barreto G, Schäfer A, Marhold J, Stach D, Swaminathan SK, Handa V, Döderlein G, Maltry N, Wu W, Lyko F, Niehrs C. Gadd45a promotes epigenetic gene activation by repair-mediated DNA demethylation. *Nature* 2007;445: 671–5.

Bestor TH, Verdine GL. DNA methyltransferases. *Curr Opin Cell Biol* 1994;6: 380–9.

Bistulfi G, Vandette E, Matsui S, Smiraglia DJ. Mild folate deficiency induces genetic and epigenetic instability and phenotype changes in prostate cancer cells. *BMC Biol* 2010;8: 6.

Brown SE, Szyf M. Epigenetic Programming of the rRNA promoter by MBD3. *Mol Cell Biol* 2007;27: 4938–52.

Chen WG, Chang Q, Lin Y, Meissner A, West AE, Griffith EC, Jaenisch R, Greenberg ME. Derepression of BDNF transcription involves calcium-dependent phosphorylation of MeCP2. *Science* 2003;302: 885–9.

Cervoni N, Szyf M. Demethylase activity is directed by histone acetylation. *J Biol Chem* 2001;276: 40778–87.

Cervoni N, Detich N, Seo SB, Chakravarti D, Szyf M. The oncoprotein Set/TAF-1beta, an inhibitor of histone acetyltransferase, inhibits active demethylation of DNA, integrating DNA methylation and transcriptional silencing. *J Biol Chem* 2002;277: 25026–31.

Detich N, Theberge J, Szyf M. Promoter-specific activation and demethylation by MBD2/demethylase. *J Biol Chem* 2002;277: 35791–4.

Detich N, Hamm S, Just G, Knox JD, Szyf M. The methyl donor S-Adenosylmethionine inhibits active demethylation of DNA: A candidate novel mechanism for the pharmacological effects of S-Adenosylmethionine. *J Biol Chem* 2003;278: 20812–20.

Dolinoy DC, Das R, Weidman JR, Jirtle RL. Metastable epialleles, imprinting, and the fetal origins of adult diseases. *Pediatr Res* 2007a;61: 30R-7R.

Dolinoy DC, Huang D, Jirtle RL. Maternal nutrient supplementation counteracts bisphenol A-induced DNA hypomethylation in early development. *Proc Natl Acad Sci U S A* 2007b;104: 13056–61.

Elliott E, Ezra-Nevo G, Regev L, Neufeld-Cohen A, Chen A. Resilience to social stress coincides with functional DNA methylation of the Crf gene in adult mice. *Nat Neurosci* 2010;13: 1351–3.

Ernst C, Deleva V, Deng X, Sequeira A, Pomarenski A, Klempan T, Ernst N, Quirion R, Gratton A, Szyf M, Turecki G. Alternative splicing, methylation state, and expression profile of tropomyosin-related kinase B in the frontal cortex of suicide completers. *Arch Gen Psychiatry* 2009;66: 22–32.

Feinberg AP, Irizarry RA. Evolution in health and medicine Sackler colloquium: Stochastic epigenetic variation as a driving force of development, evolutionary adaptation, and disease. *Proc Natl Acad Sci U S A* 2010;107: 1757–1764.

Feng J, Zhou Y, Campbell SL, Le T, Li E, Sweatt JD, Silva AJ, Fan G. Dnmt1 and Dnmt3a maintain DNA methylation and regulate synaptic function in adult forebrain neurons. *Nat Neurosci* 2010; 13: 423–30.

Flanagan JM, Popendikyte V, Pozdniakovaite N, Sobolev M, Assadzadeh A, Schumacher A, Zangeneh M, Lau L, Virtanen C, Wang SC, Petronis A. Intra- and interindividual epigenetic variation in human germ cells. *Am J Hum Genet* 2006;79: 67–84.

Francis D, Diorio J, Liu D, Meaney MJ. Nongenomic transmission across generations of maternal behavior and stress responses in the rat. *Science* 1999;286: 1155–8.

Fujita H, Fujii R, Aratani S, Amano T, Fukamizu A, Nakajima T. Antithetic effects of MBD2a on gene regulation. *Mol Cell Biol* 2003;23: 2645–2657.

Gruenbaum Y, Stein R, Cedar H, Razin A. Methylation of CpG sequences in eukaryotic DNA. *FEBS Lett* 1981;124: 67–71.

Gruenbaum Y, Cedar H, Razin A. Substrate and sequence specificity of a eukaryotic DNA methylase. *Nature* 1982;295: 620–2.

Hamm S, Just G, Lacoste N, Moitessier N, Szyf M, Mamer O. On the mechanism of demethylation of 5-methylcytosine in DNA. *Bioorg Med Chem Lett* 2008;18: 1046–1049.

Hanson MA, Gluckman PD. Developmental origins of health and disease: new insights. *Basic Clin Pharmacol Toxicol* 2008;102: 90–3.

Herbert V. The role of vitamin B12 and folate in carcinogenesis. *Adv Exp Med Biol* 1986;206: 293–311.

Ito S, D'Alessio AC, Taranova OV, Hong K, Sowers LC, Zhang Y. Role of Tet proteins in 5mC to 5hmC conversion, ES-cell self-renewal and inner cell mass specification. *Nature* 2010;466: 1129–33.

Jin SG, Guo C, Pfeifer GP. GADD45A does not promote DNA demethylation. *PLoS Genet* 2008;4: e1000013.

Jirtle RL, Skinner MK. Environmental epigenomics and disease susceptibility. *Nat Rev Genet* 2007;8: 253–62.

Kangaspeska S, Stride B, Métivier R, Polycarpou-Schwarz M, Ibberson D, Carmouche RP, Benes V, Gannon F, Reid G. Transient cyclical methylation of promoter DNA. *Nature* 2008;452: 112–5.

Levenson JM, Roth TL, Lubin FD, Miller CA, Huang IC, Desai P, Malone LM, Sweatt JD. Evidence that DNA (cytosine-5) methyltransferase regulates synaptic plasticity in the hippocampus. *J Biol Chem* 2006;281: 15763–73.

Linthorst AC, Flachskamm C, Muller-Preuss P, Holsboer F, Reul JM. Effect of bacterial endotoxin and interleukin-1 beta on hippocampal serotonergic neurotransmission, behavioral activity, and free corticosterone levels: an in vivo microdialysis study. *J Neurosci* 1995;15: 292034.

Liu D, Diorio J, Tannenbaum B, Caldji C, Francis D, Freedman A, Sharma S, Pearson D, Plotsky PM, Meaney MJ. Maternal care, hippocampal glucocorticoid receptors, and hypothalamic-pituitary-adrenal responses to stress. *Science* 1997;277: 1659–62.

McGowan PO, Sasaki A, Huang TC, Unterberger A, Suderman M, Ernst C, Meaney MJ, Turecki G, Szyf M. Promoter-wide hypermethylation of the ribosomal RNA gene promoter in the suicide brain. *PLoS ONE* 2008;3: e2085.

McGowan PO, Sasaki A, D'Alessio AC, Dymov S, Labonté B, Szyf M, Turecki G, Meaney MJ. Epigenetic regulation of the glucocorticoid receptor in human brain associates with childhood abuse. *Nat Neurosci* 2009;12: 342–8.

Métivier R, Gallais R, Tiffoche C, Le Péron C, Jurkowska RZ, Carmouche RP, Ibberson D, Barath P, Demay F, Reid G, Benes V, Jeltsch A, Gannon F, Salbert G. Cyclical DNA methylation of a transcriptionally active promoter. *Nature* 2008;452: 45–50.

Miller CA, Sweatt JD. Covalent modification of DNA regulates memory formation. *Neuron* 2007;53: 857–69.

Murgatroyd C, Patchev AV, Wu Y, Micale V, Bockmühl Y, Fischer D, Holsboer F, Wotjak CT, Almeida OF, Spengler D. Dynamic DNA methylation programs persistent adverse effects of early-life stress. *Nat Neurosci* 2009;12: 1559–66.

Ng HH, Zhang Y, Hendrich B, Johnson CA, Turner BM, Erdjument-Bromage H, Tempst P, Reinberg D, Bird A. MBD2 is a transcriptional repressor belonging to the MeCP1 histone deacetylase complex. *Nat Genet* 1999;23: 58–61.

Oberlander TF, Weinberg J, Papsdorf M, Grunau R, Misri S, Devlin AM. Prenatal exposure to maternal depression, neonatal methylation of human glucocorticoid receptor gene (NR3C1) and infant cortisol stress responses. *Epigenetics* 2008;3: 97–106.

Pelizzola M, Koga Y, Urban AE, Krauthammer M, Weissman S, Halaban R, Molinaro AM. MEDME: An experimental and analytical methodology for the estimation of DNA methylation levels based on microarray derived MeDIP-enrichment. *Genome Res* 2008;18: 1652–9.

Popp C, Dean W, Feng S, Cokus SJ, Andrews S, Pellegrini M, Jacobsen SE, Reik W. Genome-wide erasure of DNA methylation in mouse primordial germ cells is affected by AID deficiency. *Nature* 2010;463: 1101–5.

Poulter MO, Du L, Weaver IC, Palkovits M, Faludi G, Merali Z, Szyf M, Anisman H. GABAA receptor promoter hypermethylation in suicide brain: implications for the involvement of epigenetic processes. *Biol Psychiatry* 2008;64: 645–52.

Rai K, Huggins IJ, James SR, Karpf AR, Jones DA, Cairns BR. DNA demethylation in zebrafish involves the coupling of a deaminase, a glycosylase, and gadd45. *Cell* 2008;135: 1201–12.

Ramchandani S, Bhattacharya SK, Cervoni N, Szyf M. DNA methylation is a reversible biological signal. *Proc Natl Acad Sci U S A* 1999;96: 6107–12.

Razin A, Riggs AD. DNA methylation and gene function. *Science* 1980;210: 604–10.

Razin A, Szyf M, Kafri T, Roll M, Giloh H, et al. Replacement of 5-methylcytosine by cytosine: a possible mechanism for transient DNA demethylation during differentiation. *Proc Natl Acad Sci U S A* 1986;83: 2827–31.

Roth TL, Lubin FD, Funk AJ, Sweatt JD. Lasting epigenetic influence of early-life adversity on the BDNF gene. *Biol Psychiatry* 2009;65: 760–769.

Ruppenthal GC, Arling GL, Harlow HF, Sackett GP, Suomi SJ. A 10-year perspective of motherless-mother monkey behavior. *J Abnorm Psychol* 1976;85: 341–9.

Shen JC, Rideout WMd, Jones PA. High frequency mutagenesis by a DNA methyltransferase. *Cell* 1992;71: 1073–80.

Sinclair KD, Lea RG, Rees WD, Young LE. The developmental origins of health and disease: current theories and epigenetic mechanisms. *Soc Reprod Fertil Suppl* 2007;64: 425–43.

Suomi SJ, Collins ML, Harlow HF, Ruppenthal GC. Effects of maternal and peer separations on young monkeys. *J Child Psychol Psychiatry* 1976;17: 101–112.

Szyf M, Eliasson L, Mann V, Klein G, Razin A. Cellular and viral DNA hypomethylation associated with induction of Epstein-Barr virus lytic cycle. *Proc Natl Acad Sci U S A* 1985;82: 8090–4.

Unterberger A, Szyf M, Nathanielsz PW, Cox LA. Organ and gestational age effects of maternal nutrient restriction on global methylation in fetal baboons. *J Med Primatol* 2009;38: 219–27.

Waddington CH. Canalization of development and genetic assimilation of acquired characters. *Nature* 1959;183: 1654–5.

Wade PA, Gegonne A, Jones PL, Ballestar E, Aubry F, Wolffe AP. Mi-2 complex couples DNA methylation to chromatin remodelling and histone deacetylation. *Nat Genet* 1999;23: 62–6.

Waterland RA, Jirtle RL. Transposable elements: targets for early nutritional effects on epigenetic gene regulation. *Mol Cell Biol* 2003;23: 5293–300.

Weaver IC, Cervoni N, Champagne FA, D'Alessio AC, Sharma S, Seckl JR, Dymov S, Szyf M, Meaney MJ. Epigenetic programming by maternal behavior. *Nat Neurosci* 2004;7: 847–54.

Weaver IC, Champagne FA, Brown SE, Dymov S, Sharma S, Meaney MJ, Szyf M. Reversal of maternal programming of stress responses in adult offspring through methyl supplementation: altering epigenetic marking later in life. *J Neurosci* 2005;25: 11045–54.

Weaver IC, D'Alessio AC, Brown SE, Hellstrom IC, Dymov S, Sharma S, Szyf M, Meaney MJ. The transcription factor nerve growth factor-inducible protein a mediates epigenetic programming: altering epigenetic marks by immediate-early genes. *J Neurosci* 2007;27: 1756–68.

Zhou Z, Hong EJ, Cohen S, Zhao WN, Ho HY, Schmidt L, Chen WG, Lin Y, Savner E, Griffith EC, Hu L, Steen JA, Weitz CJ, Greenberg ME. Brain-specific phosphorylation of MeCP2 regulates activity-dependent Bdnf transcription, dendritic growth, and spine maturation. *Neuron* 2006;52: 255–69.

Zingg JM, Shen JC, Jones PA. Enzyme-mediated cytosine deamination by the bacterial methyltransferase M.MspI. *Biochem J* 1998;332: 223–30.

20 Toward a unifying concept on perinatal programming: *Vegetative imprinting* by environment-dependent biocybernetogenesis

Andreas Plagemann

Life is a process of permanent environment-dependent development. Developmental origins of health and disease are framed throughout life but are particularly sustainable if shaped during critical periods of early life. This fundamental principle has a long history, but it was hidden in a niche during the past decades of gene myopia in biomedicine. Fortunately, the field meanwhile prospers enormously, but there still seems to be a lack of a general, overall concept that fulfills practicable semantic purposes and covers the whole spectrum of phenomena and underlying mechanisms, appropriately.

Attempting a synthesizing, general concept and semantics it is proposed here that "adaptive, predictive responses" (APRs) during critical developmental periods in pre- and early postnatal life lead to a *perinatal programming* of affected life functions. In this concept, APRs are mechanistically realized by a passive epigenomic and/or microstructural conditioning of the organism, leading to a homeostatic calibration of functional and tolerance ranges at the subcellular, cellular, and up to the organismic level according to the environmental conditions experienced during critical developmental periods. This basic process of *biocybernetogenesis* in terms of a developmental vegetative *training* or *learning* serves to optimize the self-organization of an organism in order to cope with the environmental conditions and challenges throughout later life. Programming by APRs generally occurs normative as a basic mechanism of ontogenesis. By alterations of the pre- and neonatal environmental conditions it may become disadvantageous or even harmful for the long-term individual health and reproductive fitness, what should be called *malprogramming* due to *dysbiocybernetogenesis*. Programming or malprogramming, as basically acquired modes of function, can even pass through generations of the maternal line by offering the resultant (altered) homeostatic milieu by mothers (affected females) to the next generation *in utero*, and so on. Thereby, over generations all of this may even affect phylogenesis and, consequently, evolution.

The most important and sustainable effects of perinatal programming occur if the main regulatory instances of the organism are affected, that is, the genome and/or the brain. Indeed, exactly this has meanwhile been shown for all fundamental life functions (metabolism, growth, and body weight regulation; stress response; immunity and neuroendocrine-immune interaction; information processing and behavior; reproduction).

For instance, pre- and/or neonatal overfeeding (maternal diabetes/obesity, neonatal overfeeding/rapid neonatal weight gain) have been shown epidemiologically, clinically, and experimentally to induce epigenomic and microstructural malprogramming of the hypothalamo-adipo-pancreatic system, leading to long-term increased metabolic syndrome risk, which is then intergeneratively transmitted through the maternal line to subsequent generations but, most of all, is preventable by normalization of perinatal food supply.

In summary, environment-dependent biocybernetogenesis and perinatal programming are critical and essential parts of ontogenesis, affecting health and disease risks for the whole life span in terms of a basal, initial conditioning. In biomedicine, this opens enormous chances and challenges of a genuine prophylaxis to the benefit of individuals and societies.

20.1 Historical and semantic notes

During recent years, the traditional understanding of the origins of health and diseases is fundamentally changing. It is becoming clear that the interaction between genes and environmental factors is not a static, independent process. Rather, during critical developmental periods, an environment-dependent *conditioning* of the biological *hardware* occurs, especially during the fetal period and in the newborn. This early programming sustainably determines the long-term fate of an organism in terms of health and/or disease dispositions. The process has been introduced as *perinatal programming* and seems to be the most important developmental cause of diseases, beyond classical teratogenesis and aging processes (Plagemann, 2004, 2010). As this opens new possibilities of a primary prevention, it likely not only leads to fundamental paradigmatic changes in developmental biology and medicine but opens new chances and challenges for public health policies.

Important roots of the field were planted at the Charité in Berlin by the endocrinologist Günter Dörner, who already in the 1970s proposed hormone-dependent pre- and neonatal preprogramming of long-term disease risks and a respective concept of *functional teratogenesis* (Dörner, 1974a, 1974b, 1975). Already in 1974, published in 1975, at an international Neurobiology Conference in Chapel Hill, Dörner formulated the following:

> Experimental and clinical data suggest that homeostatic variables, such as hormones, metabolites and neurotransmitters, . . . during the critical organization phase of an organism are capable of "preprogramming" the responsiveness of their own central nervous controllers and hence the functional and tolerance ranges of their self-organizing systems.

By this proposal, for the first time a general, mechanistic principle on the long-term impact of environment-dependent *programming* during critical periods of early life was formulated, covering all elementary life functions.

Although this was a milestone, possibly even the natal hour of today's perinatal programming field, one should consider that the overall idea of developmental origins has a much longer history (▶Tab. 20.1). Considering the actual discussion on epigenetic inheritance, it is closely related to the concepts of Lamarck (1809) and Waddington (1942) and regarding the fundamental impact of the external and internal environment for early ontogenesis to the work and achievements of Saint-Hilaire (1837) and Haeckel (1866). Essential mechanistic contributions then came from Stockard (1921), Spemann (Spemann and Mangold, 1924), and Ashby (1947). Particularly influential were the observations by Konrad Lorenz (1935) on behavioral imprinting during critical periods of early life.

All of this pioneer work during the 19th century and first half of the 20th century found a conceptual and semantic continuation during the 1960s, initially by Werboff and

Tab. 20.1: Historical conceptual and semantic milestones in developmental biology, medicine, and perinatal programming.

Author(s), Year	Term or Concept
Lamarck, 1809	Inheritance of Acquired Conditions
Saint-Hilaire, 1837	Teratology (teratomorphogenesis)
Haeckel, 1866	Ecology
Stockard, 1921	Critical Period
Spemann, 1924	Organizer Effect in Embryogenesis
Lorenz, 1935	Behavioral Imprinting
Waddington, 1942	Epigenetics
Ashby, 1947	Principle of Biological Self-Organization
Werboff and Gottlieb, 1963	Behavioral Teratology
Dubos, 1966	Biological Freudianism
Dörner, 1974/1975	Pre- and Neonatal Preprogramming Functional Teratology
Burchfield, 1979	Predictive Adaptive Response
Freinkel, 1980	Fuel-mediated Teratogenesis
Lucas, 1991	Nutritional Programming
Hales and Barker, 1992	Thrifty Phenotype Hypothesis (small baby syndrome)
Gluckman and Hanson, 2004	Match–Mismatch Hypothesis

Gottlieb (1963), focusing on behavior, and Dubos, focusing on body weight regulation (Dubos, Savage, and Schaedler, 1966). It seems reasonable, however, to credit Dörner for having framed the concept in an overall, fundamental way. By introducing *functional teratology* he suggested a new, explanatory terminology, proposed hormone-mediated epigenetic organization by the environment as a general mechanism, addressed the whole spectrum of life functions, and drew far-reaching practical conclusions in terms of perinatal prevention (Dörner, 1974a, 1974b, 1975, 1976, 1980). Already in this context and at this time, gestational diabetes as a paradigm of prenatal mal- and overnutrition came into the focus of the field, especially by fuel-mediated teratogenesis introduced by Freinkel and Metzger (1979; Freinkel, 1980), as well as by the observation of "gestational diabetes as a perinatally acquired condition", described by the group of André van Assche (Aerts and Van Assche, 1979).

However, all of this was hidden in a niche until the early 1990s. Then, to the merit of epidemiologist David Barker and biochemist Nicholas Hales, the overall approach attracted more and more attention, and nowadays it belongs to the "hot topics" in developmental biology and medicine. In this regard, points of origin were and still are the observations and hypotheses of permanently increased disease dispositions in underweight newborns (Hales and Barker, 1992). Finally, the field gained a remarkable mechanistic and conceptual input by the "match–mismatch" hypothesis introduced by Gluckman and Hanson during recent years (▶Tab. 20.1). These authors postulated a general, even phylogenetically and evolutionary-orientated hypothesis regarding the observations of increased vulnerability for diseases of civilization after low birth weight or detrimental prenatal conditions (Gluckman and Hanson, 2006, 2008; Gluckman et al., 2008).

20.2 A main current focus: The "small baby syndrome" and the "match–mismatch" hypotheses

The *small baby syndrome* hypothesis was formulated by Hales and Barker (1992) against a background of studies that showed that individuals with a low birth weight had an increased risk of developing symptoms of the metabolic syndrome, type 2 diabetes, and cardiovascular diseases in later life. The respective *thrifty phenotype hypothesis* contains the following two premises: first, low birth weight is an indicator for maternal and subsequent fetal undernutrition, and second, phenotypical characteristics that lead to energy saving should be beneficial for the individual. Barker and Hales proposed that prenatal undernutrition induces decreased insulin secretion along with insulin resistance, which then stays for a lifetime and first goes along with decreased fetal growth. Also in later life, this *in utero* acquired phenotype should be "thrifty", thereby leading to a survival advantage under restrictive nutritional conditions. However, this advantage, as they state, turns into its opposite under conditions of abundance, as is the case in modern Western industrial societies, thus leading to the metabolic syndrome, type 2 diabetes, and cardiovascular diseases (Hales and Barker, 1992).

Later on, Gluckman and Hanson widened mainly the evolutionary aspect of the hypothesis, proclaiming a mechanistic impact of "predictive-adaptive responses" (Gluckman and Hanson, 2006, 2008; Gluckman et al., 2008), a semantic that formerly has been suggested in developmental psychology (Burchfield, 1979). Following Hanson and Gluckman, the fetus performs reactive adaptations to the intrauterine environment, for example, to prenatal undernutrition, the adaptive value of which is primarily not an immediate one, but would especially be realized in later life. Signals that trigger such fetal responses are claimed to be anticipatory predictors of the postnatal environment, in other words, of those conditions that will surround the individual after birth and confront him or her for a lifetime. If the *prediction* of the later environment is correct, then, according to Hanson and Gluckman, the respective adaptations lead to an advantage in survival and reproductive fitness. If incorrect, the adaptations would rather be disadvantageous, ultimately leading to disease dispositions. In this sense, Gluckman and Hanson generalized their hypothesis by proposing the *match–mismatch* theory. This theory, or the match–mismatch paradigm, says that a *mismatch* between prenatal developmental conditions and the environment in later life increases disease risks, while a *match* would be preventive because of beneficial adaptations to later life conditions (Gluckman and Hanson, 2004, 2006, 2008; Gluckman et al., 2008).

Already during the 1990s, we and others (Dörner and Plagemann, 1994; Lucas, Fewtrell, and Cole, 1999) raised objections against the original version of this theoretical framework, the thrifty phenotype hypothesis. In particular, we asked whether the empirical background of the hypotheses, that is, the underlying data, were analyzed and interpreted correctly.

Firstly, most of the studies that investigated the small baby syndrome hypothesis did not or not adequately consider the potential role of confounders and/or media-tors in the association between low birth weight and later diseases (Plagemann and Harder, 2005a). In most of the studies, nearly without exception, no adjustments for confounders were made, such as, for example, gestational age, parental body weights, and maternal diseases during pregnancy. By using absolute cut-offs for low birth weight (e. g., < 2,500g), differences resulting from ethnic origin were often neglected. The same applies to differences resulting from body composition, while it became clear that even low birth weight babies' risk may result from increased fatness (Yajnik et al., 2003). Finally, the potential role of neonatal overnutrition in underweight newborns, which appears very probable, was not considered (Plagemann and Harder, 2005a; Plagemann, Rodekamp, and Harder, 2004).

One main problem thus results from the fact that obesity is the decisive risk factor for the metabolic syndrome, type 2 diabetes, and cardiovascular consequences, that is, those outcomes, which are linked to low birth weight. Consequently, and accord-ing to the thrifty phenotype hypothesis, one would expect that low birth weight is an independent risk factor for obesity in later life. Although consequently proclaimed, this, however, is not the case: a systematic review of the literature has shown that up to now a linear inverse relation between birth weight and later overweight risk has never been found. Instead, 89% of all studies show a linear *positive* association, which means that the higher the birth weight, the higher the overweight risk in later life (Harder et al., 2007b). A linear inverse relation between birth weight and later type 2 diabetes, which is one of the most important predictions of the thrifty phenotype hypothesis, does not exist either. By meta-analysis, it could be shown that this relation is U-shaped instead, which means that both low as well as high birth weight are associated with increased type 2 diabetes risk (Harder et al., 2007a; Plagemann and Harder, 2005a, 2009a).

Concerning the thrifty phenotype hypothesis, a further problem is that up to now no experimental model exists that convincingly shows that neonatal underweight after ma-ternal/prenatal undernutrition is an *independent* risk factor for the whole spectrum of dis-turbances of the metabolic syndrome in later life, as described in epidemiological studies. The opposite is the case; our research group and Hales's group from Cambridge could not observe adipogenic or diabetogenic alterations in terms of the metabolic syndrome in rats exposed to maternal mal-/undernutrition perinatally (Petry et al., 1997; Plage-mann, 2001). Even after dietetic provocation with high caloric cafeteria-diet in adult life, simulating modern Western lifestyle, adipogenic or diabetogenic risks were not increased (Petry et al., 1997). In this context, a general important problem in the interpretation of experimental data, which widely contributed to the establishment and acceptance of the hypothesis, is the fact that most of the experimental paradigms did not account or adjust for neonatal food supply following maternal/fetal undernutrition. In most cases, cross-fostering paradigms were not used, leading to a bias simply produced by reactive hyperphagia in dams underfed during pregnancy, which may lead *via* hypercaloric milk composition to overfeeding of suckling pups. Considering the immaturity of newborn rodents, especially concerning the central nervous system, this may lead to a completely opposite outcome and outcome interpretation, in which not prenatal undernourishment but neonatal overnourishment is the causal factor for long-term disturbances. Accordingly and worthy to note, perinatally undernourished rats have an *increased* life span, while excessive neonatal weight gain decreases life expectancy (Ozanne and Hales, 2004).

Similarly, the match–mismatch hypothesis seems to lead to discrepancies, considering epidemiological, clinical, and experimental data. For example, the exposure to maternal diabetes mellitus *in utero*, which is characterized by prenatal (glucose-) overnutrition and pathognomic increase in fetal body weight and body fat, is followed by an *increased* obesity and diabetes risk in later life, not a decreased risk (Dabelea et al., 2000; Pettitt et al., 1983; Plagemann et al., 1997a, 1997b; Silverman et al., 1991, 1995; Weiss et al., 2000). If the match–mismatch paradigm were correct, however, one would expect that children of diabetic and/or overweight mothers would be a good example for a nearly perfect *match* between prenatal exposure and later environmental conditions because these children have been exposed to excessive nutrition *in utero*, which is continued later in life. Similar results would be expected in children of overweight moms and after increased prenatal stress exposure, which often leads to preterm birth together with a low birth weight. Furthermore, these children are often exposed to additional stress in neonatal intensive care units. According to the match–mismatch paradigm, they should be adapted nearly perfectly to our modern stressful life. Unfortunately, the opposite is the case. For example, overweight newborns are far from being well-adapted to nutritional abundance. Instead, they show increased prevalences of overweight, type 2 diabetes, and cardiovascular diseases in later life, even independent of their genetic background.

With all due respect but provocatively spoken: according to the aforementioned hypotheses, the epidemically increasing overweight prevalence as well as the prevalent overnutrition in women of reproductive age should be an effective *prophylaxis* for coming generations. Similarly, the exposure to stress *in utero* and in neonatal intensive care units would be beneficial conditioning for the modern stressful life, resulting in increased tolerance and decreased stress sensitivity. Especially against the background of contrary empirical data, serious doubts have to be raised here, which bring into question the general principles of the discussed concepts.

Summarizing, there is clear evidence of a *phenomenological* relation between a low birth weight and increased risk for chronic diseases, such as, for example, the metabolic syndrome. On the other hand, neither the thrifty phenotype hypothesis nor the match–mismatch paradigm appear to be appropriate hypotheses to explain these phenomena with respect to biomedical mechanisms because they lead to obvious paradoxical, illogical conclusions. While an explanatory rationale in terms of evolutionary processes cannot be excluded, these concepts can hardly explain developmental origins of health and disease nowadays. Therefore, generalizing these concepts could lead to fatal consequences in developing preventive strategies against diseases of civilization.

20.3 An alternative, integrative, and mechanistic hypothesis on perinatal programming

Life is a process of permanent environment-dependent development. Health and disease risks are determined lifelong in an environment-dependent manner. However, during critical developmental periods this may result in lasting effects. This basic principle of developmental biology has a long history, as is reflected, for example, in the pioneer work of St. Hilaire (teratogenesis), Stockard (critical period), Spemann (organizer effect), Lorenz (behavioral imprinting), and Ashby (biological self-organization; ▶Tab. 20.1).

Unfortunately, although the field of developmental origins of health and disease (DOHaD) is prospering internationally, these fundamental concepts are often neglected. A spanning, universal theory and conception considering these theories and observations integratively is still missing. Such a concept should cover the whole spectrum of early, environment-dependently acquired characteristics and disease dispositions both in a mechanistic and semantic manner.

Attempting a general, integrative concept, considering available observations and hypotheses, it is proposed here that environment-dependent adaptive, predictive responses (APRs) during critical developmental periods lead to long-lasting epigenomic and microstructural programming of fundamental life functions, that is, to perinatal programming (Plagemann, 2004, 2005, 2008, 2010; ▶Fig. 20.1).

Note, however, in this concept the proposed APRs are not reactions in terms of an early coping strategy aiming to actively cover developmental conditions, as postulated by other authors (Gluckman and Hanson, 2006, 2008; Gluckman et al., 2008). Rather, they are passive adaptations in terms of *vegetative learning processes,* by which the developing organism is conditioned, adjusted, and trained qualitatively and quantitatively according to the actually given environmental conditions during critical periods of development. Thus, also in this concept, there is an *adaptive* as well as a *predictive* characteristic; however, not in terms of an active coping strategy and anticipation of later environmental conditions, but in terms of a passive conditioning by the given environment. A long-term disadvantage can, therefore, result both in the case of a mismatch but also a match between developmental and later life conditions, depending on their respective quality and quantity according to an optimal homeostasis. Underlying processes of vegetative adaptation and imprinting, respectively, during critical periods of self-organization lead to a predictive programming, or malprogramming, of affected life functions (programming/malprogramming by APRs).

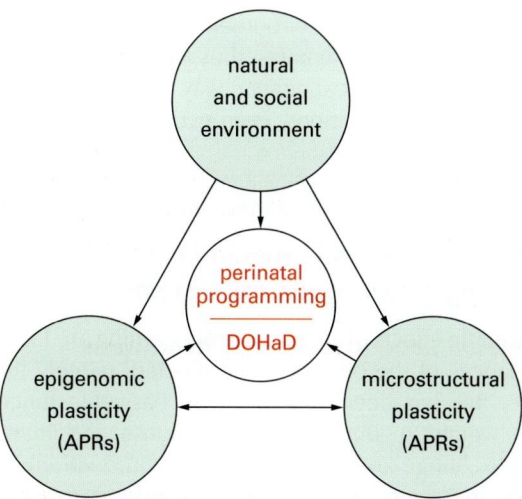

Fig. 20.1: Fundamental paradigm of perinatal programming and developmental determination of health risks (APRs – adaptive, predictive responses; DOHaD – developmental origins of health and disease; according and modified to Plagemann, 2004, 2005, 2008, 2010).

In other words, the developing organism experiences and *learns* the environmental conditions during its self-organization process through the perinatal milieu. The organism learns to handle them regulatively, takes over the regulatory *experience* from the mother, and becomes programmed accordingly. Therefore, one may also speak of a *vegetative imprinting*, thus widening Lorenz's *behavioral imprinting,* whereby the functional principles of fundamental life functions are learned and determined. The perinatal environmental conditions and stimuli are distinguished as standard and more or less fixed, accordingly. Thus, they become a measure, the *set point* or *set range,* of vegetative functions, regulations, and interactions between the individual and the environment. So, the process is more a matter of a passive programming than an active reaction of the developing individual. To a greater degree it is a kind of *trustful takeover* of vegetative regulatory standards and experiences from the maternal organism, a vegetative learning in the womb, which (seemingly) enables an optimal survival in the environment into which the organism is born.

In this concept, the causative APRs are generally realized in an epigenomic and/or microstructural manner (▶Fig. 20.1). Epigenomic and microstructural plasticity seem to be the decisive features of the self-organizational process of a developing organism. They cause a homeostatic calibration of functional and tolerance ranges at the subcellular level, the cellular level, the organ level, and up to the level of the whole organism. All this seems to take place as a physiological, normative process in ontogenesis. However, as a consequence of unphysiological, adverse, disadvantageous environmental conditions during critical developmental periods, this plasticity can also lead to a *malprogramming*. Permanent functional disturbances and disease dispositions will result in such cases, or when the developmental process results even *per se* and immediately in pathophysiologically relevant disturbances of regulatory processes.

Programming or *malprogramming* as result of functional modes perinatally acquired in that way can even be carried on intergeneratively *via* the maternal descendence (see Section 20.7). This can simply be realized by the fact that acquired functional characteristics decisively contribute to the intrauterine environment provided to the developing next generation during pregnancy of affected females, thus leading to an *inheritance* of these characteristics in an indirect, not classical genetic way. All this can consequently also influence phylogenesis and, over generations, even evolution (Plagemann, 2004, 2010; see Section 20.7).

20.4 A mechanistic clue: Developmental programming of neuro-endocrine and vegetative regulatory systems

The most important and sustainable effects of perinatal programming are likely to occur if the decisive regulatory instances of the organism are affected, namely the genome and/or the brain. Meanwhile, this has been shown for all basic life functions (metabolism, growth, and body weight regulation; stress response and immune reactions; information processing/exchange and neurobehavior; reproduction). First of all, hormone-dependent programming seems to be of essential importance here (glucocorticoids, sexual steroids, insulin, leptin, etc.), potentially causing a malprogramming both in case of deficiency or excess of these internal effectors and intercellular mediators during critical developmental periods (Plagemann and Harder, 2009b). Deleterious consequences of both increased as well as reduced levels of hormones, resulting from altered conditions of the external and internal environment during critical developmental periods, might also explain the common phenomenon of a U-shaped curve in the relationship between perinatal and later outcome (see Section 20.7; ►Fig. 20.7). In general, this indicates that hormones, acting as endogenous effectors and mediators of environmental signals, may function as "ontogenes" during development.

A respective pioneering conception of mechanisms of perinatal programming and malprogramming has been introduced in the context of Dörner's *functional teratology* (Dörner, 1975). According to this concept, the regulation of all fundamental life processes, for example, reproduction, information processing, immunity, and metabolism, is realized by the neuro-endocrine-immune system (NEIS) in its entirety, with different subsystems controlling elementary life functions. The central regulator is the brain, while hormones, neurotransmitters, and cytokines (as immune cell hormones) act as intercellular mediators within this complex system, as well as between the organism and the environment (Dörner, 1974a, 1974b, 1975).

According to this concept, the functional and tolerance ranges of neuro-endocrine regulatory systems (set point/set range) are determined primarily through the genetic material in the neurons of the respective central nervous regulator. This phylogenetically preset determination, however, can decisively be influenced and modified by the environmentally induced quantity of the relevant, later on regulated, hormones in critical developmental periods. In other words, according to this concept, during early ontogenesis a self-organization of neuro-endocrine regulatory systems of the organism, or, respectively, of central nervous regulatory centers – namely in the hypothalamus – takes place in dependence of the quantity of hormones, neurotransmitters, and cytokines present during the critical window of development. These effects of hormones as functional organizers in the processes of differentiation and maturation are considered to be more or less irreversible, leading to a programming of the gene expressibility of the developing neurons. The capacity of transcription and/or the ability of subsequent translation were proposed to be preprogrammed during critical periods of neuronal development through hormones and neurotransmitters for the lifetime functional period in an epigenetic sense (Dörner, 1974a, 1974b, 1975). Accordingly, the classical science of *teratology*, as the discipline of exogeneously induced macroscopic malformations (St. Hilaire, 1837), should be supplemented by the science of *functional teratology*, as the discipline of prenatally acquired malfunctions (Dörner, 1975).

Extending and integrating this, former, and current concepts, it should be considered that similar mechanisms seem to apply to substrates, metabolites, vitamins, and even trace elements, as well as intracellular transcription factors. All their environment-dependent quantities may also contribute to the epigenomic, microstructural, and lastly cybernetic adjustment of functional and tolerance ranges of an organism and its regulatory subsystems (►Fig. 20.2). Moreover, although the sustainability and importance for lasting dysfunctions may particularly result from malprogramming of central nervous regulators, similar mechanisms may also occur in peripheral cells, thereby also influencing the functional and tolerance ranges of affected life processes. The more so, as even maintenance of acquired epigenomic alterations during later cell division cycles becomes more and more probable (Law and Jacobson, 2010). Finally and accordingly, not only do neuro-endocrine and brain-periphery interaction and regulation seem to be the subjects of these developmental principles but so, too, are the regulatory processes

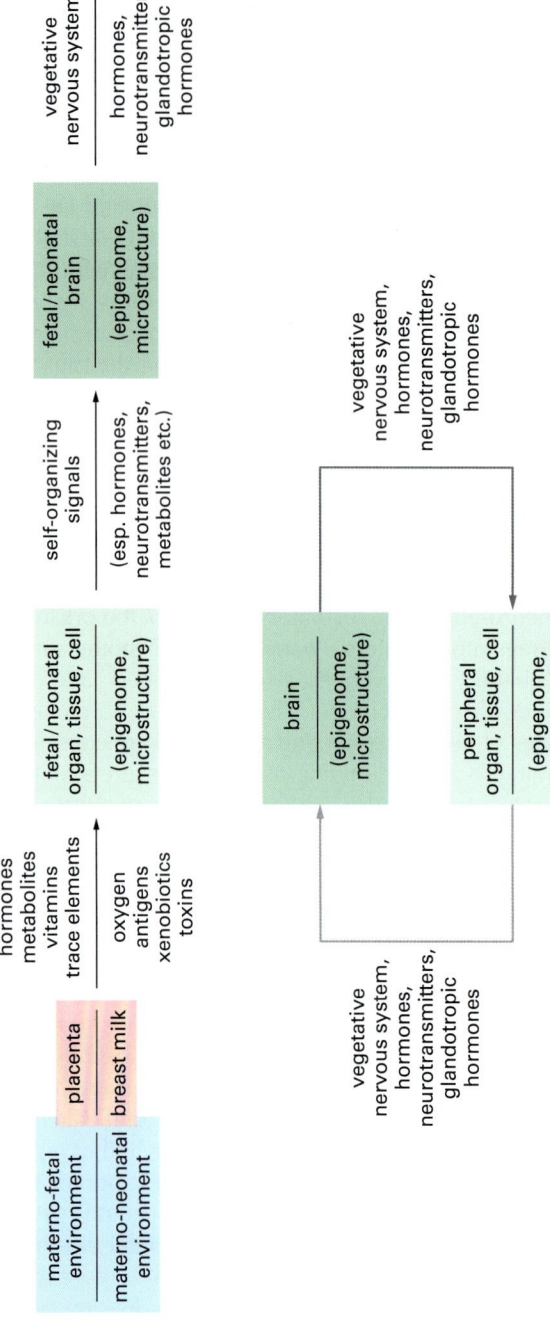

Fig. 20.2: General basic principle of self-organization of homeostatic regulatory systems of the organism (adapted, modified, and extended according to Dörner, 1975).

During critical phases of perinatal development of the brain and neuro-endocrine-immune network, primary linear, open-loop regulatory systems develop to secondarily closed, cybernetic feedback control systems (*transformation rule*). During this process the functional and tolerance ranges of central regulators are preprogrammed especially by the primary quantity of respective hormones, which are the secondarily regulated variables. Thereby, hormones act as ontogens, adjusting their own regulatory systems for lifetime functions (*determination rule*). Similar may be realized by the quantity of relevant metabolites, vitamins, trace elements, and so forth, and/or by interacting environmental substances and noxes.

of single cells, both in the brain and periphery, leading to an adjustment of cellular and subcellular functions in terms of cell integrity and/or vulnerability. In other words, environment-depending self-organization may determine the functionality from the subcellular up to the level of the whole organism during critical developmental periods. All this is likely to form the basis of the complex self-organization of an organism, in which the genome functions as hardware, while the complex functional program, the software, is finally determined by the environmental conditions during critical periods of development.

Proposing an alternative semantic, one might therefore also speak of the whole process as *biocybernetogenesis*, considering and contributing to the science of biological cybernetics, which currently mainly focuses on higher neuronal and cognitive functions. However, very similar to the proposed supplementation of behavioral imprinting (Lorenz, 1935) by vegetative imprinting, biological cybernetics should in the future include more fundamental vegetative life functions and, most of all, should be extended to and focused on the *development* and establishment of cybernetic regulatory systems. This process of biocybernetogenesis can be proposed to take place from the cellular up to the organismic level in order to ensure an optimal integrative functionality. Hereby, the scientific approach of biological cybernetics (Ashby, 1947; Wiener, 1948) would be and should be extended in terms of the environment-dependent developmental process that leads to the functionality, for example, of elementary homeostatic, vegetative regulations. Disturbances of this self-organizing process might be called dysbiocybernetogenesis. By altered or disadvantageous environmental conditions during critical periods of biological self-organization, dysbiocybernetogenesis of fundamental regulatory functions seems to be possible from the cellular up to the organismic level, finally leading to a malprogramming of respective life functions.

20.5 Epigenomic plasticity as a key mechanism in perinatal programming

The specific molecular mechanisms of perinatal programming processes are largely unknown and a matter of intensive research. In a general manner, potential mechanisms have meanwhile been postulated. Among them is the environment-dependent determination of clonal selection processes in early ontogenesis, as well as of cell numbers, cell sizes, and of the organ structures (especially innervation, vascularization, and growth). Overall, this contains microstructural adaptations, as well as acquired modes of gene expression and gene expressibility (epigenomics). In terms of a lasting influence on the functioning of homeostatic systems, first of all, the latter seems to be a mechanism that has to be regarded as very probable; however, its details are still not clarified.

But how could a lasting environmentally induced epigenomic programming or malprogramming of gene expressibility during critical developmental periods be realized and fixed for the long term? Against the background of current data on mechanisms of lasting DNA modification, one potential and particularly probable and specific mechanism of epigenomic perinatal programming shall be outlined briefly in the following (Plagemann, 2004, 2005; Plagemann et al., 2009, 2010).

The bases of the DNA helix can be modified covalently. Mammalian DNA contains 5′ methyl cytosine, which has a methyl group at its 5th carbon atom. Methylated cytosines are primarily found within dinucleotide sequences together with guanine, bound to it *via* phosphate groups (CpG; Jaenisch, 1997). These CpGs are not randomly distributed in the genome, but they are, considering the frequency of occurrence of guanine and cytosine, about fivefold underrepresented and reach their statistically expected frequency only in so-called CpG islands (Larsen et al., 1992). In the form of so-called non-CpG-methylation, also cytosines outside of CpGs can occur in a methylated form, for example, in cytosine/adenine-dinucleotides (Clark, Harrison, and Frommer, 1995). From an evolutionary point of view, DNA methylation is a relatively old process in the mammalian line (Cooper and Krawczak, 1989). DNA methylation is performed by DNA methyltransferases. In turn, methyl groups can also be removed by demethylases from the DNA sequence (Bhattacharya et al., 1999), especially during early embryogenesis. Here, general demethylation of the genomic DNA takes place, followed by a differentiated *de-novo* methylation (Razin and Shemer, 1995). The resulting DNA methylation patterns are considered to be tissue-specific and persisting (Newell-Price, King, and Clark, 2001).

At least three arguments legitimate the hypothesis that DNA methylation, as an ontogenetically acquired permanent modification of the DNA structure and function, is a molecular mechanism of perinatal programming processes.

First, methylation of the DNA can lead to permanent, thus lasting changes of gene expression. CpG-rich areas of the genome, prone to methylation, are found primarily at the 5′-terminal of coding sequences, thus in the promoter region of genes (Bird and Wolffe, 1999). It is well-known that the extent of DNA methylation in promoter regions is strictly inversely correlated to the expression of the upstream gene (Andria and Simon, 1999). In this context, it can be expected and postulated that during critical periods of early programming processes the actual binding of transcription factors, which depends on the given environmental conditions, can affect methylation pattern at the respective transcription factor binding sites simply by influencing their accessibility. In turn, this may contribute to complex epigenomic organization and, thus, programming or malprogramming of the respective promoter. This may establish the promoter activity for the long term.

Second, and in accordance with the first point, the methylation of DNA sequences is known to be environment-dependently inducible. Patterns of DNA methylation can be influenced by exogenous factors or, respectively, changes of the internal/intrauterine milieu. Especially, it is known that nutritive changes can lead to changes/alterations of the DNA methylation state. One possible mechanism may be that due to nutritional conditions, methyl groups are simply available in different amounts. These methyl groups, however, can induce DNA methyltransferases or increase their enzyme activity (Rees et al., 2000), thereby increasing methylation in DNA sequences.

Third, a possible role of DNA methylation in programming processes is supported by the fact that it is considered to be more or less irreversible after cell differentiation is completed (Razin and Shemer, 1995). A characteristic and decisive feature of programming processes is, however, that their consequences persist for the long term. This should naturally be of special importance for tissues and cells that are no longer (or not to a considerable amount) divisible in later life (terminal cells), such as, for example, neurons in the central nervous system (CNS), which functions as the decisive regulatory center of all fundamental life functions after perinatal development.

Indeed, during recent years first observations addressing and confirming the proposition of epigenomic changes resulting from environmental influences in fetal and neonatal life were reported from experimental investigations, including their functional relevance for later life. Pioneer work came from the group of Meaney, showing altered methylation pattern in the promoter of the glucocorticoid receptor and estrogen receptor in the rat hypothalamus and hippocampus due to altered rearing conditions, obviously predisposing to altered stress response and behavioral changes later on (Champagne et al., 2006; Weaver et al., 2004). Moreover, blood pressure regulation could be linked to acquired promoter methylation in genes of the adrenal gland, liver, and heart of prenatally malnourished rats (Bogdarina et al., 2007, Burdge et al., 2007; Ding et al., 2010). Recently, we could demonstrate acquired modifications of hypothalamic gene promoters involved in metabolism and body weight regulation in neonatally overfed rats (Plagemann et al., 2009, 2010, see section 20.6).

Summarizing, it can be postulated that epigenomic plasticity and respective adjustment of gene structure and function is a fundamental mechanism of environment-dependent genomic self-organization during critical developmental periods. Note, acquired microstructural alterations may also occur through epigenetic changes, and both mechanisms should be considered to be dynamically linked during the complex process of self-organization (▶Fig. 20.1). Furthermore, also microstructural adaptations to early environmental conditions may be of enduring functional relevance. Lasting consequences of microstructural dysorganization may especially apply to cases in which several organs or organ systems within a fundamental regulatory system are affected as, for example, in metabolic regulations, and/or if tissues of limited postnatal cell divisibility are affected (terminal cells), such as central neurons or adipocytes. Thus, perinatally acquired hypoplasia or hyperplasia, for example, in regulatory centers of the brain or in adipose tissue, can permanently influence the cybernetic balance and the functional and tolerance ranges in respective regulatory systems, thereby preconditioning the ability to compensate exposures in later life, with the consequence of increased or decreased disease dispositions.

20.6 For example: Fetal and neonatal overnutrition – a paradigm with practical relevance

Mechanistic evidence for the existence of the biomedical phenomenon of perinatal programming originated mainly from the fields of reproductive behavior and stress (Dörner 1975, 1976, 1980; Meaney et al., 1996; Francis and Meaney, 1999), with research addressing the significance of altered concentrations of the respective steroid hormones (sex steroids, gluco- and mineralocorticoids) during critical periods of perinatal development for a permanent malprogramming of the affected subsystems of the NEIS. However, the results of clinical investigations and animal experiments on the long-term effects of maternal diabetes, neonatal overnourishment, and thereby, perinatal overfeeding and hyperinsulinism for the development of the offspring have for a long time provided key support for the general concept. Therefore, the previously postulated hypotheses and mechanisms on perinatal programming shall shortly be illustrated in this almost historical paradigm, namely concerning the consequences of pre- and neonatal overnutrition for the long-term regulation of body weight and metabolism.

20.6.1 Epidemiological and clinical observations

Pregnancy is a diabetogenic situation *per se*. Women with gestational diabetes (GD), just as pregravid diabetic women, are classified as risk pregnancies, and their offspring show increased perinatal morbidity and mortality. The disturbances manifested during the neonatal period, apart from a tendency to develop hypoglycemia, hyperbilirubinemia, neonatal respiratory distress syndrome, and so forth, are characterized above all by an increased prevalence of macrosomia. This is caused by the virtually pathognomic fetal and perinatal hyperinsulinism, which arises from materno-fetal hyperglycemia and consequent overstimulation of the fetal pancreatic B cells when maternal diabetes is either not diagnosed or treated inadequately (Freinkel, 1980; Pedersen, Bojsen-Moller, and Poulsen, 1954).

Similar fetal overfeeding and consequences occur in the case of maternal overweight and maternal overnutrition *in graviditate* (Catalano 2003; Catalano et al., 2009). In all these cases, the nutritive and hormonal milieu of the developing fetus during critical developmental periods is disturbed in an adipogenic and diabetogenic manner. With the concept of malprogramming in mind, it should therefore be a source of serious concern that meanwhile about one-third of the women at reproductive age are overweight, and more than 10% of all pregnant women develop gestational diabetes, which in most cases is not diagnosed and thus not treated. Respectively, it can hardly be a simple coincidence that the common diabetes and obesity epidemic meanwhile affects not only adults, but also children and even newborns. Mean birth weight and the prevalence of macrosomia have increased alarmingly during recent decades (Plagemann and Dudenhausen, 2010; Plagemann et al., 2008; Rooth, 2003). For many years, however, epidemiological, clinical, and experimental studies have shown that affected offspring develop a permanently increased risk to develop overweight, diabetes, and components of the metabolic syndrome, even independent of or in addition to genetic dispositions (Claussen et al., 2008, 2009; Dabelea et al., 2000; Dörner et al., 1984, 1985; Dörner, Plagemann, and Reinagel, 1987; Pettitt et al., 1983; Plagemann et al., 1997a, 1997b; Silverman et al., 1991; Weiss et al., 2000). Similar results seem to apply to increased neonatal weight gain accompanied by excessive fat deposition (Dörner, Grychtolyk, and Julitz, 1977; Stettler et al., 2002), which regularly should be the consequence of neonatal overnutrition.

But how does all this fit with the small baby syndrome hypothesis on increased metabolic syndrome risk due to prenatal *under*feeding and *low* birth weight?

Noteworthy, even in the Pima Indian study, a long-term investigation of a North American population with a particularly high disposition to diabetes and obesity, it was shown very early after introduction of the Barker hypothesis that type 2 diabetes associated with overweight in adulthood was more prevalent in patients who had been overweight at birth, but also in those who were neonatally underweight (McCance et al., 1994). By means of meta-analysis of all respective studies beyond that in Pima Indians we could confirm these observations (Harder et al., 2007a), leading to the postulation that, in fact, not a linear-inverse but a U-shaped relationship exists between birth weight and later diabetes and obesity risk.

Whereas the pathogenetic context seems more or less obvious for fetal overfeeding and neonatal overweight, no clear etiopathogenetic link appears to be established between reduced perinatal weight and later metabolic syndrome (Dörner and Plagemann, 1994; Lucas et al., 1999; Plagemann, 2006). In particular, it should be emphasized that no independent causal link has been shown between low birth weight and subsequent obesity, that is, the pathophysiological key for diabetes and cardiovascular diseases (CVD) in terms of the metabolic syndrome. It therefore remains to be clarified whether fetal growth restriction and underweight at birth, *per se*, or rather the quality and quantity of early postnatal nutrition and resulting weight gain in early infancy are of pathophysiological significance for the prospective risk. The central pathogenetic importance of later overweight is clear, especially within the context of the metabolic syndrome, but though a positive correlation has frequently been demonstrated between weight at birth and weight or overweight in later life, an independent inverse relationship has never been shown (Harder et al., 2007b). Increased weight gain in neonatal life, on the other hand, leads to increased disposition for obesity in later life (Dörner et al., 1977; Stettler et al., 2002). It also seems remarkable that increased weight gain in early childhood, in particular in underweight newborns, leads to early manifestation of insulin resistance (Crowther et al., 2000; Fewtrell et al., 2000). Finally, it has been variously shown that increased weight gain in early childhood is a predictive factor for a disposition to the metabolic syndrome and cardiovascular risk in adulthood, in particular in the case of low birth weight (Eriksson et al., 1999; Forsén et al., 1999; Vanhala et al., 1999).

However, do all these phenomena and associations express an acquired obesity and diabetes disposition due to perinatal overfeeding and consequent malprogramming?

Already in the 1970s it was shown in a cohort of 4,000 diabetic patients that type 2 diabetes was *inherited* more frequently through the mother than the father (Dörner and Mohnike, 1976). The offspring of a mother with diabetes during pregnancy shows an increased tendency to become overweight or obese already in childhood (Plagemann et al., 1997a), accompanied by disturbances of glucose tolerance, insulin secretion, and insulin sensitivity (Silverman et al., 1995; Plagemann et al., 1997b). It is particularly noticeable that these alterations may occur even independently from genetic influences and the type of maternal gestational hyperglycemia (Dabelea et al., 2000; Pettitt et al., 1983; Plagemann et al., 1997a, 1997b). However, they do show marked correlations with fetal metabolic alterations, especially the degree of fetal and perinatal hyperinsulinism (Harder et al., 2001b; Kohlhoff and Dörner, 1990; Plagemann et al., 1997b; Silverman et al., 1995). In particular, a positive correlation was found between the level of amniotic fluid insulin or perinatal hyperinsulinemia and an increase in relative body weight and the risk of impaired glucose tolerance (IGT) in later life for children of diabetic mothers (Plagemann et al., 1997b; Silverman et al., 1995). Moreover, normalization of fetal insulin led to normalization of later diabetic risk (Silverman et al., 1995). This strongly indicates a persisting influence of fetal hyperinsulinism on the long-term outcome, in the sense of a hormonally initiated malprogramming.

20.6.2 Experimental observations

Food intake, body weight, and metabolism are decisively regulated by hypothalamic nuclei (▶Fig. 20.3A) and neuropeptides, which are expressed there under control of the circulating satiety signals insulin and leptin (▶Fig. 20.4A). Studies in experimental models of maternal gestational diabetes and neonatal overnutrition have shown that this regulatory system realizes complex microstructural and epigenomic adaptations to perinatal overnutrition, with the consequence of permanently increased obesity and diabetes disposition (*diabesity*), even independent of genetic risk. Thus, in the sense of microstructural plasticity and malprogramming, for example, a persisting neuronal hypoplasia of the ventromedial hypothalamic nucleus (VMN) occurs, which functions as a satiety center, and simultaneously pancreatic B-cell hyperplasia and adipocyte hyperplasia are induced (▶Fig. 20.4C; Aerts and Van Assche, 1979; Aerts, Vercruysse, and Van Assche, 1997; Dörner and Plagemann, 1994; Harder et al., 2001a, 2003; Knittle and Hirsch, 1968). Moreover, this is accompanied by relevant epigenomic alterations, induced through perinatal overnutrition (▶Fig. 20.4B; Plagemann et al., 2009, 2010). Exemplarily, these consequences of perinatal overnutrition for the acquired phenotype and function of the hypothalamo-adipo-pancreatic system shall be briefly outlined and discussed in the following.

Animal experiments have confirmed early that maternal gestational hyperglycemia and subsequent fetal hyperinsulinism may lead to overweight, impaired glucose tolerance, hyperinsulinemia, and insulin resistance in the juvenile and adult offspring, even irrespective of any genetic disposition (Aerts and Van Assche, 1979; Aerts, Holemans,

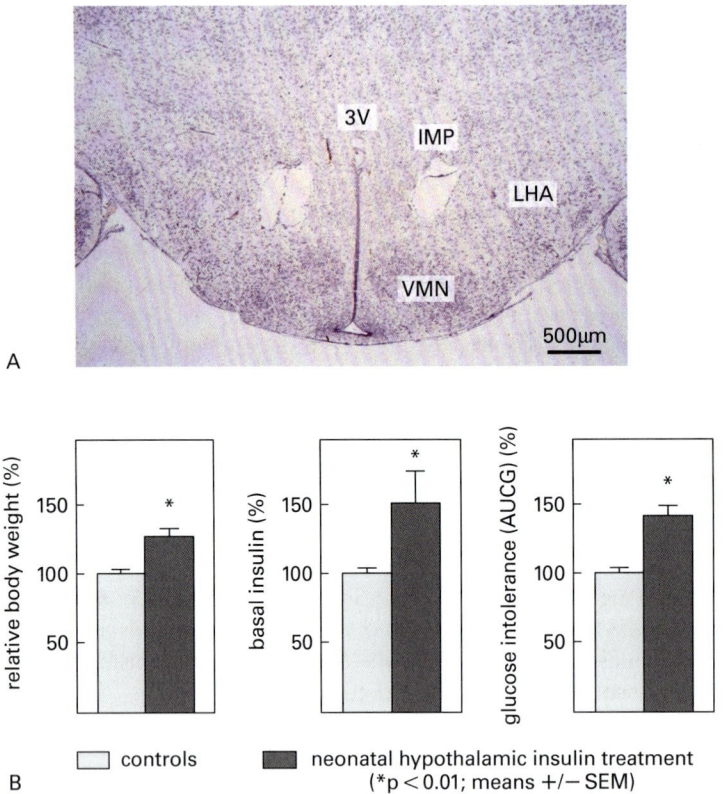

Fig. 20.3: Long-term consequences of temporary intrahypothalamic insulin excess in newborn rats. (A) In the hypothalamus of newborn rats, insulin was applied by implants immediately neighboring nuclei, which regulate body weight throughout later life (3V, 3rd ventricle; IMP, implant; LHA, lateral hypothalamic area; VMN, ventromedial hypothalamic nucleus), while in controls the insulin-free vehicle was applicated only. (B) Intrahypothalamic insulin treatment led to overweight, hyperinsulinemia, and impaired glucose tolerance in adulthood (*p < 0.01; **p < 0.001; modified according to Plagemann et al., 1992).

and Van Assche, 1990; Dörner et al., 1988; Dörner and Plagemann, 1994; Oh et al., 1991). Experiments using maternal and/or neonatal glucose and/or insulin infusion to rodents and primates (Bihoreau et al., 1986; Cha, Gelardi, and Oh, 1987; Susa et al., 1992), and even embryo transfer experiments (Gill-Randall et al., 2004), have clearly corroborated these observations.

A permanent influence on the differentiation and function of pancreatic B cells through perinatal overstimulation has been proposed, on the one hand, as an etiopathogenetic mechanism of this prenatally acquired malprogramming. In particular, hyperplasia and hyperactivity could be demonstrated in the offspring, leading in the long term to impairment of insulin secretion (Aerts et al., 1990). On the other hand, studies have shown that permanent alterations of neuroendocrine and vegetative functional systems play a key etiopathogenetic role here (Dörner et al., 1988; Dörner and Plagemann, 1994; Plagemann, 2004, 2005, 2008; Plagemann et al., 1998, 1999b). Thus, the experimental induction of gestational hyperglycemia leads not only to perinatal hyperinsulinemia but also to increased insulin concentrations within the immature brain, especially the hypothalamus, that is, the key regulator of body weight, food intake, and metabolism (Plagemann et al., 1998). Intrahypothalamic elevation of insulin also occurs in neonatally overfed rats (Plagemann et al., 1999c). In both models, this is followed by morphological characteristics of permanent, that is, lifelong dysplasia of neuropeptidergic hypothalamic controllers of metabolism and body weight (Plagemann et al., 1998, 1999c). In particular, this affects the ventromedial hypothalamic nucleus (VMN), which develops a permanent dysplasia, neuronal hypotrophy, and disturbed function as a result of the exposure to increased insulin concentrations during critical periods of early development (Davidowa and Plagemann, 2001; Dörner and Plagemann, 1994; Dörner et al., 1988; Heidel, Plagemann, and Davidowa, 1999; Plagemann et al., 1999a). Furthermore, as an expression of perinatally acquired hypothalamic resistance to the peripheral satiety signals insulin and leptin, there is a permanent dysorganization and malfunction of specific neuropeptidergic neurons in the arcuate hypothalamic nucleus (ARC). Particularly important seems to be an increased activity and number of neurons that express the orexigenic peptides galanin and neuropeptide Y (Plagemann et al., 1998, 1999d), while the number and function of anorexigenic neuropeptidergic neurons becomes permanently decreased (Davidowa, Li, Plagemann, 2003; Franke et al., 2005). All this is accompanied by and correlated to a permanently increased disposition to diabetes and obesity, hyperphagia, overweight, basal hyperinsulinemia, insulin resistance, and IGT. Noteworthy, similar alterations have been observed in offspring of rat dams with diet-induced obesity during pregnancy (Kirk et al., 2009). It should be emphasized that both clinically and experimentally these disturbances occur even independently of the birth weight and can also be observed in animals experimentally treated with insulin in neonatal life, applicated either peripherally or only intrahypothalamically (Dörner and Plagemann, 1994; Dörner et al., 1988; Harder et al., 1998; Plagemann, 2008; Plagemann et al., 1992a, 1992b; ▶Fig. 20.3).

Even type 1 diabetes susceptibility is increased after exogenous insulin treatment of newborn rats (Plagemann et al., 1992a, 1992b), as well as in the offspring of diabetic mothers. Multiple low dose streptozotocin (STZ) treatment is a well-known model for type 1–like diabetes in rats, accompanied by cell-mediated immune responses that closely resemble the autoimmune processes associated with infantile type 1 diabetes in the human. In offspring of gestational diabetic mother rats, basal hyperinsulinemia

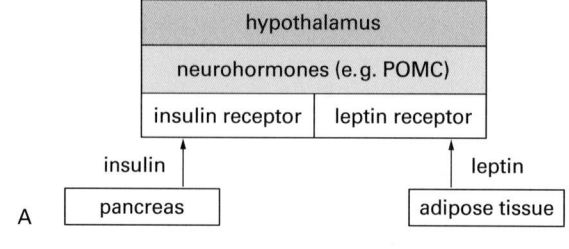

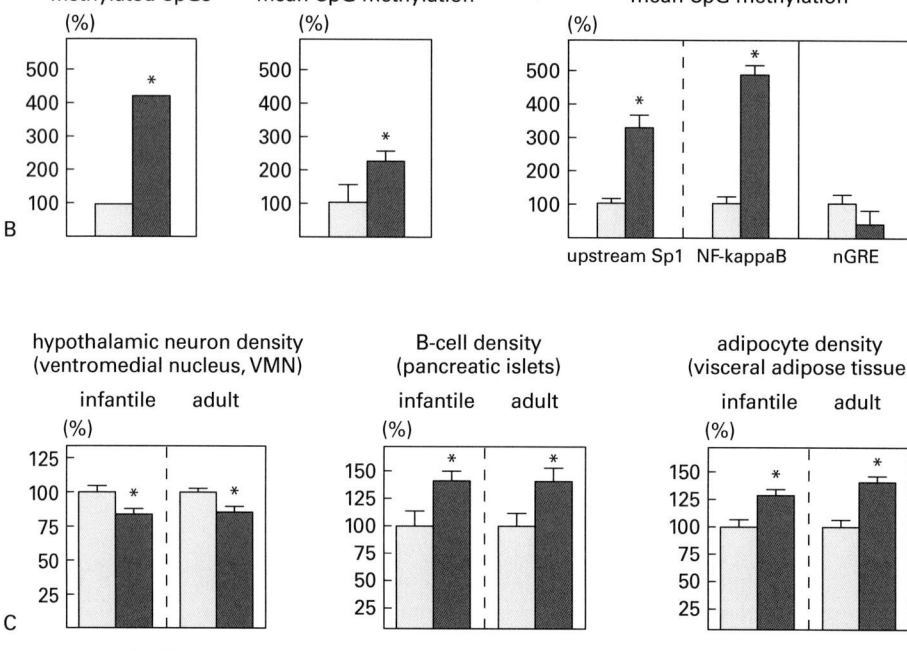

Fig. 20.4: For example – The hypothalamo-adipo-pancreatic system (A). Due to overnutrition during critical periods of early neonatal development, permanent epigenomic (B) and microstructural (C) alterations are induced: acquired hypermethylation of catabolic/anorexigenic gene promoters in central regulatory centres (B); acquired neuronal hypoplasia in central satiety centers (hypothalamic ventromedial nucleus, VMN), and, simultaneously, pancreatic B-cell hyperplasia and adipocyte hyperplasia (C; references and explanations: see text).

from birth into adulthood, indicating persisting basal overstimulation of the pancreatic B cells and, most important, a severe insulin-deficient type 1–like diabetes after a single low dose STZ treatment were observed (Dörner et al., 1988). Confirmingly, the offspring of mother rats with gestational diabetes responded to multiple low dose STZ treatment with increased spleen cell cytotoxicity to syngeneic B cells (Dörner et al., 1990).

All this points toward a hormonally and nutritionally induced complex malprogramming, induced due to pre- and neonatal overfeeding, hyperglycemia, and hyperinsulinemia, of the neuro-vegetative control system of body weight and metabolism, occurring independent of the genetic background, irrespective of birth weight, and leading to an overall increased metabolic risk in terms of diabesity.

Again, however, the question arises: how does all of this fit with the Barker hypothesis and the match–mismatch paradigm?

With respect to the thrifty phenotype hypothesis, investigations on the small baby syndrome frequently use animal models of maternal underfeeding during gestation and lactation, which experimentally leads to intrauterine and neonatal growth restriction in the offspring (Petry et al., 1997). However, it should be noted that even under extreme famine conditions in humans birth weight is hardly affected (Stanner et al., 1997; Stein et al., 2004). Moreover, detailed examination of the results on long-term effects obtained with animal models indicates that no consistent congruence with the observations after low birth weight in humans exists (Neitzke, Harder, and Plagemann, 2011). Thus, for example, animal experiments have shown that offspring born to rat dams that were malnourished during gestation and lactation do not become overweight later on but rather show a lifelong persistence of low weight. This is associated with a permanently reduced food intake (Petry et al., 1997). The animals predominantly show increased instead of decreased glucose tolerance. In contrast to the metabolic syndrome in humans, hyperinsulinemia and insulin resistance do not occur, but rather lower insulin secretion. All these findings persist even after dietary provocation in later life (Moura et al., 1997; Petry et al., 1997). Moreover, in this animal model an increased life span was observed (Ozanne and Hales, 2004), which hardly fits with the proposed increase in metabolic and cardiovascular risk (Plagemann, 2006). However, if rapid neonatal weight gain was induced, a reduced life expectancy could be observed (Ozanne and Hales, 2004).

Accordingly, we have postulated that transition from fetal undernutrition to early postnatal overfeeding could play a key role in the etiopathogenesis of the small baby syndrome (Dörner and Plagemann, 1994), especially because it seems quite possible that low weight neonates, also in the crucial epidemiological studies, had been overfed and possibly even fattened in neonatal life. Similar hypotheses on the possible significance of the early postnatal nutrition and rapid neonatal weight gain for the long-term outcome of underweight neonates have since been formulated by many other authors, including Hales and Barker (1992; Eriksson et al., 1999; Fewtrell et al., 2000). Meanwhile, rapid neonatal weight gain, which mainly seems to be attributable to absolute or relative overnourishment, is an established risk factor to explain the small baby syndrome (Monteiro and Victora, 2005; Stettler et al., 2002), thereby confirming our earlier data and concepts (Dörner and Plagemann, 1994).

The influence of early postnatal overnutriton on later metabolism and body weight has often been investigated using the small litter model. Rats that are overfed in the early postnatal period by reduction of the primary litter size show phenotypic alterations through juvenile age into adulthood, such as overweight, hyperphagia, glucose intolerance, hyperinsulinemia, dyslipidemia, and increased blood pressure, which correspond in critical aspects to those of the metabolic syndrome in humans (Boullu-Ciocca et al., 2005; Plagemann et al., 1992b, 1999c). This is all the more remarkable because clinical findings suggest that early postnatal overfeeding in humans also predisposes for an increased risk of diabesity and the metabolic syndrome in later life (Dewey et al., 1993;

Dörner et al., 1977; Harder et al., 2005; Plagemann and Harder, 2005b, 2011). But here too the pathophysiological causes and mechanisms are not clear.

As mentioned, neuropeptidergic hypothalamic centers play a key role in the regulation of food intake, body weight, and metabolism (Bouret, 2010). Note, very similar to offspring of diabetic dams, neonatally overfed rats show persisting dysorganization and malprogramming of these regulatory systems, including malfunction of the VMN and resistance of the ARC to the circulating satiety signals insulin and leptin (Davidowa and Plagemann, 2000, 2001, 2007), possibly explaining their neonatally acquired long-term risk in terms of a neuro-vegetative malprogramming (Plagemann, 2004, 2005, 2008; Plagemann et al., 1999c, 1999d).

Moreover, neonatally acquired hypothalamic leptin and insulin resistance seems to be, at least in part, due to nutritionally induced alterations of DNA methylation patterns of the promoter regions of genes encoding critical players in the respective hypothalamic circuits (▶Fig. 20.4B). Especially, we could show increased methylation of the insulin receptor promoter in the hypothalamus of neonatally overfed rats (Plagemann et al., 2010). In parallel, a specifically changed methylation pattern was found in the promoter of the most important anorexigenic neuropeptide, proopiomelanocortin (POMC). Here, activating transcription factor binding sites became hypermethylated (upstream Sp1, NF-kappaB), while inactivating transcription factor binding sites were found to be hypomethylated (nGRE), leading to a lack of upregulation of POMC expression despite marked hyperleptinemia and hyperinsulinemia. The extent of hypermethylation was shown to depend upon neonatal glucose levels (Plagemann et al., 2009). This specific constellation indicates a methylation pattern acquired through overnutrition and elevated glucose during the critical neonatal developmental period. Similar was observed for the insulin receptor promoter (Plagemann et al., 2010). For the first time, by these observations epigenomically induced alterations due to nutritional changes and overfeeding in perinatal life could be demonstrated. Especially important seems to be the observed correlation with the degree of glycemia for acquired methylation patterns. Note, in vitro studies have demonstrated induction of DNA-methyltransferases by high glucose concentrations (Chiang et al., 2009). Therefore, early hyperglycemia might initiate an intraindividual vicious circle by causing increased promoter methylation, especially of insulinergic genes, finally leading to further increase of glucose levels, and so on (▶Fig. 20.6A). Hypothetically, this could be an important mechanism in the pathogenesis of insulin resistance over the life span. Accordingly, these data are of paradigmatic pilot character regarding epigenetic mechanisms, which may initiate and mediate long-term consequences of an altered perinatal milieu and, moreover, an altered environmental milieu throughout life leading to epigenomic causes of diabesity pathogenesis. This might have wide-ranging paradigmatic implications not only for perinatal programming but also etiopathogenesis and the aging processes, in general (Plagemann et al., 2009, 2010).

Thus, complex epigenomic and microstructural malprogramming acquired due to perinatal overfeeding may predispose an individual to permanent hyperphagia, obesity, hyperleptinemia, hyperinsulinemia, impaired glucose tolerance, and insulin resistance, that is, all decisive components of the metabolic syndrome. These observations could provide mechanistic explanation for epidemiological–clinical phenomena, both regarding consequences of maternal diabetes/obesity as well as neonatal overfeeding in terms of excessive fat deposition (▶Fig. 20.5).

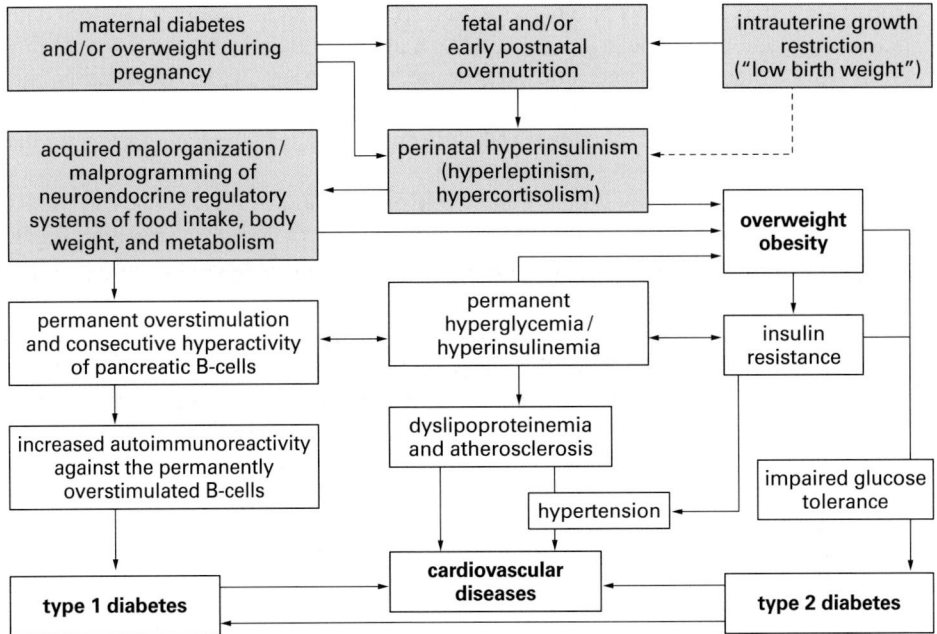

Fig. 20.5: Proposal of a pathogenetic framework, mechanisms, and consequences of perinatal malprogramming, showing the etiological significance of pre- and neonatal overfeeding and hyperinsulinism for excess weight gain, obesity, diabetes mellitus (type 2 as well as type 1), and subsequent cardiovascular diseases (CVD) in later life. Adapted, modified, and extended according to Dörner and Plagemann (1994).

20.6.3 Conclusions

Altogether, these observations, interpreted critically and integratively, show that over-nutrition during pre- and neonatal development can lead to a complex microstructural and epigenomic malprogramming in terms of the triggering noxa (overnutrition), and to a respective conditioning according to this exposure. Overnutrition and the accompanying metabolic and hormonal alterations seem to be recognized as a standard by the developing organism. A respective programming, in this case *mal*programming, occurs. This observation seems to be of paradigmatic relevance for an overall understanding of perinatal programming phenomena and mechanisms, which may lead to a passive conditioning, fixing the early experiences in terms of respective homeostatic regulations for the long term (see Section 20.2).

Note, even increased disposition to insulin-dependent type 1 diabetes may be prepro-grammed in this way (Dörner and Plagemann, 1994; Dörner et al., 1984, 1985, 1987, 2000). Here, once again the complex malprogramming of the NEIS is probably of causal significance. Acquired malfunction of the VMN and neuro-vegetative hypothalamo-pancreatic axis, along with basal hyperglycemia, may lead to permanent basal over-stimulation of the pancreatic B cells. Permanent basal B-cell overstimulation, however, not only contributes to hyperinsulinemia but also to increased autoimmune reactivity to the constantly hyperactive B cells, as typical for endocrine cells (Bottazzo et al., 1988;

Nerup et al., 1988). Especially in otherwise predisposed individuals and/or together with exposure to additional noxae (e.g., viruses), this may result in an increased susceptibility even to type 1 diabetes (Dörner and Plagemann, 1994; ▶Fig. 20.5). Remarkably, this early proposal has been supported in recent years, especially by acknowledging accelerated growth and overweight in infancy and early childhood as pathogenic factors for the manifestation of type 1 diabetes (Wilkin, 2001).

Given that gestational diabetes has meanwhile reached a prevalence surely in excess of 10% in the developed industrialized countries, while maternal overweight affects more than one-third of pregnancies, it therefore seems urgently necessary that all pregnant women are screened for glucose intolerance and adequately treated, as a measure of genuine primary prevention.

Furthermore, there is clear *phenomenological* evidence for a link between reduced birth weight and subsequently increased risk in terms of the metabolic syndrome. A critical integration of epidemiological, clinical, and experimental observations, however, may cast doubts on a causal relationship. Anyway, neonatal overfeeding and rapid early weight gain together with increased fat deposition and its hormonal consequences (hyperinsulinemia, hyperleptinemia, etc.) seem to be of long-term pathophysiological importance and appear particularly probable in underweight newborns. Therefore, prophylactic recommendations should focus on the recognition, avoidance, and optimal treatment of the causes of intrauterine growth restriction (nicotine, alcohol, stress, infections, gestosis, etc.), and also on the avoidance of neonatal overfeeding, rapid neonatal weight gain, and accompanying metabolic and hormonal alterations.

20.7 Intergenerative transmission and prevention of perinatally acquired characteristics

From the above discussed phenomena, observations, and mechanisms it seems obvious that the perinatal (periconceptional, embryonic, fetal, and neonatal) environment codetermines the self-organization, functional phenotype, and long-term fate of an organism (perinatal programming). Therefore, the important question arises on potential consequences for subsequent generations and how a malprogramming can be prevented, occasionally.

First, it should be considered and critically addressed here that there are obvious discrepancies between the various observations and explanations currently provided, with generally both decreased as well as increased birth weight, under- as well as overfeeding, and so forth, and generally both decreased as well as increased materno-fetal environmental stimuli and developmental challenges, that were linked with a deleterious long-term outcome (see Section 20.2).

For instance, pre- and neonatal under- as well as overfeeding, going along with perinatal hypo- or hyperglycemia, have both been found to predispose for later diabetes risk (see previous discussion). Both low as well as high protein supply, pre- as well as neonatally, have also been linked with a diabetogenic long-term outcome (Daenzer et al., 2002; Petry et al., 1997). Accordingly, both perinatal hypo- as well as hyperinsulinemia and hypo- as well as hyperleptinemia have been demonstrated to malorganize and malprogram hypothalamic circuits regulating metabolism, food intake, and body weight, thereby predisposing for *diabesity* later on (Bouret, 2010; Bouret, Draper, and

Simerly, 2004; Dörner and Plagemann, 1994; Plagemann, 2008; Plagemann et al., 1992a, 1999c). Furthermore, both increased as well as decreased exposure to stress-like experiences during neonatal life of rats, accompanied by respective activation of the hypothalamo-pituitary-adrenal (HPA) axis, lead to altered stress response later in life. Similar applies to and goes along with increased or decreased neurobehavioral stimuli, realized by neonatal rearing conditions and maternal care (Boullu-Ciocca et al., 2005; Champagne and Meaney, 2007; Francis and Meaney, 1999; Liu et al., 1997; Spencer and Tilbrook, 2009; Van den Bergh et al., 2008). Accordingly, with regard to immuno-logical stimuli, human studies suggest that both increased as well as decreased perinatal exposure to antigens/allergens may permanently alter allergy risk (Douwes et al., 2008). For instance, delayed exposure to allergens, as in the case of late introduction of solid food, was shown to increase allergy risk later in childhood (Nwaru et al., 2010). On the other hand, increased allergen exposure, as in the case of early cow milk protein consumption, may also predispose to allergy and atopic disease later in life (Gdalevich et al., 2001).

All these observations speak in favor of a U-shaped relationship between the quantity of perinatal developmental stimuli and later functionality, in general. Both decreased as well as increased exposure to homeostatic stimuli and variables may lead to a malpro-gramming. However, there is no contradiction between these seemingly opposite ob-servations. To the contrary, a common developmental principle seems to underly these phenomena, explainable by the necessity of an *adequate* stimulation by environmental conditions and homeostatic variables during self-organization, to ensure adequate adjustment of functionality and regulatory integrity later on.

Mechanistic explanations for similar outcomes following opposite perinatal expo-sures may include the time point, the critical window, during which a deficiency or excess of the respective stimulus occurs (Tzschentke and Plagemann, 2006). Accom-panying, sequence and combination of developmental exposures are of critical impor-tance, that is, whether or not a prenatal deficit is followed by a neonatal overflow, for example, according to nutrition. Moreover, a general explanation might be that in terms of a conditioning, a training, both insufficient as well as overstimulation may lead to a disturbed function, with finally similar deleterious outcomes. A decreased stimulation, conditioning, and training, may result in an insufficient functional capacity, whereas overstimulation may result in a functional *injury*, that is, a disruption of functionality, also leading to an insufficient function. For instance, both decreased insulin secretion, acquired by understimulation of developing B cells (undernutrition, low glucose, low amino acids), as well as increased insulin secretion, acquired by early overstimulation (overfeeding, glucose mast) and, consequently, insulin resistance at target cells, may both result in a diabetogenic disposition. Similarly, both increased as well as decreased early stimulation and activity of the HPA axis may lead to an inadequate stress response, with very similar vegetative and accompanying disturbances. Both increased as well as insufficient exposure to antigens/allergens during critical periods of tolerance induction may result in a disturbed immune function and auto-immunity, and so on.

It appears plausible that acquired alterations of the regulatory activity of homeostatic effectors may result from decreased stimulation and conditioning in early life, on the one hand, or acquired resistance to an overflow of regulatory effectors in consequence of overstimulation during critical developmental periods. Both circumstances may lead to respective dysfunctions. Exemplarily, hormonal malprogramming seems to play a critical role if a respective hormone excess or deficiency occurs, for example, of glucocorticoids, sex steroids, insulin, leptin, and so forth, during critical developmental periods. Note, as a classical and fundamental paradigm, both decreased secretion of as well as decreased sensitivity (resistance) to hormones lead to similarly disturbed functions in terms of hypoactivity and ineffectiveness of the affected system. The same, however, may apply to any kind of endogenous effectors involved in the regulation of fundamental life functions (hormones, neurotransmitters, metabolites, transcription factors, etc.), from the subcellular up to the organismic level. Hereby, a fundamental principle of perinatally acquired malfunctions can be proposed, and a fundamental explanation is provided for the common phenomenon of a U-shaped distribution in the relationship between perinatal exposures, respective concentrations of developmental signals, organizers, and ontogens, and the later outcome.

Also, multidirectional programming and malprogramming and, respectively, multiple disorders and multimorbidity have to be considered here. It must be noted that, for example, perinatal overfeeding may affect not only later diabesity risk but directly and indirectly also reproductive and mental health, behavior, cardiovascular health, aging, and even cancer risk (Boullu-Ciocca et al., 2005; Harder, Plagemann, and Harder, 2008, 2010; Ozanne and Hales, 2004; Plagemann, Tönjes, and Dörner, 1988; Plagemann et al., 1992b, 1999c; Van Assche et al., 2010). Similar seems to apply to perinatal undernourishment, stress exposure, infections, exposure to environmental toxins, and so forth, all of which have been linked to a number of long-term outcomes and disease dispositions. Altogether, this implicates the complexity of early environment-dependent self-organization, biocybernetogenesis, and long-term programming of fundamental life functions. The process is obviously realized in a complex way, by setting an individual profile of interacting homeostatic functional and tolerance ranges, in terms of a microstructural and epigenomic *fingerprint* and functional individuality, aiming to integrate environmental challenges according to the experiences during critical periods of early self-organization.

Special importance and current attention applies to the question whether programming or malprogramming, especially epigenomically, through environmental influences is restricted to early developmental periods, or may occur throughout life. This question seems to be of critical importance for the whole approach of perinatal programming. While there is overwhelming evidence of lasting consequences resulting from exposures during critical periods of early development (Stockard, 1921; Tzschentke and Plagemann, 2006), epigenomic alterations resulting from later, lifelong gene–environment interaction cannot be excluded and seem very plausible, especially as a mechanism of aging processes (McGowan and Szyf, 2010; Szyf, this volume). This, however, does not affect the long-term impact of early epigenomic and microstructural conditioning, leading anyway to long-term predispositions that may initiate and/or increase later vulnerability but, most of all, allow a primary, genuine prevention of respective alterations acquired during circumscribed time windows of early development.

Again, a fundamental paradigm results here from insights into metabolic development and regulation. While hyperglycemia during critical periods of early life has been shown epidemiologically, clinically, and experimentally to predispose for later diabesity (see previous discussion), increased glucose levels have been linked to hypermethylation (Chiang et al., 2009). Acquired alterations of insulinergic promoter sequences have been observed after perinatal hyperglycemia (Plagemann et al., 2009, 2010). The resulting diabetogenic predisposition may subsequently lead to an intraindividual vicious circle, with hyperglycemia causing increased methylation of insulinergic promoters, finally further increasing glucose levels, and in turn, again increasing promoter methylation, and so on (▶Fig. 20.6A). Hypothetically, this could be an important mechanism underlying not only perinatal programming but progredient pathogenesis of insulin resistance over the life time, thereby potentially providing a new explanation for diabetes pathogenesis, in general (Plagemann et al., 2010).

Moreover, beyond such an *intra*individual vicious circle, even an epigenetic *intergen*erative vicious circle can be suggested (▶Fig. 20.6B). For instance, overfeeding during

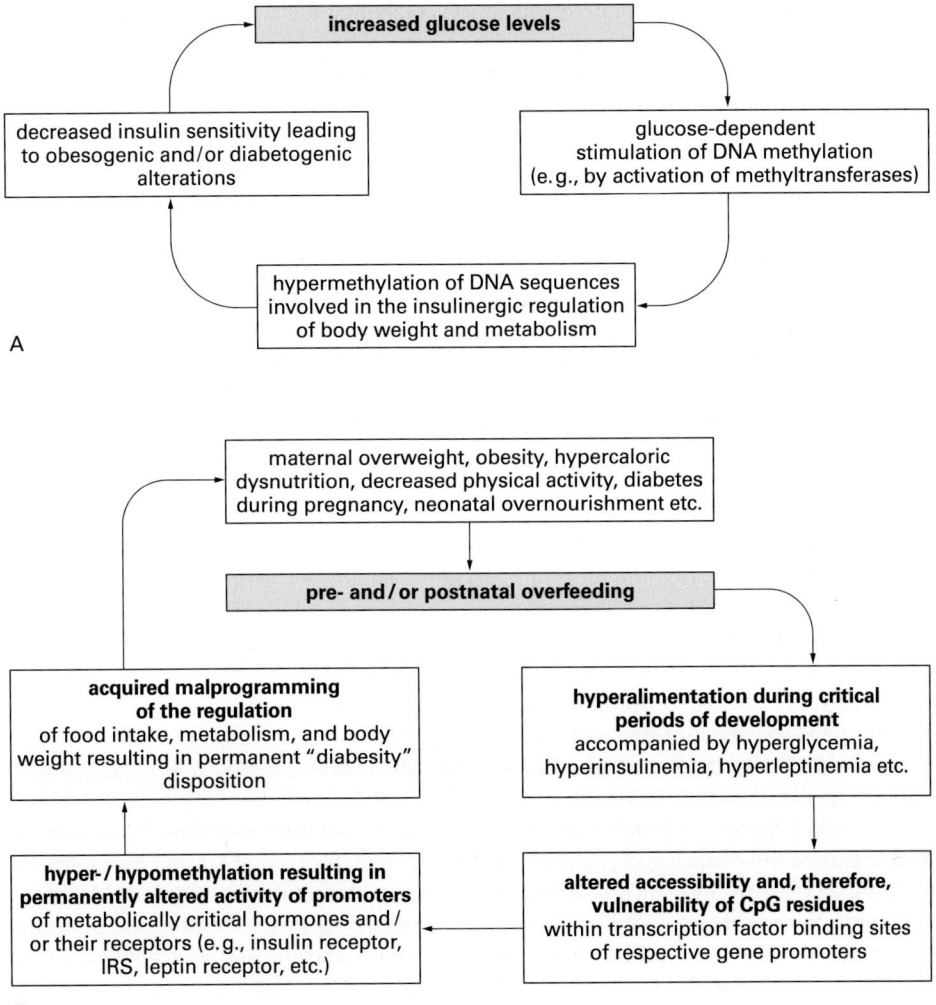

Fig. 20.6: Proposal and general concept of nutrition-dependent epigenomic malprogramming leading (A) by hyperglycemia to an *intra*individual vicious circle, and (B) an *inter*individual vicious circle of epigenetic diabesity programming and intergenerative transmission through the maternal line. Prevention appears to be possible by normalization of food supply in early life.

critical periods of development leads to an altered accessibility and, thereby, vulnerability of CpG dinucleotides within promoters of genes critically involved in the regulation of food intake, body weight, and metabolism. Initially, the resulting alterations in promoter methylation must not necessarily lead to altered transcription but might become pathogenic over time due to additional, synergistically acting adverse exposures, such as, for example, hypercaloric nutrition, and so forth. The resulting alterations of methylation pattern of respective promoters will ultimately alter their activity and gene transcription. Consequently, the affected regulatory systems become functionally ineffective, leading to an increased disposition toward obesity, diabetes, and associated disorders. If females affected in that way enter reproductive age and become pregnant, by being or becoming *in graviditate* obese and/or diabetic they will expose their offspring again in a similar way to a hypercaloric/hyperglycemic environment during pre- and perinatal life that they were exposed to themselves, thereby closing a vicious intergenerative circle, leading to an acquired epigenetic disposition to obesity and diabetes in the next generation again, and so on (▶Fig. 20.6B). Such epigenetic mechanisms might, therefore, substantially contribute to the global epidemics of diabesity.

Moreover, from these experimentally and empirically founded proposals, a number of respective observations, and considering biological plausibility, it can be proposed that perinatally acquired conditions and disease dispositions may not only affect the F1 generation, but can even be transmitted over several generations of the maternal line. Because functional characteristics acquired perinatally may consequently also affect hormonal, metabolic, immunological, cardiovascular, neurobehavioral, and so forth, function and vulnerability during a pregnancy, it appears rather self-evidently that these acquired conditions may also affect subsequent generations of the maternal line simply by affecting in a respective way their developmental conditions *in utero*, again. Therefore, it is no surprise that a number of observations in humans and experimental animals have shown an intergenerative transmission of acquired conditions through the maternal line.

For instance, for many years materno-fetal transmission of acquired diabesity predisposition has been documented, accordingly. Female F1 offspring of gestationally diabetic F0 dams spontaneously develop gestational hyperglycemia. In the F2 offspring, thereby exposed *in utero*, this in turn leads to diabetogenic disturbances in later life again; therefore, an epigenetic materno-fetal transmission of increased diabetes disposition is possible through a number of generations in sequence, without any "classical" genetic predisposition (Aerts and Van Assche, 1979; Aerts et al., 1990; Dörner and Plagemann, 1994; Dörner et al., 1988; Plagemann, 2004, 2005, 2008; Plagemann, Harder, and Dudenhausen, 2008).

Even type 1 diabetes susceptibility can be acquired and intergeneratively transmitted in that way in the offspring of diabetic mothers. In maternal-side F1 and F2 offspring of gestational diabetic mother rats (F0) spontaneous gestational diabetes, basal hyperinsulinemia from birth into adulthood, indicating persisting basal overstimulation of the pancreatic B cells that predisposes for auto-immunity, and, most importantly, a severe insulin-deficient type 1–like diabetes after low dose STZ treatment were observed, in contrast to the F2 offspring of control mothers and grandmothers, respectively (Dörner and Plagemann, 1994; Dörner et al., 1988, 1990). These experimental data were confirmed by clinical and epidemiological observations, indicating transmission of increased diabetes risk, even of type 1 diabetes susceptibility, over several generations of the maternal line (Dörner and Plagemann, 1994; Dörner et al., 1987).

Remarkably, it has also been demonstrated that perinatally acquired neurobehavioral and accompanying stress–response phenotypes can be transmitted through the maternal line in a "nongenetic" way to the F2 generation (Francis and Meaney, 1999). Perinatally acquired predisposition to reproductive malfunction has also been proposed to pass through the maternal descendence (Plagemann et al., 1988). Similarly, it has been suggested that a perinatally acquired increased risk of atopy can be transmitted via altered breast milk composition to the maternal-line offspring of the next (F2) generation (Huurre et al., 2008).

Taken together, animal experiments as well as human studies speak in favor of the possibility and probability that perinatally acquired characteristics and disease dispositions, resulting from the environmental conditions during critical periods of early life, can be transmitted through the maternal line in a nonclassical, nongenetic way of epigenetic inheritance, simply by decisively determining the *in utero* and perinatal conditions of subsequent generations (▶Fig. 20.7). Obesity, diabetes, cardiovascular disorders, atopy, behavioral alterations, stress vulnerability, and so forth, have been shown to follow and are attributable to these mechanisms. An intergenerative transmission *via* several generations of the maternal line of perinatally acquired characteristics is thereby possible, without involvement of classical genetic inheritance (▶Fig. 20.7).

Most recently, however, epigenetic transmission has been proposed to occur even trough the paternal line. While materno-fetal transmission by repeated *in utero* exposures over generations to *in utero* acquired conditions seems biologically plausible, and mechanistically verified, intergenerative transmission of acquired conditions through the paternal line remains questionable, and rather unexplainable today. At least regarding the transmission of acquired diabetes risk, experimental data are controversial here (Dörner et al., 1988; Dörner and Plagemann, 1994), as well as epidemiological observations (Dörner et al., 1987). On the other hand, recent experimental and epidemiological data seem to support an epigenetic transmission of acquired metabolic risks even through the paternal line (Ng et al., 2010; Kaati, Bygren, and Edvinsson, 2002; Pentinat et al., 2010). Responsible mechanisms have not been suggested but would necessarily imply and require epigenomic modification of the germ cell line and subsequent transmission and expression of respective alterations in the offspring, phenotypically. Whether and how this may be realized remains to be verified. Interestingly enough, however, paternal body weight and diet, for example, have been suggested to affect the offspring risk over generations of developing obesity and associated metabolic disturbances in rodents (Ferguson-Smith and Patti, 2011). Obesity in humans has been shown to affect sperm quality and the likelihood of DNA damage (Kasturi, Tannir, and Brannigan, 2008), while a paternal high fat diet in rodents has been observed to affect B-cell function in the offspring, accompanied by some epigenomic alterations (Ng et al., 2010). Whether and by which epigenomic mechanisms an intergenerative transmission of acquired characteristics may pass through the paternal line remains to be established.

Howsoever, here, at the latest, considering the variety of observations on inter- and multigenerative transmission of acquired conditions, the question arises on whether these processes may influence beyond ontogenesis even phylogenesis, and evolution. And the answer appears to be yes. Because perinatal programming may affect the phenotype and health risks for generations, at least of the maternal line, an influence over generations for phylogenesis appears rather self-evidently. Moreover, all critical and basic principles of the synthetic evolutionary theory seem to be covered by the

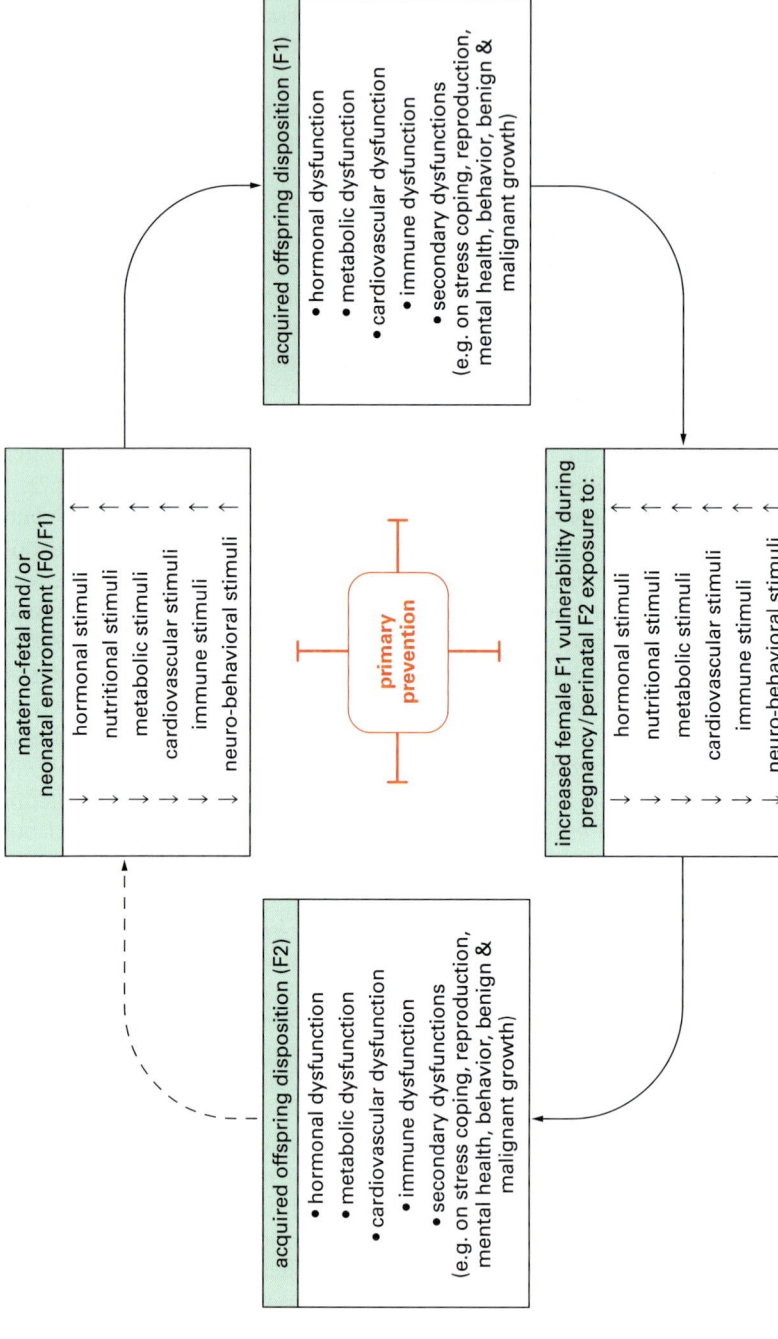

Fig. 20.7: General proposal of a vicious circle of materno-fetal induction and transmission of acquired disease dispositions over several generations, induced by altered environmental conditions and developmental challenges during critical periods of perinatal life.

processes, mechanisms, and outcomes realized through perinatal programming, that is, environment-dependent determination and selection of phenotype and genotype, affecting, realized by, and transmitted trough reproduction and, thereby, contributing to an intergenerative transmission of characteristics (Mayr, 1942).

Interpreting and considering these aspects integratively, it seems mandatory to propose that the processes of perinatal environment-dependent development and programming, representing gene – environmental interaction in a fundamental and sustainable way for generations, may contribute even to the process of natural selection and, thereby, evolution (Darwin, 1859). Consequently, however, the proposal of *inheritance of acquired conditions* (Lamarck, 1809) should be re-estimated in the light of these recent observations and mechanistic insights in perinatal programming and epigenetics. If these phenomena and mechanisms are verified, this will lead to a fundamental extension of not only developmental medicine and perinatology but also developmental biology, in general. Occasionally, implications go back to Lamarck (1809), whose concepts did originally not only decisively influence the work and theories of Darwin (1859) but also seem to gain now a mechanistic dimension, possibly leading to a renaissance of these so far unexplainable ideas and concepts.

Finally, from the previously illustrated and discussed aspects, the important question arises on practical consequences for human health, especially in terms of prevention. Worthy to note, already in 1974/1975, repeated and redefined since then continuously, general thesis and recommendations on pre- and neonatal prevention of perinatally acquired health risks have been suggested by Dörner in a pioneer manner (Dörner, 1974a, 1975, 1976, 1980, 2000). In essence and summarized (Plagemann, 2004, 2005; Plagemann and Dudenhausen, 2008), these include the following major points, recommending the avoidance and/or adequate correction/treatment during critical developmental periods of

- quantitative and/or qualitative malnutrition,
- infection and/or inadequate immune challenges,
- cardiovascular challenges and/or disorders,
- distress and/or maternal deprivation,
- exposure to drugs and disrupting medication, and
- exposure to environmental toxins, xenobiotica, radiation, and environmental chemicals.

Although appearing rather general, these seemingly very common recommendations imply a number of concrete approaches for basic research and, already today, very concrete and substantial recommendations of improvement and implementation of respective public health measures and policies in perinatal medicine (▶Fig. 20.7).

Exemplarily, once again, exposure to hyperglycemia and overfeeding, pre- as well as neonatally, have been convincingly shown to increase diabesity risk for generations. Even genetically determined risks have been shown to be decisively modified by early nutritional conditions. While beneficial rearing conditions are capable of reducing genetic burden, genetically inconspicuous traits may become pathogenic through perinatal overfeeding (Gorski et al., 2006; Levin, 2000, 2010; Reifsnyder, Churchill, and Leiter, 2000; Schmidt et al., 2000, 2001). Thus, perinatally acquired dispositions probably decisively contribute to the global increase in overweight, diabetes, metabolic syndrome, and subsequent cardiovascular diseases, which are hardly explainable by classical genetic dispositions. However, in contrast to classical genetic dispositions, accessibility to a genuine, primary prevention becomes possible here. Avoiding overweight already before conception, avoiding overweight and overfeeding during pregnancy, ensuring adequate physical activity during pregnancy, diagnosing and adequately treating glucose intolerance in pregnant women on the basis of a universal diabetes screening *in graviditate*, as well as avoiding neonatal overnutrition, especially by providing exclusive breast-feeding during the first 4 to 6 months of life, are simple as well as appropriate measures of perinatal primary prevention and, therefore, should strongly be recommended, promoted, enabled, and practiced (Dörner and Plagemann, 1994; Plagemann, 2004, 2008; Plagemann and Dudenhausen, 2010; Plagemann, Harder, and Dudenhausen, 2008; Plagemann et al., 2008).

Accordingly, a number of respective epidemiological, clinical, and experimental data have been accumulated, clearly demonstrating the possibility, effectiveness, and mechanistic explanations of preventive measures to avoid long-term malprogramming and resulting health risks. By elegant epidemiological studies it could be convincingly demonstrated that avoiding and/or adequately correcting maternal overweight (Kral et al., 2006; Smith et al., 2009) and maternal diabetes during pregnancy effectively prevents increased diabesity risk in the offspring, even of several generations, including type 1 diabetes susceptibility (Dörner et al., 1984, 1985, 1987, 2000; Dörner, Rodekamp, and Plagemann, 2008). Prevention of fetal hyperinsulinism was demonstrated to be of critical importance (Silverman et al., 1995). All of this could be confirmed in experimental models, and prevention of hormonal malorganization of hypothalamic regulatory systems has been shown in a variety of approaches to be crucial for preventive effects (Bouret et al., 2004; Davidowa, Ziska, and Plagemann, 2006; Franke et al., 2005; Harder et al., 2001a, 2003; Vickers et al., 2005). Accordingly, prevention of neonatal overfeeding has been demonstrated to be of long-term benefit for metabolic health, both by clinical–epidemiological studies (Dörner et al., 1977, 2008; Harder et al., 2005; Plagemann and Harder, 2005b, 2011) as well as mechanistically by respective experimental models (Fahrenkrog et al., 2004; Gorski et al., 2006; Patterson et al., 2010). Similar preventive effects and mechanisms should be regarded concerning cardiovascular, immune, neurobehavioral, and so forth, challenges and dysfunctions, including reproduction, cognition, behavior, and even malignant growth (▶Fig. 20.7).

Beyond famine in the third world and developing countries, absurdly, obesity is probably the most challenging health problem in the developed world at the beginning of the 21st century. Overweight is the most important cause of the metabolic syndrome, including a number of accompanying and subsequent health problems. Approximately one-third of adult humans in the highly developed Western countries are suffering from the metabolic syndrome and its components. Accordingly, about one-third of women at reproductive age are overweight, while surely more than 10% are suffering from gestational diabetes. However, most gestational diabetics are not adequately treated, with deleterious consequences for the health of mother and child, simply for the fact that no universal screening to diagnose glucose intolerance is considered and performed according to respective public health policies. Considering, on the other hand, that the overall costs of obesity have been estimated to exceed US$ 140 billion per year in the United States in 2008 (Finkelstein et al., 2009), while the sex- and age-adjusted risk of developing diabetes and obesity was found to be increased up to 7-fold in offspring of mothers with diabetes during pregnancy (Claussen et al., 2008; Dabelea et al., 2000;

Pettitt et al., 1983; Plagemann et al., 1997a, 1997b; Silverman et al., 1995; Weiss et al., 2000), the potential dimensions resulting from disadvantageous developmental conditions during critical periods of early life become impressively obvious, considering only this very prominent and challenging entity and example. Chances and challenges of perinatal medicine by implementing and providing primary preventive measures become exemplarily clear here.

Summarizing, *perinatal programming* is a critical and essential part of ontogenesis, affecting health and disease risks for the whole life span. Perinatally acquired characteristics can even be transmitted to subsequent generations. In biomedicine, this opens enormous chances and challenges of a genuine perinatal prophylaxis to the benefit of individuals and societies. In a politically sensible, responsible, and even pragmatic way this should start to be realized now, on the basis of an integrative interdisciplinary evaluation and estimation of relevant perinatal risk factors acting globally during perinatal life, for example, famine, overfeeding, infection, exposure to xenobiotica and environmental toxins, materno-fetal distress, and so forth. This could and should immediately be practically reflected, concerning the fate of future generations.

Already in the 1980s, it was paradigmatically shown that the long-term deleterious consequences of exposure to a diabetic intrauterine environment may run over several generations of the maternal line - and can be prevented. From these data, accompanied by respective experimental observations, in 1987 we proposed that "an epigenetic transmission of acquired conditions appears to be possible over several generations (epigenetic transmission rule)" (Dörner et al., 1987) and, most of all, appears to be accessible to primary prevention by providing an improved perinatal environment and/or adequate correction and normalization of perinatal developmental conditions. Meanwhile, these early proposals seem to have been verified, confirmed, extended in a variety of important aspects, and even generalized.

20.8 Synopsis

Today, the field of perinatal programming prospers enormously, and international research activities are increasing rapidly. Epidemiological, clinical, and experimental studies from a number of well- and newly established working groups, departments, and institutions nearly worldwide are aiming to identify long-term health risks resulting from the prenatal and neonatal environmental conditions. Many disadvantageous or even harmful conditions have been identified, spanning, for example, from pre- and periconceptional maternal nutritional and body weight dysbalance through materno-fetal exposure to stress, infection, xenobiotica, and cardiovascular dysregulation up to influences of peripartal and neonatal medication, rearing conditions, and mal- or overnutrition. Increased offspring risk may result, to develop metabolic, cardiovascular, allergic, mental, reproductive, and even malignant diseases, especially those that are related to the modern Western life style. All this appears to be a fundamental mechanism and reflection of gene–environment-dependent phenotype establishment during critical periods of early biocybernetogenesis and, respectively, development-dependent determination of disease risks, which may occur in addition to, interacting with, or even independent of classical genetic dispositions (▶Fig. 20.8).

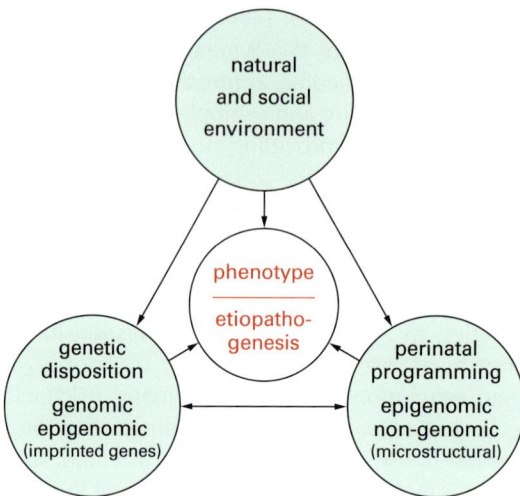

Fig. 20.8: Proposal of a fundamental biomedical paradigm of the determination of phenotype and etiopathogenesis (according and modified to Plagemann, 2004, 2005, 2008, 2010).

Accordingly, it appears legitimate and necessary to propose a supplementation of the general etiopathology, which should include environment-dependent determination of the functional phenotype during critical periods of life as a third, distinct aspect and burden in the determination of diseases and disease dispositions, beyond and in addition to environmental and genetic factors acting *per se* throughout life (Plagemann, 2004, 2005, 2006, 2008, 2010) (►Fig. 20.8). Most importantly, in contrast to classical genetic diseases and dispositions, resulting from mutations and so forth, here we may find chances of implementing a primary, genuine prevention for the long term through detecting, avoiding, and/or adequately treating relevant exposures and disturbances during critical developmental periods. This unravels important new challenges for perinatal medicine and health policies, which should be seized to the benefit of future generations. Finally, already today it can be predicted that these and further findings in developmental biomedicine, epigenetics, and environment-dependent programming of genotype and phenotype will probably revolutionize our classical view on ontogenesis, phylogenesis, and even evolution.

Acknowledgment

The concepts, ideas, and hypotheses cursorily formulated here are a result of years of epidemiological, clinical, experimental, and theoretical–conceptual research work. It is my urgent desire to give warm thanks to all who have accompanied me on the way and decisively contributed to it. I am deeply indebted and would like to express my particular gratitude to my academic teacher, Günter Dörner, who introduced the topic to me, and I would like to thank him for the early scientific "programming" that I experienced essentially by him. I am particularly grateful to Dr. Thomas Harder, MScE, for years of both trustful and indispensible scientific cooperation and support. K. Melchior, U. Richter (†), E. Rodekamp, J.C. Rückert, K. Schellong, U. Schramme, J. Stupin, and T. Ziska are gratefully acknowledged for decisive contributions to our joint work on a vision – against all odds here at the Charité in Berlin. I would like to cordially thank L. Aerts, H. Davidowa, R. Kohlhoff, I. Schmidt, B. Tzschentke, and F. A. Van Assche for years of intensive, productive, and friendly collaboration. Special thanks must go to Joachim W. Dudenhausen, who insisted in trusting in our work and consequently enabled and supported it under worsening conditions. Underlying studies were continuously supported especially by the German Research Foundation (Deutsche Forschungsgemeinschaft, DFG) and by the German Federal Ministry of Education and Research since 1992.

References

Aerts L, Van Assche FA. Is gestational diabetes an acquired condition? *J Dev Physiol* 1979;1: 219–25.

Aerts L, Holemans K, Van Assche FA. Maternal diabetes during pregnancy: Consequences for the offspring. *Diabetes Metab Rev* 1990;6: 147–67.

Aerts L, Vercruysse L, Van Assche FA. The endocrine pancreas in virgin and pregnant offspring of diabetic pregnant rats. *Diab Res Clin Pract* 1997;38: 9–19.

Andria ML, Simon EJ. Localization of promotor elements in the human mu-opioid receptor gene and regulation by DNA methylation. *Mol Brain Res* 1999;70: 54–65.

Ashby WR. Principles of the self-organizing dynamic system. *J Gen Psychol* 1947;37: 125–8.

Bhattacharya SK, Ramchandani S, Cervoni N, Szyf M. A mammalian protein with specific demethylase activity for mCpG DNA. *Nature* 1999;397: 579–83.

Bihoreau MT, Ktorza A, Kinebanyan MF, Picon L. Impaired glucose homeostasis in adult rats from hyperglycaemic mothers. *Diabetes* 1986;35: 979–84.

Bird A, Wolffe AP. Methylation-induced repression – belts, braces, and chromatin. *Cell* 1999;99: 451–4.

Bogdarina I, Welham S, King PJ, Burns SP, Clark AJ. Epigenetic modification of the renin-angiotensin system in the fetal programming of hypertension. *Circ Res* 2007;100: 520–6.

Bottazzo GF, Bosi E, Todd J, Belfiore A, Pujol-Borvell R. Inappropriate HLA class II expression on epithelial cells: Basis for new interpretation of HLA association in autoimmune endocrine disorders. In: Farid NR, ed. *Immunogenetics of Endocrine Disorders.* London: Alan R Liss Inc; 1988: 133–43.

Boullu-Ciocca S, Dutour A, Guillaume V, Achard V, Oliver C, Grino M. Postnatal diet-induced obesity in rats upregulates systemic and adipose tissue glucocorticoid metabolism during development and in adulthood: its relationship with the metabolic syndrome. *Diabetes* 2005;54: 197–203.

Bouret SG, Draper SJ, Simerly RB. Trophic action of leptin on hypothalamic neurons that regulate feeding. *Science* 2004;304: 108–10.

Bouret SG. Neurodevelopmental actions of leptin. *Brain Res* 2010;350: 2–9.

Burchfield SR. The stress response: a new perspective. *Psychosomatic Med* 1979;41: 661–72.

Burdge GC, Slater-Jefferies J, Torrens C, Phillips ES, Hanson MA, Lillycrop KA. Dietary protein restriction of pregnant rats in the F0 generation induces altered methylation of hepatic gene promoters in the adult male offspring in the F1 and F2 generations. *Br J Nutr* 2007;97: 435–9.

Catalano PM. Obesity and pregnancy – the propagation of a viscous cycle? *J Clin Endocrinol Metab* 2003;88: 3505–6.

Catalano P, Presley L, Minium J, De Mouzon SH. Fetuses of obese mothers develop insulin resistance in utero. *Diabetes Care* 2009;32: 1076–80.

Cha CJ, Gelardi NL, Oh W. Accelerated growth and abnormal glucose tolerance in young female rats exposed to fetal hyperinsulinemia. *Pediatr Res* 1987;21: 83–7.

Champagne FA, Weaver IC, Diorio J, Dymov S, Szyf M, Meaney MJ. Maternal care associated with methylation of the estrogen receptor-alpha1b promoter and estrogen receptor-alpha expression in the medial preoptic area of female offspring. *Endocrinology* 2006;147: 2909–15.

Champagne FA, Meaney MJ. Transgenerational effects of social environment on variations in maternal care and behavioural response to novelty. *Behav Neurosci* 2007;121: 1353–63.

Chiang EP, Wang YC, Chen WW, Tang FY. Effects of insulin and glucose on cellular metabolic fluxes in homocysteine transsulfuration, remethylation, S-adenosylmethionine synthesis, and global deoxyribonucleic acid methylation. *J Clin Endocrinol Metab* 2009;94: 1017–25.

Clark SJ, Harrison J, Frommer M. CpNpG methylation in mammalian cells. *Nat Genet* 1995;10: 20–7.

Claussen TD, Mathiesen ER, Hansen T, et al. High prevalence of type 2 diabetes and pre-diabetes in adult offspring of women with gestational diabetes mellitus or type 1 diabetes: the role of intrauterine hyperglycemia. *Diabetes Care* 2008;31: 340–6.

Claussen TD, Mathiesen ER, Hansen T, et al. Overweight and the metabolic syndrome in adult offspring of women with diet-treated gestational diabetes mellitus or type 1 diabetes. *J Clin Endocrinol Metab* 2009; 94: 2464–70.

Cooper DN, Krawczak M. Cytosine methylation and the fate of CpG dinucleotides in vertebrate genomes. *Hum Gen* 1989;83: 181–8.

Crowther NJ, Trusler J, Cameron N, Toman M, Gray IP. Relation between weight gain and beta-cell secretory activity and non-esterified fatty acid production in 7-year-old african children: results from the birth to ten study. *Diabetologia* 2000;43: 978–85.

Dabelea D, Hanson RL, Lindsay RS, et al. Intrauterine exposure to diabetes conveys risks for type 2 diabetes and obesity: a study of discordant sibships. *Diabetes* 2000;49: 2208–11.

Daenzer M, Ortmann S, Klaus S, Metges CC. Prenatal high protein exposure decreases energy expenditure and increases adiposity in young rats. *J Nutr* 2002;132: 142–4.

Darwin C. *On the Origin of Species by Means of Natural Selection, or the Preservation of Favoured Races in the Struggle for Life*. London: John Murray; 1859.

Davidowa H, Plagemann A. Decreased inhibition by leptin of hypothalamic arcuate neurons in neonatally overfed young rats. *Neuroreport* 2000;11: 2795–8.

Davidowa H, Plagemann A. Inhibition by insulin of hypothalamic VMN neurons in rats overweight due to postnatal overfeeding. *Neuroreport* 2001;12: 3201–4.

Davidowa H, Li Y, Plagemann A. Altered responses to orexigenic (AGRP, MCH) and anorexigenic (alpha-MSH, CART) neuropeptides of paraventricular hypothalamic neurons in early postnatally overfed rats. *Eur J Neurosci* 2003;18: 613–21.

Davidowa H, Ziska T, Plagemann A. GABA receptor antagonists prevent abnormalities in leptin, insulin and amylin actions on paraventricular hypothalamic neurons of overweight rats. *Eur J Neurosci* 2006;23: 1248–54.

Davidowa H, Plagemann A. Insulin resistance of hypothalamic arcuate neurons in neonatally overfed rats. *Neuroreport* 2007;18: 521–4.

Dewey KG, Heinig MJ, Nommsen LA, Peerson JM, Lönnerdal B. Breast-fed infants are leaner than formula-fed infants at 1 y of age: the DARLING study. *Am J Clin Nutr* 1993;57: 140–5.

Ding Y, Lv J, Mao C, et al. High-salt diet during pregnancy and angiotensin-related cardiac changes. *J Hypertens* 2010;28: 1290–7.

Dörner G. Environment-dependent brain differentiation and fundamental processes of life. *Acta Biol Med Germ* 1974a;33: 129–48.

Dörner G. Problems and terminology of functional teratology. *Acta Biol Med Germ* 1974b;34: 1093–5.

Dörner G. Perinatal hormone levels and brain organization. In: Stumpf W, Grant LD, eds. *Anatomical Neuroendocrinology*. Basel: Karger; 1975: 245–52.

Dörner G. *Hormones and Brain Differentiation*. Amsterdam, Oxford, New York: Elsevier; 1976.

Dörner G, Mohnike A. Further evidence for a predominantly maternal transmission of maturity-onset type diabetes. *Endokrinologie* 1976;68: 121–4.

Dörner G, Grychtolyk H, Julitz M. Überernährung in den ersten drei Lebensmonaten als entscheidender Risikofaktor für die Entwicklung von Fettsucht und Folgeerkrankungen. *Dt Gesundhw* 1977;32: 6–9.

Dörner G. Die Ontogenese des neuroendokrinen Systems als kinetischer Prozess. *Nova Acta Leopoldina Neue Folge* 1980;51: 279–91.

Dörner G, Steindel E, Thoelke H, Schliack V. Evidence for a decreasing prevalence of diabetes mellitus in childhood apparently produced by prevention of hyperinsulinism in the foetus and newborn. *Exp Clin Endocrinol* 1984;84: 134–42.

Dörner G, Steindel E, Kohlhoff R, et al. Further evidence for a preventive therapy of insulin- dependent diabetes mellitus in the offspring by avoiding maternal hyperglycaemia during pregnancy. *Exp Clin Endocrinol* 1985;86: 129–40.

Dörner G, Plagemann A, Reinagel H. Familial diabetes aggregation in type I diabetics: gestational diabetes an apparent risk factor for increased diabetes susceptibility in the offspring. *Exp Clin Endocrinol* 1987;89: 84–90.

Dörner G, Plagemann A, Rückert JC, et al. Teratogenetic maternofoetal transmission and prevention of diabetes susceptibility. *Exp Clin Endocrinol* 1988;91: 247–58.

Dörner G, Köhler E, Friedrichs J, Götz F, Rohde W, Kürschner U. Increased cell-mediated cytotoxicity against beta-cells in streptozotocin-treated offspring of mother animals with gestational hyperglycaemia. *Exp Clin Endocrinol* 1990;95: 4–10.

Dörner G, Plagemann A. Perinatal hyperinsulinism as possible predisposing factor for diabetes mellitus, obesity and enhanced cardiovascular risk in later life. *Horm Metab Res* 1994;26: 213–21.

Dörner G. Ten ontogenetic theses for promotion of health and primary prevention of important diseases by a prenatal and early postnatal neuro-endocrine-immune prophylaxis. *Neuro Endocrinol Lett* 2000;21: 265–7.

Dörner G, Plagemann A, Neu A, Rosenbauer J. Gestational diabetes as risk factor for type I childhood-onset diabetes in the offspring. *Neuroendocrinol Lett* 2000;21: 355–9.

Dörner G, Rodekamp E, Plagemann A. Maternal deprivation and overnutrition in early postnatal life and their primary prevention: historical reminiscence of an "ecologic experiment" in Germany. *Hum Ontogenet* 2008;2: 51–9.

Douwes J, Cheng S, Travier N, et al. Farm exposure in utero may protect against asthma, hay fever and eczema. *Eur Respir J* 2008;32: 603–11.

Dubos R, Savage D, Schaedler R. Biological freudianism: lasting effects of environmental influences. *Pediatrics* 1966;38: 789–800.

Eriksson JG, Forsén T, Winter PD, Osmond C, Barker DJP. Catch-up growth in childhood and death from coronary heart disease: longitudinal study. *BMJ* 1999;318: 427–31.

Fahrenkrog S, Harder T, Stolaczyk E, et al. Cross-fostering to diabetic rat dams affects early development of mediobasal hypothalamic nuclei regulating food-intake, body weight, and metabolism. *J Nutr* 2004;134: 648–654.

Ferguson-Smith AC, Patti ME. You are what your dad ate. *Cell Metab* 2011;13: 115–7.

Fewtrell MS, Doherty C, Cole TJ, Stafford M, Hales CN, Lucas A. Effects of size at birth, gestational age and early growth in preterm infants on glucose and insulin concentrations at 9–12 years. *Diabetologia* 2000;43: 714–7.

Finkelstein EA, Trogdon JG, Cohen JW, Dietz W. Annual medical spending attributable to obesity: payer- and service-specific estimates. *Health Aff* (Millwood) 2009;28: w822–31.

Forsén T, Eriksson JG, Tuomilehto J, Osmond C, Barker DJP. Growth in utero and during childhood among women who develop coronary heart disease: longitudinal study. *BMJ* 1999;319: 1403–7.

Francis DD, Meaney MJ. Maternal care and the development of stress response. *Curr Opin Neurobiol* 1999;9: 128–34.

Franke K, Harder T, Aerts L, et al. Programming of orexigenic and anorexigenic hypothalamic neurons in offspring of treated and untreated diabetic mother rats. *Brain Res* 2005;1031: 276–83.

Freinkel N, Metzger, BE. Pregnancy as a tissue culture experience: the critical implications of maternal metabolism for fetal development. In: *Pregnancy Metabolism, Diabetes, and the Fetus.* Ciba Foundation Symposium 63. Amsterdam: Excerpta Medica; 1979: 3–23.

Freinkel N. Of pregnancy and progeny. Banting lecture 1980. *Diabetes* 1980;29: 1023–35.

Gdalevich M, Mimouoni D, David M, Mimouni M. Breast-feeding and the onset of atopic dermatitis in childhood: a systematic review and meta-analysis of prospective studies. *J Am Acad Dermatol* 2001;45: 520–7.

Gill-Randall R, Adams D, Ollerton RL, Lewis M, Alcolado JC. Type 2 diabetes mellitus – genes or intrauterine environment? An embryo transfer paradigm in rats. *Diabetologia* 2004;47: 1354–9.

Gluckman PD, Hanson ME. Living with the past: evolution, development, and patterns of disease. *Science* 2004;305: 1733–6.

Gluckman PD, Hanson MA. The conceptual basis for the developmental origins of health and disease. In: Gluckman PD, Hanson MA, eds. *Developmental Origins of Health and Disease.* Cambridge: University Press; 2006: 33–50.

Gluckman PD, Hanson MA. *Mismatch: The Lifestyle Diseases Timebomb.* Oxford: University Press; 2008.

Gluckman PD, Hanson MA, Cooper C, Thornburg KL. Effect of in utero and early-life conditions on adult health and disease. *N Engl J Med* 2008;359: 61–73.

Gorski J, Dunn-Meynell AA, Hartman TG, Levin BE. Postnatal environment overrides genetic and prenatal factors influencing offspring obesity and insulin resistance. *Am J Physiol* 2006;291: R768–78.

Haeckel E. *Generelle Morphologie der Organismen. Allgemeine Grundzüge der organischen Formen-Wissenschaft, mechanisch begründet durch die von Charles Darwin reformirte Descendenz-Theorie.* Vol 2. Berlin: G. Reimer; 1866.

Hales CN, Barker DJP. Type 2 (non-insulin-dependent) diabetes mellitus: the thrifty phenotype hypothesis. *Diabetologia* 1992;35: 595–601.

Harder T, Plagemann A, Rohde W, Dörner G. Syndrome X-like alterations in adult female rats due to neonatal insulin treatment. *Metabolism* 1998;47: 855–62.

Harder T, Aerts L, Franke K, Van Bree R, Van Assche FA, Plagemann A. Pancreatic islet transplantation in diabetic pregnant rats prevents acquired malformation of the ventromedial hypothalamic nucleus in their offspring. *Neurosci Lett* 2001a;299: 85–8.

Harder T, Kohlhoff R, Dörner G, Rohde W, Plagemann A. Perinatal "programming" of insulin resistance in childhood: Critical impact of neonatal insulin and low birth weight in a risk population. *Diabetic Med* 2001b;18: 634–9.

Harder T, Franke K, Fahrenkrog S, et al. Prevention by maternal pancreatic islet transplantation of hypothalamic malformation in offspring of diabetic mother rats is already detectable at weaning. *Neurosci Lett* 2003;352: 163–6.

Harder T, Bergmann R, Kallischnigg G, Plagemann A. Duration of breastfeeding and risk of overweight: a meta-analysis. *Am J Epidemiol* 2005;162: 397–403.

Harder T, Rodekamp E, Schellong K, Dudenhausen JW, Plagemann A. Birth weight and subsequent risk of type 2 diabetes: a meta-analysis. *Am J Epidemiol* 2007a;165: 849–57.

Harder T, Schellong K, Stupin J, Dudenhausen JW, Plagemann A. Where is the evidence that low birthweight leads to obesity? (letter) *Lancet* 2007b;369: 1859.

Harder T, Plagemann A, Harder A. Birth weight and subsequent risk of childhood primary brain tumors: a meta-analysis. *Am J Epidemiol* 2008;168: 366–73.

Harder T, Plagemann A, Harder A. Birth weight and risk of neuroblastoma: a meta-analysis. *Int J Epidemiol* 2010;39: 746–56.

Heidel E, Plagemann A, Davidowa H. Increased response to NPY of hypothalamic VMN neurons in postnatally overfed juvenile rats. *Neuroreport* 1999;10: 1827–31.

Huurre A, Laitinen K, Rautava S, Korkeamäki M, Isolauri E. Impact of maternal atopy and probiotic supplementation during pregnancy on infant sensitization: a double-blind placebo-controlled study. *Clin Exp Allergy* 2008;38: 1342–8.

Jaenisch R. DNA methylation and imprinting: why bother? *Trends Gen* 1997;13: 323–9.

Kaati G, Bygren LO, Edvinsson S. Cardiovascular and diabetes mortality determined by nutrition during parents' and grandparents' slow growth period. *Eur J Hum Gent* 2002;10: 682–8.

Kasturi SS, Tannir J, Brannigan RE. The metabolic syndrome and male infertility. *J Androl* 2008;29: 251–9.

Kirk SL, Samuelsson AM, Argenton M, et al. Maternal obesity induced by diet in rats permanently influences central processes regulating food intake in offspring. *PLoS One* 2009;4: 5870.

Knittle JL, Hirsch J. Effect of early nutrition on the development of rat epididymal fat pads: cellularity and metabolism. *J Clin Invest* 1968;47: 2091–8.

Kohlhoff R, Dörner G. Perinatal hyperinsulinism and perinatal obesity as risk factors for hyperinsulinaemia in later life. *Exp Clin Endocrinol* 1990;96: 105–8.

Kral JG, Biron S, Simard S, et al. Large maternal weight loss from obesity surgery prevents transmission of obesity to children who were followed for 2 to 18 years. *Pediatrics* 2006;118:e1644–9.

Lamarck JB. *Philosophie Zoologique, ou exposition des Considérations relatives à l'histoire naturelle des Animaux; à la diversité de leur organisation et des facultés qu'ils en obtiennent.* Paris: Dentu et l'Auteur; 1809.

Larsen F, Gundersen G, Lopez R, Prydz H. CpG islands as gene markers in the human genome. *Genomics* 1992;13:1095–7.

Law JA, Jacobson SE. Establishing, maintaining and modifying DNA methylation patterns in plants and animals. *Nat Rev Genet* 2010;11: 204–20.

Levin BE. The obesity epidemic: metabolic imprinting on genetically susceptible neural circuits. *Obes Res* 2000;8: 342–7.

Levin BE. Developmental gene x environment interactions affecting systems regulating energy homeostasis and obesity. *Front Neuroendocrinol* 2010;31: 270–83.

Liu D, Diorio J, Tannenbaum B, et al. Maternal care, hippocampal glucocorticoid receptors, and hypothalamic-pituitary-adrenal responses to stress. *Science* 1997;277: 1659–62.

Lorenz K. Der Kumpan in der Umwelt des Vogels: Der Artgenosse als auslösendes Moment sozialer Verhaltensweisen. *Journal für Ornithologie* 1935;1: S83.

Lucas A, Fewtrell MS, Cole TJ. Fetal origins of adult disease – the hypothesis revisited. *BMJ* 1999;319: 245–9.

Mayr E. *Systematics and the Origin of Species from a Viewpoint of a Zoologist.* Boston: Harvard University Press; 1942.

McCance DR, Pettitt DJ, Hanson RL, Jacobsson LTH, Knowler WC, Bennett PH. Birth weight and non-insulin dependent diabetes: thrifty genotype, thrifty phenotype, or surviving small baby genotype? *BMJ* 1994;308: 942–5.

McGowan PO, Szyf M. Environmental epigenomics: understanding the effects of parental care on the epigenome. *Essays Biochem* 2010;48: 275–87.

Meaney MJ, Diorio J, Francis D, et al. Early environmental regulation of forebrain glucocorticoid receptor gene expression : implications for adrenocortical responses to stress. *Dev Neurosci* 1996;18: 49–72.

Monteiro POA, Victora CG. Rapid growth in infancy and childhood and obesity in later life – a systematic review. *Obes Rev* 2005;6: 143–54.

Moura AS, De Souza CFJ, De Freitas MPC, De Sa CCNF. Insulin secretion impairment and insulin sensitivity improvement in adult rats undernourished during early lactation. *Res Comm Mol Pathol Pharmacol* 1997;96: 179–92.

Neitzke U, Harder T, Plagemann A. Intrauterine growth restriction and developmental programming of the metabolic syndrome: a critical appraisal. *Microcirculation* 2011;18: 304–11.

Nerup J, Mandrup-Poulsen T, Molvig J, Helquist S, Wogensen L, Egeberg J. Mechanisms of pancreatic ß-cell destruction in type I diabetes. *Diabetes Care* 1988;11 Suppl 1: 16–23.

Newell-Price J, King P, Clark AJL. The CpG island promotor of the human proopiomelanocortin gene is methylated in nonexpressing normal tissue and tumors and represses expression. *Mol Endocrinol* 2001;15: 338–48.

Ng SF, Lin RC, Laybutt DR, Barres R, Owens JA, Morris MJ. Chronic high-fat diet in fathers programs beta-cell dysfunction in female rat offspring. *Nature* 2010;467: 963–6.

Nwaru BI, Erkkola M, Ahonen S, et al. Age at the introduction of solid foods during the first year and allergic sensitization at age 5 years. *Pediatrics* 2010;125: 50–9.

Oh W, Gelardi NL, Cha CJM. The cross-generation effect of neonatal macrosomia in rat pups of streptozotocin-induced diabetes. *Pediatr Res* 1991;29: 606–10.

Ozanne SE, Hales CN. Lifespan: catch-up growth and obesity in male mice. *Nature* 2004;427: 411–2.

Patterson CM, Bouret SG, Park S, Irani BG, Dunn-Meynell AA, Levin BE. Large litter rearing enhances leptin sensitivity and protects selectively bred diet-induced obese rats from becoming obese. *Endocrinology* 2010;151: 4270–9.

Pedersen J, Bojsen-Moller B, Poulsen H. Blood sugar in newborn infants of diabetic mothers. *Acta Endocrinol* 1954;15: 33–52.

Pentinat T, Ramon-Krauel M, Cebria J, Diaz R, Jimenez-Chillaron JC. Transgenerational inheritance of glucose intolerance in a mouse model of neonatal overnutrition. *Endocrinology* 2010;151: 5617–23.

Petry CJ, Ozanne SE, Wang CL, Hales CN. Early protein restriction and obesity independently induce hypertension in 1-year-old rats. *Clin Sci* 1997;93: 147–52.

Pettitt DJ, Baird HR, Aleck KA, Bennett PA, Knowler PC. Excessive obesity in offspring of Pima Indian women with diabetes during pregnancy. *N Engl J Med* 1983;308: 242–5.

Plagemann A, Tönjes R, Dörner G. Impairment of sexual behaviour in female rats with impaired glucose tolerance due to streptozotocin treatment of their maternal grandmothers. *Exp Clin Endocrinol* 1988;91: 369–72.

Plagemann A, Heidrich I, Götz F, Rohde W, Dörner G. Lifelong enhanced diabetes susceptibility and obesity after temporary intrahypothalamic hyperinsulinism during brain organization. *Exp Clin Endocrinol* 1992a;99: 91–5.

Plagemann A, Heidrich I, Götz F, Rohde W, Dörner G. Obesity and enhanced diabetes and cardiovascular risk in adult rats due to early postnatal overfeeding. *Exp Clin Endocrinol* 1992b;99: 154–8.

Plagemann A, Harder T, Kohlhoff R, Rohde W, Dörner G. Overweight and obesity in infants of mothers with long-term insulin-dependent diabetes or gestational diabetes. *Int J Obes* 1997a;21: 451–6.

Plagemann A, Harder T, Kohlhoff R, Rohde W, Dörner G. Glucose tolerance and insulin secretion in children of mothers with pregestational insulin-dependent diabetes mellitus or gestational diabetes. *Diabetologia* 1997b;40: 1094–1100.

Plagemann A, Harder T, Rake A, et al. Hypothalamic insulin and neuropeptide Y in the offspring of gestational diabetic mother rats. *NeuroReport* 1998;9: 4069–73.

Plagemann A, Harder T, Janert U, et al. Malformations of hypothalamic nuclei in hyperinsulinaemic offspring of gestational diabetic mother rats. *Dev Neurosci* 1999a;21: 58–67.

Plagemann A, Harder T, Melchior K, Rake A, Rohde W, Dörner G. Elevation of hypothalamic neuropeptide Y-neurons in adult offspring of diabetic mother rats. *NeuroReport* 1999b;10: 3211–6.

Plagemann A, Harder T, Rake A, et al. Perinatal increase of hypothalamic insulin, acquired malformation of hypothalamic galaninergic neurons, and syndrome X-like alterations in adulthood of neonatally overfed rats. *Brain Res* 1999c;836: 146–55.

Plagemann A, Harder T, Rake A, et al. Observations on the orexigenic hypothalamic neuropeptide Y-system in neonatally overfed weanling rats. *J Neuroendocrinol* 1999d;11: 541–6.

Plagemann A. Fetale Programmierung und Funktionelle Teratologie: Ausgewählte Mechanismen und Konsequenzen. In: Gortner L, Dudenhausen JW, eds. *Vorgeburtliches Wachstum und gesundheitliches Schicksal: Störungen-Risiken-Konsequenzen*. Frankfurt/Main: Med. Verl.-Ges. Umwelt & Medizin; 2001: 65–78.

Plagemann A. "Fetal programming" and "functional teratogenesis": on epigenetic mechanisms and prevention of perinatally acquired lasting health risks. *J Perinat Med* 2004;32: 297–305.

Plagemann A, Rodekamp E, Harder T. To: Hales CN, Ozanne SE (2003) For Debate: Fetal and early postnatal growth restriction lead to diabetes, the metabolic syndrome and renal failure. *Diabetologia* 46:1013–1019 (letter). *Diabetologia* 2004;47: 1334–5.

Plagemann A. Fetale Programmierung und Funktionelle Teratologie. In: Ganten D, Ruckpaul K, Wauer R, eds. *Molekulare Medizin Bd.14: Molekularmedizinische Grundlagen von fetalen und neonatalen Erkrankungen.* Berlin, Heidelberg, New York: Springer; 2005: 325–44.

Plagemann A, Harder T. Premature birth and insulin resistance (letter). *N Engl J Med* 2005a;352: 939–40.

Plagemann A, Harder T. Breast feeding and the risk of obesity and related metabolic diseases in the child. Metabolic Syndrome 2005b;3: 192–202.

Plagemann A. Perinatal nutrition and hormone-dependent programming of food intake. *Horm Res* 2006;65 Suppl 3: 83–9.

Plagemann, A. A matter of insulin: Developmental programming of body weight regulation. *J Mat Fet Med* 2008;21: 143–8.

Plagemann A, Dudenhausen JW. Weichenstellung im Mutterleib. *Humboldt-Spektrum* 2008;1:1–8.

Plagemann A, Harder T, Dudenhausen JW. The diabetic pregnancy, macrosomia, and perinatal programming. In: Barker DJP, Bergmann R, eds. *The First 24 Months. A Window of Opportunity.* Nestle Nutrition Workshop Series 61. Basel: Karger; 2008: 91–102.

Plagemann A, Harder T, Rodekamp E, Schellong K, Stupin J, Dudenhausen JW. Ernährung und frühe kindliche Prägung. In: Deutsche Gesellschaft für Ernährung, ed. *Ernährungsbericht.* Mekkenheim: DGE-Medienservice; 2008: 271–300.

Plagemann A, Harder T. Birth weight and risk of type 2 diabetes. (letter) *JAMA* 2009a;301: 1540.

Plagemann A, Harder T. Hormonal programming in perinatal life – leptin and beyond. (Commentary) *Br J Nutr* 2009b;101: 151–2.

Plagemann A, Harder T, Brunn M, et al. Hypothalamic POMC promoter methylation becomes altered by early overfeeding: An epigenetic model of obesity and the metabolic syndrome. *J Physiol* 2009;587: 4963–76.

Plagemann A. Toward a unifying concept on "perinatal programming." *J Perinat Med* 2010; Suppl. 1, doi: 10.1515/JPM.2010.199.

Plagemann A, Dudenhausen JW, eds. *Adipositas als Risiko in der Perinatalmedizin.* München: Springer; 2010.

Plagemann A, Roepke K, Harder T, et al. Epigenetic malprogramming of the insulin receptor promoter due to developmental overfeeding. *J Perinat Med* 2010;38: 393–400.

Plagemann A, Harder T. Fuel-mediated teratogenesis and breastfeeding (editorial). *Diabetes Care* 2011;34: 779–81.

Razin A, Shemer R. DNA methylation in early development. *Hum Mol Gen* 1995;4: 1751–5.

Rees WD, Hay SM, Brown DS, Antipatis C, Palmer RM. Maternal protein deficiency causes hypermethylation of DNA in livers of rat fetuses. *J Nutr* 2000;130: 1821–6.

Reifsnyder PC, Churchill G, Leiter EH. Maternal environment and genotype interact to establish diabesity in mice. *Genome Res* 2000;10: 1568–78.

Rooth G. Increase in birthweight: a unique biological event and an obstetrical problem. *Eur J Obstet Gynecol Reprod Biol* 2003;106: 86–7.

Saint-Hilaire IG. *Histoire générale et particulière des anomalies de l'organisation chez l'homme et le animaux ou traité de tératologie.* Brussels: Baillière, Haumann and Cattoir; 1832–1837.

Schmidt I, Schoelch C, Ziska T, Schneider D, Simon E, Plagemann A. Interaction of genetic and environmental programming of the leptin system and of obesity disposition. *Physiol Genomics* 2000;3: 113–20.

Schmidt I, Fritz A, Schoelch C, Schneider D, Simon E, Plagemann A. The effect of leptin treatment on the development of obesity in overfed suckling Wistar rats. *Int J Obes* 2001;25: 1168–74.

Silverman BL, Rizzo T, Green OC, Metzger BE. Long-term prospective evaluation of offspring of diabetic mothers. *Diabetes* 1991;40: 121–5.

Silverman BL, Metzger BE, Cho NH, Loeb CA. Impaired glucose tolerance in adolescent offspring of diabetic mothers. *Diabetes Care* 1995;18: 611–7.

Smith J, Cinaflone K, Biron S, et al. Effects of maternal surgical weight loss in mothers on intergenerational transmission of obesity. *J Clin Endocrinol Metab* 2009;94: 4275–83.

Spemann H, Mangold H. Über Induktion von Embryonalanlagen durch Implantation artfremder Organisatoren. *Arch Mikr Anat Entw* 1924;100: 599–638.

Spencer SJ, Tilbrook A. Neonatal overfeeding alters adult anxiety and stress responsiveness. *Psychoneuroendocrinology* 2009;34:1133–43.

Stanner SA, Bulmer K, Andres C, et al. Does malnutrition in utero determine diabetes and coronary heart disease in adulthood? Results from the Leningrad siege study, a cross sectional study. *BMJ* 1997;315: 1342–8.

Stein AD, Zybert PA, van de Bor M, Lumey LH. Intrauterine famine exposure and body proportions at birth: the Dutch Hunger Winter. *Int J Epidemiol* 2004;33: 831–6.

Stettler NS, Zemel BS, Kumanyika S, Stallings VA. Infant weight gain in a multicenter, cohort study. *Pediatrics* 2002;109: 194–9.

Stockard CR. Developmental rate and structural expression: an experimental study of twins, "double monsters" and single deformities, and the interaction among embryonic organs during their origin and development. *Am J Anat* 1921;28: 115–263.

Susa JB, Boylan JM, Seghal P, Schwartz R. Persistence of impaired insulin secretion in infant rhesus monkeys that had been hyperinsulinemic in utero. *J Clin Endocrinol Metab* 1992;75: 265–9.

Tzschentke B, Plagemann A. Imprinting and critical periods in early development. *World's Poult Sci J* 2006;62: 627–38.

Van Assche FA, Devlieger R, Harder T, Plagemann A. Mitogenic effect of insulin and developmental programming. (letter) *Diabetologia* 2010;53: 1243.

Van den Bergh BRH, Van Calster B, Smits T, Van Huffel S, Lagae L. Antenatal maternal anxiety is related to HPA-axis dysregulation and self-reported depressive symptoms in adolescence: A prospective study on the fetal origins of depressed mood. *Neuropsychopharmacology* 2008;33: 536–45.

Vanhala MJ, Vanhala PT, Keinänen-Kiukaanniemi SM, Kumpusalo EA, Takala JK. Relative weight gain and obesity as a child predict metabolic syndrome as an adult. *Int J Obes* 1999;23: 656–9.

Vickers MH, Gluckman PD, Coveny AH, et al. Neonatal leptin treatment reverses developmental programming. *Endocrinology* 2005;146: 4211–6.

Waddington CH. Canalisation of development and the inheritance of acquired characters. *Nature* 1942;150: 563–4.

Weaver IC, Cervoni N, Champagne FA, et al. Epigenetic programming by maternal behaviour. *Nat Neurosci* 2004;7: 847–54.

Weiss PAM, Scholz HS, Haas J, Tamussino KF, Seissler J, Borkenstein MH. Long-term follow-up of infants of mothers with type 1 diabetes. Evidence for hereditary and nonhereditary transmission of diabetes and precursors. *Diabetes Care* 2000;23: 905–11.

Werboff J, Gottlieb JS. Drugs in pregnancy: behavioural teratology. *Obstet Gynecol Surv* 1963;18: 420–3.

Wiener N. *Cybernetics or Control and Communication in the Animal and the Machine.* Boston: MIT Press; 1948.

Wilkin TJ. The accelerator hypothesis: weight gain is the missing link between Type I and Type II diabetes. *Diabetologia* 2001;44: 914–22.

Yajnik CS, Fall CH, Coyaji KJ, et al. Neonatal anthropometry: the thin-fat Indian baby. The Pune Maternal Nutrition Study. *Int J Obes* 2003;27: 173–80.

Author index

Leona Aerts
Department of Obstetrics and Gynecology
University of Leuven
Belgium
Chapter 14

Kristian Almstrup
Department of Growth and Reproduction
Rigshospitalet Copenhagen
Denmark
kristian@almstrup.net
Chapter 18

Ernst Beinder
Clinic of Obstetrics
University of Zurich
Switzerland
and
Clinic of Obstetrics
Charité University Medicine Berlin
Germany
Chapter 6

Angelica B. Bernal
The Liggins Institute
The University of Auckland and the
National Research Centre for Growth
and Development
Auckland
New Zealand
Chapter 7

Karl E. Bergmann
Clinic of Obstetrics
Charité University Medicine Berlin
Germany
Chapter 17

Renate L. Bergmann
Clinic of Obstetrics
Charité University Medicine Berlin
Germany

renate.bergmann@charite.de
Chapter 17

Sebastien G. Bouret
The Saban Research Institute
Childrens Hospital Los Angeles
University of Southern California
Los Angeles, California
USA
and
Inserm, Jean-Pierre Aubert Research
Center
University Lille 2
Lille
France
sbouret@chla.usc.edu
Chapter 11

Tilo Burkhardt
Clinic of Obstetrics
University of Zurich
Switzerland
Chapter 6

Patrick M. Catalano
Department of Obstetrics and
Gynecology
MetroHealth Medical Center
Case Western Reserve University
Cleveland, Ohio
USA
pcatalano@metrohealth.org
Chapter 10

Tine Dalsgaard Clausen
Center for Pregnant Women with Diabetes
Departments of Endocrinology and
Obstetrics
Rigshospitalet, The Juliane Marie Centre
Faculty of Health Sciences
University of Copenhagen
Denmark
Chapter 13

Peter Damm
Center for Pregnant Women with Diabetes
Departments of Endocrinology and
Obstetrics
Rigshospitalet, The Juliane Marie Centre
Faculty of Health Sciences
University of Copenhagen
Denmark
pdamm@dadlnet.dk
Chapter 13

Urmila S. Deshmukh
King Edward Memorial Hospital and
Research Centre
Pune, Maharashtra
India
Chapter 8

Günter Dörner
Institute of Experimental Endocrinology
Charité University Medicine Berlin
Germany
g.doerner@yahoo.de
Chapter 2

Jörg Dötsch
Clinic of Pediatrics
University of Cologne
Germany
Chapter 5

Joachim W. Dudenhausen
Clinic of Obstetrics
Charité University Medicine Berlin
Germany
joachim.dudenhausen@charite.de
Chapter 1

Joram Feldon
Laboratory of Behavioral Neurobiology
Swiss Federal Institute of Technology (ETH)
Zurich
Switzerland
feldon@behav.biol.ethz.ch
Chapter 15

Chantal A. A. Heppolette
Institute of Metabolic Science
University of Cambridge
United Kingdom
Caah2@cam.ac.uk
Chapter 3

Mark B. Hampton
Free Radical Research Group
Department of Pathology
University of Otago
Christchurch
New Zealand
Chapter 7

Thomas Harder
Division of Experimental Obstetrics
Clinic of Obstetrics
Charité University Medicine Berlin
Germany
thomas.harder@charite.de
Chapter 14

Graham J. Howie
The Liggins Institute
The University of Auckland and the
National Research Centre for Growth and
Development
Auckland
New Zealand
Chapter 7

Louise Kelstrup
Center for Pregnant Women with Diabetes
Departments of Endocrinology and
Obstetrics
Rigshospitalet, The Juliane Marie Centre
Faculty of Health Sciences
University of Copenhagen
Denmark
Chapter 13

Simon C. Langley-Evans
Division of Nutritional Sciences
School of Biosciences
University of Nottingham
United Kingdom
Simon.Langley-Evans@nottingham.ac.uk
Chapter 4

Barry E. Levin
Neurology Service
Veterans Administration Medical Center
Department of Neurology and
Neurosciences
New Jersey Medical School
Newark, New Jersey
USA
levin@umdnj.edu
Chapter 12

Elisabeth R. Mathiesen
Center for Pregnant Women with Diabetes
Departments of Endocrinology and Obstetrics
Rigshospitalet, The Juliane Marie Centre
Faculty of Health Sciences
University of Copenhagen
Denmark
Chapter 13

Urs Meyer
Laboratory of Behavioral Neurobiology
Swiss Federal Institute of Technology (ETH)
Zurich
Switzerland
urmeyer@ethz.ch
Chapter 15

Eva Nüsken
Clinic of Pediatrics
University of Cologne
Germany
Chapter 5

Kai-Dietrich Nüsken
Clinic of Pediatrics
University of Cologne
Germany
kai-dietrich.nuesken@uk-koeln.de
Chapter 5

Susan E. Ozanne
Institute of Metabolic Science
University of Cambridge
United Kingdom
Chapter 3

Donald Palmer
Royal Veterinary College
London
United Kingdom
Chapter 3

Andreas Plagemann
Division of Experimental Obstetrics
Clinic of Obstetrics
Charite University Medicine Berlin
Germany
andreas.plagemann@charite.de
Chapters 14, 20

Lucilla Poston
Maternal and Fetal Research Unit

Division of Women's Health
King's College London
United Kingdom
lucilla.poston@kcl.ac.uk
Chapter 9

Ewa Rajpert-De Meyts
Department of Growth and
Reproduction
Rigshospitalet Copenhagen
Denmark
Chapter 18

Manfred Rauh
Clinic of Pediatrics
University of Erlangen
Germany
Chapter 6

Leonhard Schäffer
Clinic of Obstetrics
University of Zurich
Switzerland
Chapter 6

Niels E. Skakkebæk
Department of Growth and Reproduction
Rigshospitalet Copenhagen
Denmark
Chapter 18

Deborah M. Sloboda
The Liggins Institute
The University of Auckland and the
National Research Centre for Growth and
Development
Auckland
New Zealand
Chapter 7

Sophie M. Steculorum
The Saban Research Institute
Childrens Hospital Los Angeles
University of Southern California,
Los Angeles, California
USA
and
Inserm, Jean-Pierre Aubert Research Center
University Lille 2
Lille
France
Chapter 11

Moshe Szyf
Department of Pharmacology and Therapeutics
Sackler Program for Epigenetics
and Psychobiology
McGill University
Montreal
Quebec
Canada
mszyf@pharma.mcgill.ca
Chapter 19

Maren Tomaske
Department of Pediatric Cardiology
University of Zurich
Switzerland
Chapter 6

Anja Tzschoppe
Clinic of Pediatrics
University of Erlangen
Germany
Chapter 5

F. André Van Assche
Department of Obstetrics and Gynecology
University of Leuven
Belgium
Chapter 14

Bea R. H. Van den Bergh
Developmental Psychology
Tilburg University
The Netherlands
Bea.vdnBergh@uvt.nl
Chapter 16

Mark H. Vickers
The Liggins Institute
The University of Auckland and the
National Research Centre for Growth and
Development
Auckland
New Zealand
Chapter 7

Chittaranjan S. Yajnik
King Edward Memorial Hospital
and Research Centre
Pune, Maharashtra
India
diabetes@vsnl.com
Chapter 8

Index